Personalized Medicine in Oncology

Personalized Medicine in Oncology

Editor

Ari VanderWalde

MDPI • Basel • Beijing • Wuhan • Barcelona • Belgrade • Manchester • Tokyo • Cluj • Tianjin

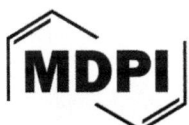

Editor
Ari VanderWalde
Emeritus Director of Clinical
Research
West Cancer Center and
Research Institute
Memphis
United States

Editorial Office
MDPI
St. Alban-Anlage 66
4052 Basel, Switzerland

This is a reprint of articles from the Special Issue published online in the open access journal *Journal of Personalized Medicine* (ISSN 2075-4426) (available at: www.mdpi.com/journal/jpm/special issues/personalized_oncology).

For citation purposes, cite each article independently as indicated on the article page online and as indicated below:

LastName, A.A.; LastName, B.B.; LastName, C.C. Article Title. *Journal Name* **Year**, *Volume Number*, Page Range.

ISBN 978-3-0365-2821-2 (Hbk)
ISBN 978-3-0365-2820-5 (PDF)

© 2022 by the authors. Articles in this book are Open Access and distributed under the Creative Commons Attribution (CC BY) license, which allows users to download, copy and build upon published articles, as long as the author and publisher are properly credited, which ensures maximum dissemination and a wider impact of our publications.

The book as a whole is distributed by MDPI under the terms and conditions of the Creative Commons license CC BY-NC-ND.

Contents

About the Editor vii

Ari VanderWalde
Personalized Medicine in Oncology; a Special Issue of the *Journal of Personalized Medicine*
Reprinted from: *J. Pers. Med.* **2021**, *11*, 632, doi:10.3390/jpm11070632 1

Matthew K. Stein, Oluchukwu Oluoha, Kruti Patel and Ari VanderWalde
Precision Medicine in Oncology: A Review of Multi-Tumor Actionable Molecular Targets with an Emphasis on Non-Small Cell Lung Cancer
Reprinted from: *J. Pers. Med.* **2021**, *11*, 518, doi:10.3390/jpm11060518 5

Sandra Ríos-Arrabal, Jose D. Puentes-Pardo, Sara Moreno-SanJuan, Ágata Szuba, Jorge Casado, María García-Costela, Julia Escudero-Feliu, Michela Verbeni, Carlos Cano, Cristina González-Puga, Alicia Martín-Lagos Maldonado, Ángel Carazo and Josefa León
Endothelin-1 as a Mediator of Heme Oxygenase-1-Induced Stemness in Colorectal Cancer: Influence of p53
Reprinted from: *J. Pers. Med.* **2021**, *11*, 509, doi:10.3390/jpm11060509 39

Laura Cortesi, Claudia Piombino and Angela Toss
Germline Mutations in Other Homologous Recombination Repair-Related Genes Than BRCA1/2: Predictive or Prognostic Factors?
Reprinted from: *J. Pers. Med.* **2021**, *11*, 245, doi:10.3390/jpm11040245 57

Vittorio Branchi, Benedict Jürgensen, Laura Esser, Maria Gonzalez-Carmona, Tobias J. Weismüller, Christian P. Strassburg, Jonas Henn, Alexander Semaan, Philipp Lingohr, Steffen Manekeller, Glen Kristiansen, Jörg C. Kalff, Marieta I. Toma and Hanno Matthaei
Tumor Infiltrating Neutrophils Are Frequently Found in Adenocarcinomas of the Biliary Tract and Their Precursor Lesions with Possible Impact on Prognosis
Reprinted from: *J. Pers. Med.* **2021**, *11*, 233, doi:10.3390/jpm11030233 67

Jinkook Kim, Eunjeong Ji, Kwangrok Jung, In Ho Jung, Jaewoo Park, Jong-Chan Lee, Jin Won Kim, Jin-Hyeok Hwang and Jaihwan Kim
Gender Differences in Patients with Metastatic Pancreatic Cancer Who Received FOLFIRINOX
Reprinted from: *J. Pers. Med.* **2021**, *11*, 83, doi:10.3390/jpm11020083 79

Ari VanderWalde, Axel Grothey, Daniel Vaena, Gregory Vidal, Adam ElNaggar, Gabriella Bufalino and Lee Schwartzberg
Establishment of a Molecular Tumor Board (MTB) and Uptake of Recommendations in a Community Setting
Reprinted from: *J. Pers. Med.* **2020**, *10*, 252, doi:10.3390/jpm10040252 87

Michael A. Ulm, Tiffany M. Redfern, Ben R. Wilson, Suriyan Ponnusamy, Sarah Asemota, Patrick W. Blackburn, Yinan Wang, Adam C. ElNaggar and Ramesh Narayanan
Integrin-Linked Kinase Is a Novel Therapeutic Target in Ovarian Cancer
Reprinted from: *J. Pers. Med.* **2020**, *10*, 246, doi:10.3390/jpm10040246 97

Benjamin Miron, David Xu and Matthew Zibelman
Biomarker Development for Metastatic Renal Cell Carcinoma: Omics, Antigens, T-cells, and Beyond
Reprinted from: *J. Pers. Med.* **2020**, *10*, 225, doi:10.3390/jpm10040225 113

Loredana G. Marcu
Imaging Biomarkers of Tumour Proliferation and Invasion for Personalised Lung Cancer Therapy
Reprinted from: *J. Pers. Med.* **2020**, *10*, 222, doi:10.3390/jpm10040222 . . . . **131**

Hossein Taghizadeh, Matthias Unseld, Martina Spalt, Robert M. Mader, Leonhard Müllauer, Thorsten Fuereder, Markus Raderer, Maria Sibilia, Mir Alireza Hoda, Stefanie Aust, Stephan Polterauer, Wolfgang Lamm, Rupert Bartsch, Matthias Preusser, Kautzky-Willer A. and Gerald W. Prager
Targeted Therapy Recommendations for Therapy Refractory Solid Tumors—Data from the Real-World Precision Medicine Platform MONDTI
Reprinted from: *J. Pers. Med.* **2020**, *10*, 188, doi:10.3390/jpm10040188 . . . . **149**

Taichiro Goto
Patient-Derived Tumor Xenograft Models: Toward the Establishment of Precision Cancer Medicine
Reprinted from: *J. Pers. Med.* **2020**, *10*, 64, doi:10.3390/jpm10030064 . . . . **167**

About the Editor

Ari VanderWalde

Dr. VanderWalde's research interests include immune therapies in solid tumors and melanoma. He is Director of Research at West Cancer Center; Senior Medical Director at George Clinical; and Medical Director of Precision Medicine at OneOncology. He has collaborated and participated on advisory board with many of the nation's thought leaders and top experts in the field and previously served as United States Medical Lead and Clinical Research Medical Director with Amgen Inc., directing U.S. global development of talimogene laherparepvec, a novel viral-based immunitherapeutic that has shown efficacy in late-stage clinical trials in melanoma.

As Director of Research at West Cancer Center, Dr. VanderWalde is responsible for managing the portfolio of all clinical trials at the Cancer Center. He also serves as Medical Director of the Clinical Trials Network of Tennessee. He has been involved in research targeting therapy in a more personalized fashion based on immune markers and aberrations in cancer genetics.

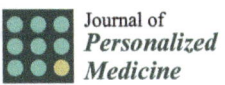

Editorial

Personalized Medicine in Oncology; a Special Issue of the *Journal of Personalized Medicine*

Ari VanderWalde

West Cancer Center and Research Institute, Memphis, TN 38138, USA; avanderw@westclinic.com

Nowhere is the explosion in comprehensive genomic testing more evident than in oncology. Multiple consensus guidelines now recommend molecular testing as part of the standard of care for most metastatic tumors. To aid in the advancement of this rapidly changing field, we intended this Special Issue of *JPM* to focus on technical developments in the genomic profiling of cancer, detail promising somatic alterations that either are, or have a high likelihood of being, relevant in the near future, and to address issues related to the pricing and value of these tests.

The last few years have seen the cost of molecular testing decrease by orders of magnitude. In 2018, we saw the first "site-agnostic" drug approvals in cancer (for microsatellite unstable cancer (PD-1 inhibitors) and NTRK-fusions (TRK inhibitors)). This has recently been followed by pan-tumor approvals for tumors that have a high tumor mutational burden. Research on targetable mutations, determination of genetic "signatures" that can use multiple individual genes/pathways, development of targeted therapy, and insight into the value of new technology remains at the cutting edge of research in this field. In this Special Issue of *JPM* we solicited papers that present new technologies to assess predictive biomarkers in cancer, conducted original research (pre-clinical or clinical) that demonstrates promise for particular targeted therapies in cancer, and articles that explore the clinical and financial impacts of this paradigmatic shift in cancer diagnostics and treatment.

In this issue, four review articles and a commentary present great depth in biomarker testing both in the clinic as well as in early science.

Two papers discuss the role of tumor biomarkers in the diagnosis and treatment of various malignancies. Stein et al. present a comprehensive review of the molecular and immunologic biomarkers that have led to approvals in more than one malignancy [1]. With a focus on US-FDA approvals as well as studies leading to those approvals, the paper serves as an overview of patient-directed therapy based upon these markers. This paper also performs a deep dive into molecular and genomic biomarkers specifically in metastatic non-small-cell lung cancer; a cancer for which over 50% of cases have a targetable molecular alteration. Miron et al. [2] perform a deep dive into renal cell cancer—another malignancy with genomic and molecular alterations that predispose to response in for both immune therapy and targeted therapy. The authors particularly discuss the development and discovery of these markers and how they are used in a real-world setting.

In addition to these clinical reviews, Cortesi and colleagues provide commentary on the role of on relatively uncommon germline mutations that effect homologous recombination repair (HRR), such as *PALB2, CHEK2, ATM*, and others [3]. The authors propose that the presence of homologous repair deficiency can often serve as a positive prognostic factor, but that the prediction of whether tumors associated with these genes respond to PARP inhibitor therapy depends on the gene and on the penetrance. The authors assert that tests that can reveal the presence of all HRR genes should be part of a standard germline panel, rather than just focusing on BRCA1 and 2.

In the basic-science realm, Dr. Tachiro Goto presents a review paper describing the role of patient-derived xenografts (PDX) in precision oncology [4]. The paper describes the preparation of PDX and the grafting of human tumor tissue into nude mice as well as much of the current advancement of the field using this model. Due to the preservation of tumor heterogeneity as well as the tumor microenvironment, the paper predicts the use of these relatively novel pre-clinical approaches to biomarker driven testing and therapeutics.

Finally, Dr. Loredana Marcu proposes a different type of biomarker useful in diagnosis and prediction of response or progression in lung cancer [5]. By focusing on the development of imaging-based radiologic biomarkers, the paper paves the way for personalized oncology focused not only on tumor-based genomic alterations, but on the ability of advanced imaging to discover the presence of pathological findings such as the presence of cancer-stem cells, apoptosis, and circulating tumor cells as well as the ability to determine proliferation kinetics.

With the context provided by these reviews and commentaries, intriguing original research is presented in this Special Issue that explores the role of novel biomarkers in specific cancer types, explores demographic "biomarkers" as keys to response to therapy, and details results of operational tests and processes that serve to integrate precision oncology into the clinic.

Two of the original research pieces look specifically at novel biomarkers in gastrointestinal cancers. Rios-Arrabal and colleagues present the role of heme oxygenase-1 (HO-1) as a marker of "stemness" in colorectal cancer [6]. The authors found that HO-1 overexpression is commonly co-expressed with endothelin converting enzyme-1, and that resistance was unrelated to the presence or absence of p53 (a poor prognosis tumor marker). Further exploration led to the conclusion that HO-1 based-therapies could be developed and preferentially used in patients with expression of these markers.

Branchi et al. explored tissue samples obtained from 27 patients with biliary tract adenocarcinomas and assessed them for the presence and density of tumor infiltrating lymphocytes (TIL) [7]. It was found that those cancers with high TIL density exhibited an overall survival almost twice as long as those with low density of TIL. As such, they propose that TIL density could serve as a potential clinical biomarker for prognosis in biliary tract cancer and suggest that this difference shows that there is a key regulator role in the immune landscape in this cancer type.

In ovarian cancer, Ulm and colleagues explore the potential role of integrin associated kinase as a biomarker in this malignancy [8]. Ovarian cancer tissue samples were pair-matched to normal adjacent ovarian tissue from 24 patients and tissue microarray was used to compare gene expression profiles which then led to the identification of molecular pathways for further analysis. Integrin-linked kinase (ILK) emerged as a commonly upregulated pathway in ovarian cancer, and it was shown to be a driver of malignancy. An ILK-1 chemical inhibitor had positive results against ILK-1 expressing tumors in xenograft models. These may serve as initial findings to justify the development of ILK-1 directed therapies in this malignancy.

While precision medicine is usually targeting molecular alterations, it is important to recognize that virtually any clinical, laboratory, or patient-reported factors may potentially serve as markers predicting for various outcomes in cancer. In this issue, Kim et al. present a retrospective study of 97 patients who received the chemotherapeutic regimen FOLFIRINOX for pancreatic cancer [9]. The authors demonstrated better outcomes for women than for men on this regimen, including a trend for improved progression-free-survival and significantly better overall survival, despite a higher median age of women as compared to men. There are of course limitations on the interpretability of this study, but it is an important step to use real-world data to identify not only molecular markers, but demographic markers as well to guide therapy in cancer.

Just as identification of biomarkers in the lab and in clinical trials is important in precision oncology, the integration of these findings into clinical practice is equally, if not more, essential. Taghizadeh and colleagues describe how their real-world precision medicine platform MONDTI (molecular oncologic diagnostics and therapy) at the Medical University of Vienna was able to identify patients with actionable molecular alterations [10]. The group used standard multi-gene next generation sequencing panels and immunohistochemistry and utilized a multidisciplinary team meeting held every other week that made recommendations for off-label use based on levels of evidence. In this retrospective study the authors evaluated what demographic or disease state characteristics were more or less likely to result in recommendations for targeted therapy among the almost 600 patients who went through the MONDTI system. They found that certain types of malignancies were more likely to result in recommendations, that certain genomic alterations were more likely to result in recommendations, and that male gender was more likely to result in recommendations.

A similar article by me and my colleagues described the implementation of a molecular tumor board in a community oncology setting [11]. Rather than focusing on characteristics associated with recommendations, we focused on the types of recommendations made and whether or not the recommendations were followed. Among 613 patients reviewed by the bi-weekly molecular tumor board, 37% of patients had standard therapy recommended, 31% had a recommendation to go onto a clinical trial, germline testing was recommended in 17% of patients, and off-label therapy was recommended in only 10%. Follow-through with recommendations depended on the type of recommendation. Only 13% of those for whom a trial was recommended were able to go onto a study. Standard therapy recommendations were followed almost 80% of the time, while germline testing recommendations were only followed in about a third of patients.

The opportunity to dedicate an entire issue to precision oncology is important. The articles in this issue represent the breadth of what is being done regarding discovery, development, measurement, and integration of precision oncology in patients. While the field has truly blossomed in the last decade, significant work remains to be done. Each of the articles in this Special Issue captures an important piece of the genomic and personalized oncology puzzle. Though some of the puzzle has been solved, what remains will provide us with mysteries to solve for years to come.

Conflicts of Interest: The author has received research support from Amgen, is a consultant for Bristol-Myers Squibb and Elsevier, and participates in advisory boards for Roche/Genentech, Mirati, and Bristol-Myers Squibb.

References

1. Stein, M.K.; Oluoha, O.; Patel, K.; VanderWalde, A. Precision Medicine in Oncology: A Review of Multi-Tumor Actionable Molecular Targets with an Emphasis on Non-Small Cell Lung Cancer. *J. Pers. Med.* **2021**, *11*, 518. [CrossRef]
2. Miron, B.; Xu, D.; Zibelman, M. Biomarker Development for Metastatic Renal Cell Carcinoma: Omics, Antigens, T-cels, and Beyond. *J. Pers. Med.* **2020**, *10*, 225. [CrossRef] [PubMed]
3. Cortesi, L.; Piombino, C.; Toss, A. Germline Mutations in Other Homologous recombination Repair-Related Genes Than BRCA1/2: Predictive or Prognostic Factors? *J. Pers. Med.* **2021**, *11*, 245. [CrossRef] [PubMed]
4. Goto, T. Patient-Derived Tumor Xenograft Models: Toward the Establishment of Precision Cancer Medicine. *J. Pers. Med.* **2020**, *10*, 64. [CrossRef] [PubMed]
5. Marcu, L.G. Imaging Biomarkers of Tumour Proliferation and Invasion for Personalised Lung Cancer Therapy. *J. Pers. Oncol.* **2020**, *10*, 222.
6. Rios-Arrabal, S.; Puentes-Pardo, J.D.; Moreno-SanJuan, S.; Szuba, A.; Casado, J.; Garcia-Costela, M.; Escudero-Feliu, J.; Verbeni, M.; Cano, C.; Gonzalez-Puga, C. Endothelin-1 as a Mediator of heme Oxygenase-1-Induced Stemness in Colorectal Cancer: Influence of p53. *J. Pers. Med.* **2021**, *11*, 509. [CrossRef]
7. Branchi, V.; Jurgensen, B.; Esser, L.; Gonzalez-Carmona, M.; Weismuller, T.J.; Strassburg, C.P.; Henn, J.; Semaan, A.; Lingohr, P.; Manekeller, S.; et al. Tumor Infiltrating Neutrophils Are Frequently Found in Adenocarcinomas of the Biliary Tract and Their Precursor Lesions with Possible Impact on Prognosis. *J. Pers. Med.* **2021**, *11*, 233. [CrossRef] [PubMed]
8. Ulm, M.A.; Redfern, T.M.; Wilson, B.R.; Ponnusamy, S.; Asemota, S.; Blackburn, P.W.; Wang, Y.; ElNaggar, A.C.; Narayanan, R. Integrin-Linked Kinase Is a Novel Therapeutic Target in Ovarian Cancer. *J. Pers. Med.* **2020**, *10*, 246. [CrossRef] [PubMed]
9. Kim, J.; Ji, E.; Jung, K.; Jung, I.H.; Park, J.; Lee, J.-C.; Kim, J.W.; Hwang, J.-H.; Kim, J. Gender Differences in Patients with Metastatic Pancreatic Cancer Who Received FOLFIRINOX. *J. Pers. Med.* **2021**, *11*, 83. [CrossRef] [PubMed]
10. Taghizadeh, H.; Unseld, M.; Spalt, M.; Mader, R.M.; Mullauer, L.; Fuereder, T.; Raderer, M.; Sibilia, M.; Hoda, M.A.; Aust, S.; et al. Targeted Therapy Recommendations for Therapy Refractory Solid Tumors—Data from the Real-World Precision Medicine Platform MONDTI. *J. Pers. Med.* **2020**, *10*, 188. [CrossRef] [PubMed]
11. VanderWalde, A.; Grothey, A.; Vaena, D.; Vidal, G.; ElNaggar, A.; Bufalino, G.; Schwartzberg, L. Establishment of a Molecular Tumor Board (MTB) and Uptake of Recommendations in a Community Setting. *J. Pers. Med.* **2020**, *10*, 252. [CrossRef] [PubMed]

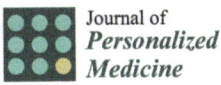

Review

Precision Medicine in Oncology: A Review of Multi-Tumor Actionable Molecular Targets with an Emphasis on Non-Small Cell Lung Cancer

Matthew K. Stein [1], Oluchukwu Oluoha [2], Kruti Patel [2] and Ari VanderWalde [3,*]

1. Missouri Baptist Medical Center, Heartland Cancer Research, NCI Community Oncology Research Program, St. Louis, MO 63131, USA; Matthew.stein@bjc.org
2. Division of Hematology and Oncology, University of Tennessee Health Science Center, Memphis, TN 38103, USA; ooluoha@westclinic.com (O.O.); kpatel@westclinic.com (K.P.)
3. West Cancer Center and Research Institute, Germantown, TN 38138, USA
* Correspondence: avanderwalde@westclinic.com

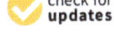

Citation: Stein, M.K.; Oluoha, O.; Patel, K.; VanderWalde, A. Precision Medicine in Oncology: A Review of Multi-Tumor Actionable Molecular Targets with an Emphasis on Non-Small Cell Lung Cancer. *J. Pers. Med.* **2021**, *11*, 518. https://doi.org/10.3390/jpm11060518

Academic Editor: Luigi Minafra

Received: 29 April 2021
Accepted: 2 June 2021
Published: 5 June 2021

Publisher's Note: MDPI stays neutral with regard to jurisdictional claims in published maps and institutional affiliations.

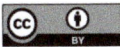

Copyright: © 2021 by the authors. Licensee MDPI, Basel, Switzerland. This article is an open access article distributed under the terms and conditions of the Creative Commons Attribution (CC BY) license (https://creativecommons.org/licenses/by/4.0/).

Abstract: Precision medicine is essential for the modern care of a patient with cancer. Comprehensive molecular profiling of the tumor itself is necessary to determine the presence or absence of certain targetable abnormalities or biomarkers. In particular, lung cancer is a disease for which targetable genomic alterations will soon guide therapy in the majority of cases. In this comprehensive review of solid tumor-based biomarkers, we describe the genomic alterations for which targeted agents have been approved by the United States Food and Drug Administration (FDA). While focusing on alterations leading to approvals in a tumor-agnostic fashion (MSI-h, TMB-h, *NTRK*) and on those alterations with approvals in multiple malignancies (*BRAF, ERBB2, RET, BRCA*, PD-L1), we also describe several biomarkers or indications that are likely to lead to an approved drug in the near future (e.g., KRAS G12C, PD-L1 amplification, HER2 overexpression in colon cancer, HER2 mutations in lung cancer). Finally, we detail the current landscape of additional actionable alterations (*EGFR, ALK, ROS1, MET*) in lung cancer, a biomarker-rich malignancy that has greatly benefitted from the precision oncology revolution.

Keywords: cancer; next-generation sequencing; targeted therapy; precision oncology; tumor-agnostic indications; solid tumors; tumor markers; FDA-approved therapeutics

1. Introduction

Precision medicine, defined as supplying the right treatment to the right patient at the right time, has become an essential element of cancer care, Taking advantage of novel technologies developed following sequencing of the human genome approximately twenty years ago, precision oncology leverages a tumor's molecular features with available and novel therapeutics [1–4]. Prior to the advancement of comprehensive tumor profiling, successful implementation of a precision oncology approach included tyrosine kinase inhibitors (TKIs) imatinib for breakpoint cluster region-Abelson (*BCR-ABL*)-rearranged chronic myeloid leukemia [5] and trastuzumab for human epidermal growth factor 2 (HER2) immunohistochemistry (IHC) overexpressed or amplified breast cancer [6,7].

Currently, molecular profiling is available to comprehensively characterize a patient's tumor within as few as two weeks and includes interrogation of anywhere from hundreds of genes to the whole exome for mutations, insertions, deletions or copy-number alterations via next-generation sequencing (NGS), gene fusions with RNA sequencing and various protein changes with IHC. The goal of such extensive testing is to unveil the genomic makeup of a patient's tumor, which can inform the most effective therapeutic approach. Oftentimes, this must be coupled with the malignancy's site-of-origin and histologic features; however, precision treatment strategies are increasingly being employed in a tissue-agnostic fashion through a growing list of pan-tumor United States Food and Drug Administration (FDA) approvals, clinical trials and off-label use when a molecular approach can be justified (e.g., through a tumor board consensus) [8].

In this review, we will outline progress in precision medicine in oncology, with an aim to summarize the current landscape of FDA-approved therapies based upon predictive molecular biomarkers in solid tumors, focusing on those markers that determine therapeutic options in more than one malignancy type. As will be seen, several pan-tumor and multi-tumor FDA approvals exist for both tumors with alterations expressing sensitivity to targeted agents (including TKIs and antibody-drug conjugates (ADCs)) as well as immune checkpoint inhibitors (ICIs). The full extent of molecular targets in cancer cannot be completely summarized in a single paper, and we will concentrate on those findings deemed DNA-based alterations by most NGS vendors.

We will conclude by switching from biomarker to malignancy, detailing present treatment options available for non-small cell lung cancer (NSCLC). NSCLC serves as a model for precision oncology where patients can benefit substantially from employment of molecular profiling.

2. Molecular Alterations with Approvals Regardless of Tumor-Site

To date, three molecular targets (microsatellite instability-high (MSI-H) or mismatch repair deficient (MSI-H/dMMR), neurotrophic tropomyosin-related kinase (*NTRK1/2/3*) fusions or high tumor mutational burden (TMB-H)), have led to four site- or tumor-agnostic approvals by the FDA. These biomarkers and drugs with corresponding FDA approvals are listed in the first part of Table 1.

Table 1. Molecular alterations guiding therapy with agents approved in multiple tumor types.

Alteration(s)	Indication	Line of Therapy	Medications	Drug Class	FDA Approval Date
MSI-h/ dMMR	Any tumor type	>2nd line metastatic	Pembrolizumab	PD-1 mAb	23 May 2017 [9]
	Colorectal cancer	2nd line metastatic	Nivolumab	PD-1 mAb	31 July 2017 [10]
		2nd line metastatic	Ipilimumab + Nivolumab	CTLA-4 mAb + PD-1 mAb	10 July 2018 [11]
		1st line metastatic	Pembrolizumab	PD-1 mAb	29 June 2020 [12]
	Endometrial cancer	Progression after platinum	Dostarlimab	PD-1 mAb	22 April 2021 [13]
TMB-h (>10 mut/Mb)	Any tumor type	>2nd line metastatic	Pembrolizumab	PD-1 mAb	16 June 2020 [14]
NTRK fusions	Any tumor type	Any line	Larotrectinib	Trk inhibitor	26 November 2018 [15]
			Entrectinib	Trk inhibitor	15 August 2019 [16]
BRAF V600 mt	Melanoma	Any metastatic line	Vemurafenib [1]	BRAF inhibitor	17 August 2011 [17]
			Dabrafenib [1]	BRAF inhibitor	29 May 2013 [18]
			Trametinib [1]	MEK inhibitor	29 May 2013 [18]
			Vemurafenib + Cobimetinib	BRAF + MEK	10 November 2015 [19]
			Dabrafenib + Trametinib	BRAF + MEK	9 January 2014 [20]
			Encorafenib + Binimetinib	BRAF + MEK	27 June 2018 [21]
		Adjuvant	Dabrafenib + Trametinib	BRAF + MEK	30 April 2018 [22]

Table 1. Cont.

Alteration(s)	Indication	Line of Therapy	Medications	Drug Class	FDA Approval Date
		1st line	Atezolizumab, Vemurafenib and Cobimetinib	PD-L1 + BRAF + MEK	30 July 2020 [23]
	NSCLC	2nd line	Dabrafenib + Trametinib	BRAF + MEK	22 June 2017 [24]
	Anaplastic thyroid	Any line	Dabrafenib + trametinib	BRAF + MEK	4 May 2018 [25]
	Colorectal	2nd line	Encorafenib + cetuximab	BRAF inh + EGFR mAb	8 April 2020 [26]
HER2 (ERBB2) overexpression	Breast [2]	Neoadjuvant, adjuvant or metastatic	Trastuzumab	Anti HER2 mAb	25 September 1998 [27]
			Pertuzumab	Anti HER2 mAb	8 June 2012 [28]
		Adjuvant or metastatic	Ado-trastuzumab emtansine (TDM-1)	Antibody drug conjugate	22 February 2013 [29]
			Neratinib	Small molecule	17 July 2017 [30]
		Metastatic	Fam-trastuzumab deruxtecan	Antibody drug conjugate	20 December 2019 [31]
			Lapatinib	Small molecule	13 March 2007 [32]
			Tucatinib	Small molecule	17 April 2020 [33]
	Gastric/GEJ	1st line metastatic	Trastuzumab	Anti HER2 mAb	20 October 2010 [34]
			Fam-trastuzumab deruxtecan	Antibody drug conjugate	15 January 2021 [35]
RET alterations	Medullary thyroid cancer (RET-mutated)	Metastatic	Selpercatinib	Small molecule RET inhibitor	8 May 2020 [36]
	Any thyroid cancer (RET fusion)	Metastatic	Selpercatinib		8 May 2020 [36]
	NSCLC (RET fusion)	Metastatic	Selpercatinib		8 May 2020 [36]
			Pralsetinib		4 September 2020 [37]
DNA repair deficiency (Either BRCA1/2 somatic mutations, BRCA1/2 germline mutations, homologous repair deficiency (HRD) or homologous recombination repair mutations (HRR)	Ovarian cancer	1st line or late-line maintenance	Olaparib (BRCA germline, somatic or HRD)	PARP inhibitor	19 December 2018 (BRCA), 8 May 2020 (HRD) [38]
			Rucaparib (initially for BRCA mutation, now regardless of biomarker status)	PARP inhibitor	19 December 2016 (BRCA) [39] 6 April 2018 (regardless of biomarker) [40]
			Niraparib (regardless of biomarker status for maintenance, late line for HRD)	PARP inhibitor	27 March 2017 (regardless of biomarker) [41] 10/23/2019 (HRD) [42]
	Breast cancer	>2nd line metastatic	Olaparib (BRCA germline only)	PARP inhibitor	12 January 2018 [43]
			Talazoparib (BRCA germline only)	PARP inhibitor	16 October 2018 [44]

Table 1. Cont.

Alteration(s)	Indication	Line of Therapy	Medications	Drug Class	FDA Approval Date
	Pancreatic cancer	Metastatic maintenance	Olaparib (BRCA germline only)	PARP inhibitor	30 December 2019 [45]
	Prostate cancer	Metastatic	Rucaparib (BRCA germline or somatic)	PARP inhibitor	15 May 2020 [46]
			Olaparib (HRR germline or somatic)	PARP inhibitor	19 May 2020 [47]

[1] No longer preferred as single agents in this disease. [2] Many HER2 agents may be used in combination with other HER2 agents or with chemotherapy, depending on the indication. Approvals given for HER2 agents are for the first approval of each drug.

2.1. MSI-h/dMMR

The first of these approvals occurred on 23 May 2017 when pembrolizumab, an ICI whose activity lies in the inhibition of programmed cell death protein 1 (PD-1), was approved for second-line or later treatment of metastatic or unresectable solid tumors in pediatric and adult patients found to be MSI-H/dMMR [9]. The basis of the approval was from 149 MSI-H/dMMR patients spanning five uncontrolled, multi-cohort, multicenter, single-arm clinical trials (KEYNOTE-012, -016, -028, -158 and -164) [9,48–51], where the overall response rate (ORR) was 40% (95% confidence interval (CI): 31.7, 47.9) and responses lasted for >6 months in 78% of responders. In this cohort, 90/149 (60%) of patients had colorectal cancer, for which prior treatment with a fluoropyrimidine, oxaliplatin and irinotecan was required; 14 other tumor types were evaluated leading up to the 2017 FDA approval.

Several other ICI agents are FDA approved for MSI-H/dMMR colorectal cancer patients. These include nivolumab following treatment with a fluoropyrimidine, oxaliplatin and irinotecan (July 2017; CheckMate 142) [52]; nivolumab and ipilimumab after a fluoropyrimidine, oxaliplatin and irinotecan (July 2018; CheckMate 142) [53]; and pembrolizumab as the first frontline approval in MSI-H/dMMR colorectal cancer (June 2020; KEYNOTE-177) [54]. While the tumor site-agnostic approval was groundbreaking, recently published data from KEYNOTE-158 showed a wide range of response rates to pembrolizumab in this setting based on primary tumor site [51], with the highest responses seen in endometrial cancer (57%) and the lowest with pancreatic (18%) and central nervous system (0%) malignancies. While larger cohorts and further study is needed into the molecular mechanisms of response [55], these findings suggest the site-agnostic model of ICI use should be evaluated thoughtfully in these and other MSI-H/dMMR solid tumors when other treatment options exist [56].

2.2. NTRK1/2/3 Fusions

NRTK fusions occur in <0.5% of all cancer types, but are enhanced in some rare cancers or those with atypical histology, including salivary carcinoma (5%), thyroid (2%), sarcoma (including uterine, 1%) and possibly glioblastoma multiforme (<1%) [57]. The FDA approved larotrectinib [15] on 26 November 2018 and entrectinib [16] on 15 August 2019 for adult and pediatric solid tumor patients whose metastatic or unresectable tumors do not contain a resistance mutation to either agent at the start of treatment. Approval of larotrectinib was based upon the efficacy observed in the first 55 patients of three multicenter, open-label, single-arm clinical trials (LOXO-TRK-14001, SCOUT, NAVIGATE), where Drilon et al. reported a response rate of 75%, which was ongoing in 71% of responders at one year [58]. Comprising a cohort of 17 different tumor types, patients harboring a TRK fusion and treated with larotrectinib primarily had grade 1 toxicities including increased liver enzymes, fatigue, nausea, vomiting and anemia. In a recent pooled analysis of a larger cohort from the same three trials, an ORR was found to be 79% for 153 evaluable patients, with 16% complete responses and a median duration of response of over 35 months [59]. Additionally, long-term toxicity data showed the safety of larotrectinib with no treatment-related deaths observed and the most frequent grade 3 or 4 toxicities were increased alanine aminotransferase levels (3%), neutropenia (2%) and anemia (2%).

The efficacy of entrectinib for patients with advanced solid tumors with NTRK fusions was likewise recently described in a combined analysis from three ongoing phase 1 and 2 clinical trials (ALKA-372-001, STARTRK-1 and STARTRK-2). Doebele and colleagues described a 57% response rate with a median duration of 10 months in a cohort of 54 patients (>60 had received prior systemic therapy) comprising 19 different histologies [60]. It should also be noted that in addition to activity against NTRK fusions, entrectinib is also FDA approved for the treatment of ROS proto-oncogene 1 (ROS1) rearranged NSCLC.

The robust efficacy of larotrectinib and entrectinib with a tolerable safety profile makes both agents attractive for NTRK fusion-positive metastatic cancer patients. Upon progression, molecular profiling should be repeated to assess for resistance mechanisms, as NTRK kinase domain mutations (involving solvent front, gatekeeper residue or xDFG motif) or off-target mutations (including Kirsten rat sarcoma viral oncogene homolog (KRAS) mutations, mesenchymal-epithelial transition (MET) amplifications and serine-threonine protein kinase B-RAF (BRAF) V600E mutations) can inform the next systemic approach [61]. If progression is restricted to a limited number of sites (termed oligometastatic), local therapy with continued NTRK inhibition can be pursued. However, if extensive progression occurs and NTRK resistance mutations are identified, next-generation TKIs repotrectinib [62,63] and seltrectinib [64] are currently being evaluated and show preliminary efficacy in this setting.

2.3. Tumor Mutational Burden

On 16 June 2020, the FDA approved pembrolizumab for its second tumor site-agnostic indication. Specifically, pembrolizumab can be considered following progression on another treatment for all metastatic or unresectable adult and pediatric solid tumor patients found to have high tumor mutational burden (TMB-H), defined as ≥ 10 mutations/megabase (mut/Mb). As a part of this approval, the FoundationOne CDx assay (Foundation Medicine, Cambridge, MA, USA) was authorized as a companion diagnostic for tissue TMB evaluation [14]. The approval was based upon recently published prospective data from 10 treatment-refractory cohorts in the phase 2 KEYNOTE-158 trial, which showed an ORR of 29% of 102 TMB-H patients to pembrolizumab, compared to 6% of those with TMB <10 mut/Mb [65].

The pan-tumor approval for TMB-H has been controversial in the oncology community. On one hand, some point to potential flaws in the study including a perceived arbitrary TMB cutoff of 10 mut/Mb, the lack of a control arm in KEYNOTE-158 and the composition of tumor types included in the 102 TMB-H patients (i.e., >60% were small cell lung, endometrial and cervical, which already have ICIs approved in some capacity; less commonly enrolled tumor types need a higher sample size to determine efficacy) [66]. To this end, McGrail and colleagues recently published retrospective data from The Cancer Genome Atlas (TCGA) which suggests a blanket TMB cutoff of 10 mut/Mb for pembrolizumab us may not be applicable in all solid tumor types. The authors first divided solid tumor patients into two categories, those with a positive versus no correlation between CD8 T-cell levels and neoantigen load, a term referring to the presumption that higher amounts of tumor mutations lead to certain antigen peptides which in turn activate the immune system. While TMB-H predicted a response to ICI in those with a correlation between CD8 T-cells and neoadjuvant load (e.g., melanoma, bladder and lung cancer), this benefit was not seen in those tumor types where no such correlation was seen (e.g., breast, prostate, glioma). In fact, the ORR for TMB-H patients in this latter subgroup was <20%, and TMB-H patients were actually found to have a lower ORR than those with low TMB (odds ratio (OR) = 0.46, 95% CI 0.24–0.88, $p = 0.02$) [67].

In contrast, advocates of utilizing TMB-H such as Subbiah and colleagues cite the durability of responses seen in KEYNOTE-158 (approximately half were for at least two years), the resultant expansion of genomic profiling to include rare tumors, improvement of pembrolizumab reimbursement and access given FDA approval, access for minority and underserved populations and overall enabling of patients and physicians to make informed clinical decisions [68]. As the careful use of TMB-H makes its way to the clinic, emerging co-occurring biomarkers, such as mutations in DNA polymerase epsilon (*POLE*) and delta 1 (*POLD1*) may help predict survival with ICI use [69], though no FDA approvals have yet been based on these alterations.

2.4. On the Horizon: PD-L1 Amplification

While requiring further study, additional biomarkers obtained from comprehensive molecular profiling may eventually be considered for predictive pan-tumor use. One such biomarker includes amplification of *PD-L1* (or *CD274*), which Goodman et al. identified in 0.7% of 118,000 profiled solid tumor patients and may predict efficacy to ICI [70]. This is in contrast to PD-L1 expression measured using immunohistochemistry, which is both more common and less predictive (see PD-L1 section below). With only limited published case reports or series to date [71–73], there does appear to be a histologic-dependent range in frequency of *PD-L1* amplifications with increased incidence in uncommon tumor types including bladder squamous cell, renal sarcomatoid, liver mixed hepatocellular and anaplastic thyroid carcinoma (all >5%) [70].

3. Molecular Alterations with Approvals in Multiple Tumor Types

While not approved in a site-agnostic fashion, a growing compendium of molecular biomarkers are susceptible to precision oncology therapies with FDA approval in more than one tumor type. The latter part of Table 1 provides a summary of the agents which are discussed below.

3.1. BRAF V600 Mutations

3.1.1. Melanoma

Mutations in the 600th amino acid position of *BRAF* activate the mitogen-activated protein (MAP) kinase pathway, leading to cancer cell growth and proliferation. These lesions, predominantly V600E or V600K, can be identified in multiple solid tumors using NGS or other sequencing panels and are targetable. The prototype for targeting *BRAF* V600 lesions is cutaneous melanoma, where BRAF mutations occur in 40–60% and the single-agent selective BRAF-inhibitor, vemurafenib, was approved a decade ago [74]. Shortly following the FDA approval of vemurafenib, the single-agent BRAF-inhibitor dabrafenib [75] and the single-agent mitogen-activated protein kinase (*MEK*)-inhibitor trametinib [76] likewise showed activity, including activity against brain metastases in the case of dabrafenib [77], and both received approval in 2013. Due to the superior efficacy of alternative combination regimens and ICIs (see below), single-agent BRAF inhibition is currently given only if other agents are contraindicated while trametinib monotherapy is no longer recommended in BRAF mutant melanoma.

Predictable resistance to single-agent *BRAF* V600 inhibitors occurs through various means of reactivation of the MAP kinase pathway including paradoxical activation of downstream MEK [78]. Therefore, dual pathway blockade with both a BRAF and a MEK inhibitor has since become the predominant targeted approach to BRAF-mutant melanoma. First-line phase 3 trials comparing BRAF/MEK combinations to single-agent targeted therapy have shown an overall survival (OS) advantage for dual therapy and have led to the FDA approvals of dabrafenib and trametinib in 2014 (COMBI-d, COMBI-v) [79–83], vemurafenib and cobimetinib in 2015 (CO-BRIM) [84,85] and encorafenib and binimetinib in 2018 (COLUMBUS) [86–88]. For example, long-term follow-up of encorafenib and binimetinib showed a 34-month median OS with this combination versus 17 months with vemurafenib, amounting to a 39% decreased risk of death (HR 0.61; 95% CI, 0.48–0.79) [88].

While all three combinations are FDA approved and have ORRs of approximately 60–70% (vs. 50% for single-agent), median PFS of 11–15 months (vs. 7–10 months), the combination of encorafenib and binimetinib may be more tolerable with reduced pyrexia, fatigue and other symptoms [89].

It should also be noted that dabrafenib and trametinib were FDA approved in 2018 for the adjuvant treatment of *BRAF* V600E or V600K mutations following resection, which was based upon the COMBI-AD phase 3 study [90]. This represents one of the first approvals of a targeted agent for early-stage disease following surgery (with the exception of HER2 therapy for breast cancer; see below). Recently, Dummer et al. showed 5-year follow-up data, noting a 49% reduction for relapse or death for patients treated with planned 12 months of adjuvant dabrafenib and trametinib versus placebo [91].

Advances in targeted therapy for BRAF-mutated melanoma occurred at the same time as the development of ICI. In light of this, several additional points should be made in the management of BRAF-mutant melanoma. First, while *BRAF* V600 mutations predict response to targeted therapy, patients are also eligible to receive ICI in either the adjuvant [92,93] or metastatic [94–98] setting regardless of *BRAF* mutation status. Additionally, the IMspire150 trial was recently published, leading to the approval of the combination of agent atezolizumab (anti-PD-L1) and the BRAF/MEK inhibitors vemurafenib and cobimetinib in first-line metastatic disease [99]. The decision of whether to treat metastatic patients with ICIs, anti-BRAF/MEK agents or a combination of the two is not standardized, but involves shared-decision making with the patient and considerations such as toxicity differences, disease aggressiveness and pace, metastatic distribution including brain metastases, lactate dehydrogenase level and other clinical factors. Finally, it should be noted that only appropriate *BRAF* mutations (namely V600, with rare exceptions) are selected for targeted therapy, as utilization of BRAF/MEK inhibitors for certain non-V600 (e.g., K601E) lesions can paradoxically activate the MAP kinase pathway and possibly result in poor outcomes [100–102].

3.1.2. Lung Cancer

In June 2017, the FDA approved the combination of dabrafenib and trametinib for metastatic NSCLC patients harboring *BRAF* V600E mutations based upon the international, multicenter, three-cohort, non-randomized, open-label BRF113928 trial [103–105]. Overall, 93 metastatic NSCLC patients were treated, with 36 receiving no prior therapy. Previously untreated patients showed an ORR of 64% with the majority partial responses; 69% had at least one grade 3–4 adverse event, including pyrexia, hypertension, increase in alanine aminotransferase and vomiting [105]. Subsequent molecular profiling of new tissue or liquid samples after progression has been described to show resistance mechanisms in MAP kinase signaling, such as MEK, KRAS and NRAS mutations [106].

3.1.3. Thyroid Cancer

BRAF V600E mutations are frequent in differentiated thyroid cancer, occurring in almost 50% of papillary disease and associated with poor prognosis, especially when co-occurring with *TERT* promoter mutations [107,108]. For metastatic differentiated thyroid cancer patients harboring *BRAF* V600E mutations who are refractory to radioactive iodine, targeted therapy with BRAF-inhibitors dabrafenib or vemurafenib can be considered [109,110]. Anaplastic thyroid carcinoma is typically highly aggressive with a 1-year survival of roughly 20% [111]. Harboring *BRAF* V600 mutations in roughly 20–50% [112], Subbiah et al. showed a promising ORR of 69% (11 of 16) with dabrafenib and trametinib [113], ultimately leading to FDA approval of this BRAF/MEK combination for unresectable anaplastic thyroid carcinoma in 2018.

3.1.4. Colorectal Cancer

Finally, on 8 April 2020, the FDA approved the doublet encorafenib and cetuximab for metastatic colorectal cancer containing a *BRAF* V600E mutation after receipt of prior therapy [114]. The approval was based on data from the randomized, phase 3 BEACON CRC trial, where both the triplet (encorafenib, cetuximab and MEK inhibitor binimetinib) and doublet (encorafenib plus cetuximab) arms similarly improved ORR, PFS and OS versus standard-of-care cetuximab plus irinotecan-based regimens. Updated analysis showed a similar median PFS of 4.5 months for the triplet arm and 4.3 months for the doublet arm, both superior to 1.5 months for control [115]. With similar efficacy and reduced toxicity including gastrointestinal and hematologic compared to the triplet, preference for FDA approval was given to doublet encorafenib and cetuximab in advanced *BRAF* V600E colorectal cancer.

3.2. ERBB2/HER2

3.2.1. Breast and Gastric Cancer

Up to 20% of breast [116] and 13% of gastric cancers [117] overexpress the HER2 protein. That HER2 expression is a negative prognostic factor in breast and gastric cancer has been long recognized [118,119]. Generally, HER2 overexpression is determined by IHC testing (defined as 3+) and confirmed by reflex in-situ hybridization (ISH) testing for tumors with equivocal (2+) IHC results. Historically, tumors with 0 or 1+ expression by IHC have been denoted HER2-negative. Since 1998, trastuzumab, a monoclonal antibody targeting the HER2 protein has been available for the treatment of metastatic disease based on a number of studies [7,120–122]. Afterward, HER2 therapy with trastuzumab expanded into the adjuvant and neoadjuvant settings [123–125].

Numerous other HER-2 directed agents are now available. For example, in the metastatic setting, lapatinib was approved by the FDA in 2007 in combination with capecitabine and also has been shown to provide a benefit when combined with trastuzumab [126,127]. Additional monoclonal antibodies (pertuzumab, based on the CLEOPATRA study) [128] as well as ADCs (ado-trastuzumab emtansine (T-DM1) based on the EMILIA study, and fam-trastuzumab deruxtecan (T-DXd) based on the DESTINY-Breast01 study) [129,130] have entered practice in the metastatic setting either alone or in combination with trastuzumab. Additional TKIs (neratinib based on the NALA trial and tucatinib based on the HER2CLIMB study) [131,132] have also been approved. Pertuzumab can be effective when combined with trastuzumab and chemotherapy in adjuvant and neoadjuvant settings [133,134]. As a whole, advances in targeted agents with improved efficacy, including superior intracranial activity [135], have greatly improved the prognosis for breast cancer expressing HER2.

In gastric cancer, trastuzumab was initially approved in the metastatic setting in 2010 based on the TOGA trial [136]. Most recently, T-DXd received FDA approval in the metastatic setting in January 2021 based on the DESTINY-gastric01 trial [137]. In this latter study, T-DXd was compared to chemotherapy for metastatic patients who had received two prior systemic lines of therapy, including trastuzumab. Both an improvement in ORR (51% vs. 14%, $p < 0.001$) and median OS were seen (12.5 vs. 8.4 months, HR 0.59). Approximately 10% of T-DXd treated patients developed interstitial lung disease or pneumonitis, although the majority were grades 1 or 2.

3.2.2. On-the Horizon: Colorectal Cancer

While no FDA approvals have occurred to date, several clinical trials have evaluated HER2-directed agents, either alone or in combination, for advances colorectal cancer patients exhibiting HER2 overexpression. Combinatorial regimens include pertuzumab and trastuzumab in the MyPathway and TRIUMPH trials [138,139]; trastuzumab and lapatinib in HERACLES-A [140]; trastuzumab and tucatinib in MOUNTAINEER [141]; and T-DM1 and pertuzumab in HERACLES-B [142]. Additionally, data for T-DXd in DESTINY-CRC01 was recently reported [143] Taken as a whole, these studies showed variable ORRs from 9% to 55% with seemingly better responses found for those patients whose tumors are KRAS wild-type.

3.2.3. On-the-Horizon: HER2 Mutations in NSCLC

In addition to HER2 overexpression discussed in breast, gastric and colorectal cancer, activating HER2 mutations are found in multiple solid tumors and are potentially druggable [144], but no approvals have occurred to date. In NSCLC, driver HER2 mutations are identified in approximately 2% of patients. In a phase II basket trial utilizing T-DM1 in mostly pre-treated metastatic NSCLC patients, 8/18 (44%) obtain a partial response [145]. Responses were seen in patients with HER2 exon 20 insertions as well as other kinase and non-kinase domain mutations. Additionally, Smit and colleagues reported data from the cohort of DESTINY-Lung01 which evaluated T-DXd in NSCLC patients with activating HER2 mutations, on which 90% were relegated to the kinase domain [146] With most patients previously receiving both chemotherapy and ICI, an impressive ORR of 62% (26/42) was seen, for which the median duration was not reached at the time of data cutoff (median follow-up eight months).

3.3. RET
Medullary Thyroid, Other Thyroid and Lung Cancers

An additional predictive molecular target with multi-tumor approved agents are *RET* alterations, with potentially sensitizing mutations seen in approximately 70% of medullary thyroid cancers (MTC), fusions in <10% of other thyroid cancers and fusions in 1–2% of NSCLC [147–149]. While 'dirty' multikinase inhibitors previously showed some activity in *RET*-altered disease, a tradeoff of significant toxicity was seen. However, in May 2020 the FDA approved selpercatinib, a selective small-molecule *RET* inhibitor for adult NSCLC patients with metastatic *RET* fusions, as well as patients $\geq$12 years old with *RET*-mutated MTC or fusion-positive thyroid cancer who require systemic therapy (and are refractory to radioactive iodine, if indicated). Approval was based upon the results of LIBRETTO-001, a multicenter, open-label, multi-cohort trial. Key findings reported in *RET* fusion-positive NSCLC include a 64% ORR of 105 consecutively enrolled and pre-treated patients, with a median duration of almost 18 months; for untreated NSCLC patients, an 85% ORR was seen [150]. Importantly, only 2% discontinued selpercatinib due to drug-related toxicity, and 91% (n = 11 of 12) with measurable central nervous system disease had an intracranial response. In *RET*-altered thyroid cancer, Wirth et al. detailed an ORR of 73% and 92% 1-year PFS of 88 untreated MTC patients harboring *RET* mutations; of 55 other MTC patients who received prior multi-kinase TKIs vandetinib and/or cabozantinib, impressive response rates and durability were still seen [151].

It should also be noted that pralsetinib was subsequently approved for *RET* fusions in advanced NSCLC in September 2020 and advanced, mutated or fusion-positive thyroid cancer patients (similar to the selpercatinib indication) in December 2020 based upon the ARROW trial. For NSCLC, a 57% ORR of 87 previously-treated patients was observed; further, an additional 27 untreated fusion-positive NSCLC patients had a 70% ORR to pralsetinib, with nearly 60% of responses extending beyond six months [37,152,153]. Clinical progression to selpercatinib (or pralsetinib) should prompt molecular testing for resistance mechanisms, which can include *RET* solvent front mutations, as well as *MET* and *KRAS* amplifications [154,155]. While some resistance mechanisms may be targetable, development of next-generation *RET* inhibitors is warranted for solvent front alterations.

3.4. DNA Damage Response/PARP Inhibition

Many loss-of-function alterations occur in genes involved in DNA repair, particularly in homologous recombination repair (HRR). BRCA1 and BRCA2 are the most common and most well-characterized genes involved in this process, but other genes such as ATM, CHEK2, PALB2 and RAD51 are also linked to HRR deficiency (HRD). Deleterious mutations in HRR can be found both in the germline setting as well as somatic alterations uncovered with tumor molecular profiling. Responses to poly(adenosine diphosphate-ribose) polymerase (PARP) inhibition have been described in several tumor types with

HRD, either by specific mutations identified in a candidate gene or via genomic instability identified during molecular profiling.

3.4.1. Ovarian Cancer

Ovarian cancer is known to be associated with germline alterations in BRCA1 or BRCA2, though somatic mutations can also occur. Olaparib was approved in 2018 for the maintenance of patients with somatic mutations in the setting of complete or partial response to first-line platinum therapy. This indication is based on the SOLO-1 trial comparing olaparib versus placebo in this setting. Progression-free survival was improved in the olaparib arm (HR 0.30; $p < 0.0001$) [156]. The indication was expanded to include a combination of olaparib with bevacizumab in 2020 based on the PAOLA-1 trial [157]. The PARP inhibitor rucaparib initially had approval only in patients with BRCA germline mutations. However, soon thereafter rucaparib was approved in the maintenance setting for ovarian cancer regardless of BRCA status. Interestingly, the PARP inhibitor rucaparib was later approved regardless of BRCA status based on the ARIEL3 trial. While this trial evaluated patients for BRCA or HRD, the overall study population showed a benefit in PFS (HR 0.36, $p < 0.0001$) [158]. In 2017, approval for the PARP inhibitor niraparib was obtained for maintenance therapy in ovarian cancer, also without the need for HRD mutations with this indication expanded to the first-line maintenance setting in 2020 based on the PRIMA trial [159]. In 2019, however, niraparib was approved again in late-line ovarian cancer for patients with HRD mutations [42]. As is clear from these approval timelines, PARP inhibitor therapy in ovarian cancer remains complex, with certain agents approved in certain settings regardless of genomic alterations, some approved only for BRCA1/2 genomic alterations and others approved for germline or somatic alterations in BRCA1/2 or HRD tumors.

3.4.2. Prostate Cancer

The approval of PARP inhibitors for somatic HRD mutations in prostate cancer was based on the PROfound study which randomized 256 patients to the PARP inhibitor olaparib and 131 patients to the investigator's choice of hormone therapy. Patients were divided into two cohorts, one with mutations in *BRCA1*, *BRCA2* or *ATM* and the other with mutations among 12 other genes in the HRR pathway. A statistically significant difference was seen in PFS among the BRCA/ATM cohort (HR 0.34, $p < 0.0001$) as well as overall across both cohorts (HR 0.49; $p < 0.0001$) [160]. Even more recently, the PARP inhibitor rucaparib was also approved in castrate-resistant prostate cancer in patients specifically with BRCA1 or two mutations, whether germline or somatic, who have failed hormone therapy and a taxane. The approval was based on the TRITON2 trial, a single-arm trial of 115 patients showing a confirmed objective response rate of 44% among the 65 patients who had measurable disease [161].

3.4.3. Breast Cancer

In January 2018, the FDA approved olaparib in metastatic HER-2 negative breast cancer patients whose tumors harbored a germline *BRCA* mutation and received prior chemotherapy based upon the results of the randomized phase 3 OlympiAD trial [162]. In this study, olaparib was found to have an ORR of 60% and a superior PFS compared to physician's choice of chemotherapy (7.0 versus 3.2 months; HR 0.58). Subsequently, talazoparib received a similar approval for germline *BRCA* mutated metastatic breast cancer, with the EMBRACA trial demonstrating a higher ORR (63% versus 27%, $p < 0.001$) and improved median PFS (8.6 versus 5.6 months; HR 0.54) when compared to chemotherapy [163].

3.4.4. Pancreatic Cancer

Germline BRCA1/2 mutations occur in approximately 5% of pancreatic cancers [164]. On 27 December 2019, olaparib was FDA approved for this subset of metastatic pancreatic cancer patients in the maintenance setting, where the agent was given after a minimum of 16 weeks of platinum-based chemotherapy. Golan and colleagues reported an improvement in median PFS (7.4 versus 3.8 months for placebo; HR 0.53); however, an interim analysis did not show a difference in OS [165].

A summary of major clinical trials leading to approvals in more than one malignancy can be seen in Table 2.

3.5. PD-L1

The use of ICI therapy, particularly anti-programmed death-1 (PD1) antibodies or anti-programmed death ligand-1 (PD-L1) antibodies, has become virtually ubiquitous in cancer. Currently, there are seven anti-PD-1 or PD-L1 therapies in use in the clinic, approved across 19 malignancies and with 77 different indications [166–172]. Being as the mechanism of action of these therapies depends upon the interaction between PD-1 and PD-L1, PD-L1 protein expression was early determined to be a potential predictor of response to ICI [173]. However, the fact that some tumors with high expression of PD-L1 do not respond to PD-(L)1 therapy, and the fact that some tumors with no or low PD-L1 expression do respond to PD-(L)1 therapy, highlights the difficulty in using this biomarker as a true surrogate of response [173]. Additionally, various companion diagnostics using different detection antibodies, methods of measuring PD-L1 expression and "positive" cutoffs have been problematic and present a barrier to the interpretation of biomarker data in clinical trials [174]. In an evaluation of the pivotal trials leading to 45 FDA approvals of PD-(L)1 inhibitors from 2015–2019, PD-L1 expression was predictive in only 29% of the approvals, while it was not predictive in 53% and not tested in 18% [175]. However, while PD-L1 expression is not always predictive, failure to include the biomarker into certain clinical trials or utilization of the wrong assay or wrong cutoff may have led to a determination of an overall lack of efficacy [176,177]. At the current time, 12 indications for PD-(L)1 therapy in seven malignancies are dependent on PD-L1 status [166–168,171]. These indications utilize different methods of determining PD-L1 status (tumor cell proportion score, immune cell proportion score or combined positive score), different thresholds for positivity and different FDA-approved companion diagnostics. Table 3 summarizes the PD-L1 based approvals that exist in lung, head and neck, bladder, gastric, esophageal, cervical and breast cancer together with the various measures of PD-L1 expression, companion diagnostics and positive thresholds. In summary, PD-L1 remains a highly imperfect biomarker, and other markers of immune responsiveness are simultaneously being tested for (e.g., MSI status, TMB-h) and studied (tumor-infiltrating lymphocytes, tumor microenvironment, etc.) to enable proper selection of treatment with ICIs [174].

Table 2. Key pivotal trials leading to FDA approval in alterations with multiple tumor indications (MSI-h, TMB-h, NTRK fusion, BRAF, HER2, RET, BRCA).

Setting/Genomic Alteration	Cancer Type, Line of Therapy	Study	Trial Phase	Number of Subjects	Line of Therapy	Agent	Comparator	Primary Outcome	Primary Outcome Results	Key Secondary Outcomes	Results (If Applicable)
MSI-h, dMMR	Pan-tumor	KEYNOTE-158 [51]	II	233	Metastatic 2nd line or greater	Pembrolizumab	None	ORR (objective response rate)	34.3% (95% CI, 28.3%, 40.8%)	Overall survival (OS)	23.5 mo (95% CI, 13.5–not reached (NR))
	Colorectal cancer	CheckMate 142 [53]	II	119	Metastatic any line	Nivolumab + Ipilimumab	None	ORR	55% (95% CI, 45.2–63.8%)	Disease control rate (DCR) >12 weeks	80%
		KEYNOTE-177 [54]	III	307	Metastatic 1st line	Pembrolizumab	Chemotherapy	Progression-free survival (PFS) (median)	16.5 v 8.2 months, hazard ratio (HR) 0.60 (95% CI, 0.45–0.8, p 0.0004)	ORR	44% vs. 33%
TMB-high	Pan-tumor	KEYNOTE-158 [65]	II	102	Metastatic 2nd line or greater	Pembrolizumab	TMB-low patients (n = 688)	ORR	29% (95% CI, 21–39%) vs. 6% (95% CI, 5–8%)	N/A	N/A
NTRK fusion	Pan-tumor	LOXO-TRK-14001, SCOUT, NAVIGATE (pooled analysis) [59]	I/II	159	Any metastatic	Larotrectinib	None	ORR	79% (95% CI, 72–85%)	Duration of response (DOR) (median)	35.2 mo (95% CI 22.8–NR)
		ALKA-372-001, STARTRK-1, STARTRK-2 (pooled analysis) [60]	I/II	54	Any metastatic	Entrectinib	None	ORR	57% (95% CI, 43–71%)	DOR (median)	10 mo (95% CI, 7.1–not estimable (NE))
BRAF V600E	Melanoma	COMBI-d [80]	III	423	Metastatic 1st line	Trametinib and Dabrafenib	Dabrafenib	PFS (median)	11.0 mo (95% CI, 8.0–13.9) vs. 8.8 mo (95% CI, 5.9–9.3)	OS (median)	25.1 v 18.7 months HR 0.71 (95% CI, 0.55–0.92, p = 0.01)
		CoBRIM [85]	III	495	Metastatic 1st line	Vemurafenib and Cobimetinib	Vemurafenib	PFS (median)	12.3 v 7.2 months HR 0.58 (95% CI, 0.46–0.72, p = <0.0001)	OS (median)	22.3 v 17.4 months HR 0.70 (95% CI, 0.55–0.90, p = 0.005)
		COLUMBUS [87]	III	383	Metastatic 2nd line or greater	Encorafenib and Binimetinib	Vemurafenib	PFS (median)	14.9 v 7.3 months HR 0.54 (95% CI, 0.41–0.71, p <0.0001)	OS (median)	33.6 v 16.9 months HR 0.61 (95% CI, 0.48–0.79, p <0.0001)
		COMBI-AD [90]	III	870	Stage III adjuvant	Dabrafenib and Trametinib	Placebo	Relapse-free survival (RFS) (three-year)	58% vs. 39%, HR 0.47 (95% CI, 0.39–0.58, p < 0.001)	OS (three-year)	86% vs. 77%, HR 0.57 (95% CI, 0.42–0.79, p = 0.0006)
	NSCLC	BRF113928 [105]	II	36	Metastatic 1st line	Dabrafenib and Trametinib	None	ORR	64% (95% CI, 46–79%)	N/A	N/A
	Anaplastic thyroid cancer	CDRB436 × 2201 [113]	II	16	Any line post-radiation or surgery	Dabrafenib and Trametinib	None	ORR	69% (95% CI, 41–89%)	DOR (median)	Not reached

Table 2. Cont.

Setting/Genomic Alteration	Cancer Type, Line of Therapy	Study	Trial Phase	Number of Subjects	Line of Therapy	Agent	Comparator	Primary Outcome	Primary Outcome Results	Key Secondary Outcomes	Results (If Applicable)
HER2 positive	Colorectal cancer	BEACON-CRC [114]	III	665	Metastatic 2nd line or greater	Encorafenib, Binimetinib and Cetuximab	Investigator choice	OS (median)	9.0 mo vs. 5.4 mo, HR 0.52 (95% CI, 0.39–0.70, $p < 0.001$)	ORR	26% (95% CI 18–35%) vs. 2% (95% CI, 0–7%)
		Slamon et al. (2001) [7]	III	469	Metastatic 1st line	Trastuzumab and chemotherapy	Placebo and chemotherapy	PFS (median)	7.4 mo vs. 4.6 mo, HR 0.51 (95% CI, 0.41–0.63, $p < 0.001$)	OS (median)	25.1 mo vs. 20.3 mo, HR 0.80 (95% CI 0.64–1.00, $p = 0.046$)
		Geyer et al. (2006) [126]	III	399	Metastatic 2nd line or greater	Lapatinib and Capecitabine	Capecitabine	Time to progression (TTP) (median)	8.4mo vs. 4.4mo, HR 0.49 (95% CI, 0.34–0.71, $p < 0.001$)	N/A	N/A
		EMILIA [130]	III	991	Metastatic 2nd line or greater	Trastuzumab emtansine (T-DM1)	Lapatinib and Capecitabine	PFS (median)	9.6 mo vs. 6.4 mo, HR 0.65 (95% CI, 0.55–0.77, $p < 0.001$)	OS (median)	30.9 mo vs. 25.1 mo, HR 0.68 (95% CI, 0.55–0.85, $p < 0.001$)
	Breast cancer	DESTINY-Breast01 [129]	II	184	Metastatic 3rd line or greater	Trastuzumab deruxtecan (T-DXd)	None	ORR	60.9% (95% CI, 53–68%)	PFS	16.4 mo (95% CI, 12.7–NR)
		CLEOPATRA [128]	III	808	Metastatic 1st line	Pertuzumab, trastuzumab and docetaxel	Trastuzumab and docetaxel	PFS (median)	18.5 mo vs. 12.4 mo, HR 0.62 (95% CI, 0.51–0.75, $p < 0.001$)	OS	HR 0.64 (95% CI, 0.47–0.88, $p = 0.005$)
		NALA [131]	III	621	Metastatic 2nd line or greater	Neratinib and Capecitabine	Lapatinib and Capecitabine	PFS	HR 0.76 (95% CI 0.63–0.93, $p = 0.0059$)	OS (co-primary endpoint)	HR 0.88 (95% CI, 0.72–1.07, $p = 0.21$)
		HER2CLIMB [132]	II	612	Metastatic 3rd line or greater	Tucatinib, trastuzumab and capecitabine	Trastuzumab and capecitabine	PFS (median)	7.8 mo vs. 5.6 mo, HR 0.54 (95% CI, 0.42–0.71, $p < 0.001$)	OS (median)	21.9 mo vs. 17.4 mo, HR 0.66 (95% CI, 0.50–0.88, $p = 0.005$)
	Gastric cancer	TOGA [136]	III	594	Metastatic 1st line	Trastuzumab and Chemotherapy	Chemotherapy	OS (median)	13.8 mo vs. 11.1 mo, HR 0.74 (95% CI, 0.60–0.91, $p = 0.0046$)	N/A	N/A
		DESTINY-Gastric01 [137]	II	187	Metastatic 3rd line or greater	T-DXd	Chemotherapy	ORR	51% vs. 14% ($p < 0.001$)	OS (median)	12.5 mo vs. 8.4 mo, HR 0.59 (95% CI 0.39–0.88, $p = 0.01$)
RET fusion	NSCLC	LIBRETTO-001 [150]	I/II	105	Metastatic previously treated	Selpercatinib	None	ORR	64% (95% CI, 54–73%)	DOR (median)	17.5 mo (95% CI, 12.0–NE)

Table 2. Cont.

Setting/Genomic Alteration	Cancer Type, Line of Therapy	Study	Trial Phase	Number of Subjects	Line of Therapy	Agent	Comparator	Primary Outcome	Primary Outcome Results	Key Secondary Outcomes	Results (If Applicable)
RET mutation	Medullary thyroid cancer	ARROW [153]	I/II	87	Metastatic previously treated	Pralsetinib	None	ORR	57% (95% CI, 46–68%)	N/A	N/A
		LIBRETTO-001 [151]	I/II	88	Metastatic 1st line	Selpercatinib	None	ORR	73% (95% CI, 62–82%)	N/A	N/A
BRCA or HRD alteration	Ovarian cancer	SOLO-1 [156]	III	391	Metastatic 1st line maintenance	Olaparib	Placebo	PFS (-three-year)	60% vs. 27%, HR 0.30 (95% CI, 0.23–0.41, $p < 0.001$)	N/A	N/A
	Castrate-resistant prostate cancer	PROfound [160]	III	245	Metastatic	Olaparib	Enzalutamide or Abiraterone	PFS (median)	7.4 vs. 3.6 mo, HR 0.34 (95% CI, 0.25–0.47, $p < 0.0001$)	OS (median)	19.1 vs. 14.7 mo, HR 0.69 (95% CI, 0.50–0.97, $p = 0.018$)
		TRITON2 [161]	II	115	Metastatic, post androgen and chemotherapy	Rucaparib	None	ORR	43.5% (95% CI, 31.0–56.7%)	Prostate-specific antigen response	54.8% (95% CI, 45.2–64.1%)
	Breast cancer	OlympiAD [162]	III	301	Metastatic, germline, no more than two prior lines	Olaparib	Chemotherapy	PFS (median)	7.0 vs. 4.2 mo, HR 0.58 (95% CI, 0.43–0.80, $p = 0.0009$)	OS (median)	19.3 vs. 17.1 mo, HR 0.90 (95% CI, 0.66–1.23)
	Pancreatic cancer	POLO [165]	III	154	Metastatic, germline, 1st line maintenance	Olaparib	Placebo	PFS (median)	7.4 vs. 3.8 mo, HR 0.53 (95% CI, 0.35–0.81, $p = 0.0035$)	ORR	23% vs. 12%

Table 3. Indications for use of PD-1 or PD-L1 antibodies dependent on PD-L1 level.

Malignancy	Line	Agent	Measurement	Positive Threshold	FDA-Approved Companion Diagnostic	FDA Approval Date
Lung cancer	1st line metastatic	Pembrolizumab	Tumor proportion score (TPS)	>1%	22c3 Ab, Dako	11 March 2019 [178]
		Nivolumab + Ipilimumab	TPS	>1%	28-8 Ab, Dako	15 May 2020 [179]
		Atezolizumab	Tumor cell proportion score (TC)	>50%	SP142 Ab, Ventana	18 May 2020 [180]
			Immune cell proportion score (IC)	>10%	SP142 Ab, Ventana	
		Cemiplimab	TPS	>50%	22c3 Ab, Dako	22 February 2021 [181]
Head and neck cancer	1st line metastatic	Pembrolizumab	TC + IC (combined positive score or CPS)	>1	22c3 Ab, Dako	10 June 2019 [182]
Bladder cancer	1st line metastatic cisplatin ineligible	Pembrolizumab	CPS	>10	22c3 Ab, Dako	19 June 2018 [183]
		Atezolizumab	IC	>5%	SP142 Ab, Ventana	19 June 2018 [183]
Gastric cancer	>3rd line metastatic	Pembrolizumab	CPS	>1	22c3 Ab, Dako	22 September 2017 [184]
Esophageal cancer (squamous)	>3rd line metastatic	Pembrolizumab	CPS	>10	22c3 Ab, Dako	30 July 2019 [185]
Cervical cancer	>2nd line metastatic	Pembrolizumab	CPS	>1	22c3 Ab, Dako	12 June 2018 [186]
Breast cancer (triple negative)	Metastatic	Atezolizumab	IC	>1%	SP142 Ab, Ventana	8 March 2019 [187]
		Pembrolizumab	CPS	>10	22c3 Ab, Dako	13 November 2020 [188]

3.6. On the Horizon—KRAS G12C

KRAS, which controls cellular signal transduction through its encoded guanosine triphosphatase activity, is the most commonly mutated oncogene in solid tumors, frequently portends a poor prognosis, is affiliated with resistance to multiple systemic treatments and thus far, its targeting has remained elusive [189–192]. Occurring in approximately 13% of NSCLC and >1% of colorectal cancer and various other solid tumors, *KRAS G12C* mutations were found to be targetable in pre-clinical studies through irreversible, covalent binding of small molecule kinase inhibitors to the mutated cysteine and nearby P2 pocket of the switch II region [193–195]. Hong et al. recently reported phase 1 data, showing promising activity of *KRAS G12C* inhibitor, sotorasib, in 129 pre-treated (median number of prior lines of therapy was 3) solid tumor patients [196]. For example, 32% of NSCLC, 7% of colorectal cancer and 14% of other solid tumor patients (including melanoma, endometrial, pancreatic and appendiceal) had an objective response. While the median PFS of responders was six months with single-agent sotorasib, future evaluation of *KRAS* inhibitors with tumor-informed precision combinations may lead to more effective targeting [197–199]. Furthermore, the efficacy of a second covalent inhibitor of *KRAS G12C*, adagrasib, was presented at the European Lung Cancer Virtual Conference in early 2021, where the multi-cohort phase I/II trial showed a 45% ORR in 51 advanced, typically pre-treated NSCLC patients [200].

4. Precision Oncology in Lung Cancer

Perhaps more than any other solid tumor, patients with lung cancer can derive benefit from therapeutic options exposed following comprehensive molecular profiling. The leading cause of cancer-related mortality worldwide [201], advanced lung cancer treated with a one-size-fits-all approach of platinum doublet chemotherapy historically resulted in relatively poor outcomes, with a limited percentage of patients achieving long-term survival [202]. However, recent evidence showed a population-level reduction in mortality of lung cancer patients from 2013–2016, attributed not only to a reduction in incidence but an early indication of the efficacy of novel precision oncology treatments in NSCLC [203].

NSCLC accounts for approximately 85% of all lung cancer; its three major histologic types include adenocarcinoma, squamous cell carcinoma and large cell carcinoma. The vast majority of lung adenocarcinoma is driven by identifiable oncogenic aberrations, with a growing number amenable to targeted therapies such that current guidelines recommend complete molecular testing for patients with metastatic disease [204]. Additionally, testing should be considered for non-adenocarcinoma NSCLC, especially those with limited smoking history or mixed histology whose samples may be enriched for targetable mutations or alterations. While testing may take several forms, up-front comprehensive molecular profiling in NSCLC should ideally consist of a broad-panel evaluation such as NGS for specific gene mutations, IHC, ISH, real-time PCR and RNA assessment to identify gene rearrangements and fusions, as well as immune biomarker appraisal with IHC for PD-L1, MSI status and TMB (see previous discussion) [205]. If available tissue is not sufficient to complete testing, liquid biopsy with plasma cell-free or circulating tumor DNA can be informative [206,207]. Unless an impending clinical scenario mandates, the treatment team should ideally wait upon receipt of comprehensive molecular data to determine if the NSCLC patient is a candidate for first-line targeted therapy. The determination of whether to begin first-line treatment with ICI or targeted therapy is of great importance, as improper initial ICI in NSCLC patients with specific oncogenic drivers can lead to significant toxicity when subsequent TKIs or targeted therapy are begun [208,209]. In addition to the aforementioned targetable alterations (BRAF V600E, *RET* fusions, as well as emerging *HER2* mutations and *KRAS* G12C), multiple other predictive molecular targets exist in NSCLC. Table 4 shows molecular alterations and their targeted agents that have been approved only in lung cancer.

Table 4. Molecular alterations leading to FDA-targeted therapy approvals only in NSCLC.

Alteration(s)	Line of Therapy	Medications	Drug Class	FDA Approval Date
EGFR (exon 19 deletions and exon 21 point mutations)	1st line metastatic	Erlotinib	EGFR TKI	14 May 2013 [210]
		Gefitinib		13 July 2015 [211]
		Afatinib		12 January 2018 [212]
		Dacomitinib		27 September 2018 [213]
		Osimertinib (also against T790M mutations)		18 April 2018 [214]
	Adjuvant	Osimertinib (also against T790M mutations)		18 December 2020 [215]
EGFR (exon 20 insertion)	2nd line metastatic	Amivantamab	EGFR, MET bispecific antibody	21 May 2021 [216]
ALK fusions	Metastatic	Crizotinib	ALK TKI	26 August 2011 [217]
		Ceritinib		29 April 2014 [218]
		Lorlatinib		2 November 2018 [219]
		Alectinib		11 December 2015 [220]
		Brigatinib		28 April 2017 [221]
ROS1 fusions	Metastatic	Crizotinib	ALK TKI	11 March 2016 [222]
		Entrectinib	Selective TKI	15 August 2019 [16]
MET exon 14 skipping mutations	Metastatic	Capmatinib	MET inhibitor	6 May 2020 [223]
		Tepotinib		3 February 2021 [224]

4.1. EGFR

Epidermal growth factor receptor (*EGFR*) is mutated in approximately 10% of Caucasian and potentially up to 50% of Asian NSCLC patients with limited or no smoking history [225]. The majority of *EGFR* mutations sensitive to targeted therapy lie within the tyrosine kinase domain, with exon 19 deletions or exon 21's L858R comprising the vast majority. Other rare lesions may also be sensitive to *EGFR* TKIs and include L861Q, G719X and S768I [226]. Current oral TKIs with FDA approved to treat advanced NSCLC patients whose tumors harbor sensitizing *EGFR* mutations include gefitinib, erlotinib (with or without ramucirumab), afatinib, dacomitinib and osimertinib.

Initially, first-generation oral TKIs gefitinib and erlotinib showed promising activity for inhibition of sensitizing *EGFR* mutations. In the randomized phase 3 trial, IPASS, first-line gefitinib was affiliated with an improved response rate versus platinum-based doublet chemotherapy (71% vs. 43%) in Asian patients with *EGFR* mutations [227]. While this agent also showed a prolonged PFS, subsequent results did not translate into an improved OS, likely due to ensuing TKI use of the chemotherapy arm upon progression [228]. These findings were also confirmed in Caucasian NSCLC patients with *EGFR* mutations [229]. Likewise, EURTAC detailed a prolonged PFS for first-line erlotinib versus chemotherapy in European *EGFR*-mutated NSCLC patients (9.7 vs. 5.2 months; HR 0.37) [230]. FDA approval was also granted in 2020 to the combination of ramucirumab, a recombinant monoclonal antibody targeting vascular endothelial growth factor (VEGF) receptors, plus erlotinib for first-line use in metastatic NSCLC patients with exon 19 deletions or L858R mutations. Approval was granted based on results of a randomized phase 3 trial, RELAY, which showed a prolonged PFS for the combination versus erlotinib monotherapy (19.4 vs. 12.4 months; HR 0.59); a similar response rate of both arms was observed (approximately 75%) [231]. However, 72% of patients in the combination arm had grade 3–4 adverse events including hypertension and transaminase abnormalities; one treatment-related death in the combination arm occurred. While FDA approved and an option to be discussed with patients, the niche of combinatorial strategies of *EGFR* TKIs with VEGF receptor inhibitors (e.g., ramucirumab or bevacizumab) [232] in the frontline setting warrants further exploration, especially when next-generation TKIs (see osimertinib below) are very efficacious and have a favorable toxicity profile.

Second-generation TKIs include afatinib and dacomitinib, which irreversibly inhibit multiple ErbB/HER receptors, including EGFR. Phase 3 LUX-Lung 3 showed an improvement of PFS in advanced lung adenocarcinoma patients with sensitizing *EGFR* mutations treated with afatinib compared to cisplatin plus pemetrexed (11.1 vs. 6.9 months). Additionally, afatinib was FDA approved in 2018 for uncommon mutations S768I, L861Q and/or G719X based upon combined analysis from the LUX-Lung 2, 3 and 6 trials [233,234]. Dacomitinib received FDA approval in 2018 following published results from the randomized phase 3 ARCHER1050 study, with updated data showing a prolongation of OS versus gefitinib in the first-line setting (median 34.1 vs. 26.8 months; HR 0.76) [235,236].

Initially FDA approved in 2017 following progression on another TKI based on its efficacy in the AURA3 trial against *EGFR* resistance mutation, T790M [237], third-generation TKI osimertinib is now considered a standard-of-care for untreated, advanced NSCLC patients with sensitizing *EGFR* aberrations based on the FLAURA study [238]. Most recently, secondary endpoint OS analysis was published, showing a significant prolongation of median OS in the osimertinib arm compared to TKIs gefitinib or erlotinib (38.6 vs. 31.8 months; HR 0.80) [239]. The attraction of osimertinib includes not only its activity against T790M, but a relatively mild toxicity profile with QT prolongation (10%, reduced cardiac ejection fraction (5%), pneumonitis (2%) and interstitial lung disease (2%) with no treatment-related deaths. Further, osimertinib can induce durable intracranial responses, including in patients with leptomeningeal disease [240,241].

The clinical utility of osimertinib in *EGFR*-mutated NSCLC is extending to other indications. For example, the agent could be considered as a possible alternative to afatinib for advanced NSCLC patients whose tumor harbors uncommon *EGFR* mutations [242,243].

Additionally, the recently-published ADAURA trial [244] showed an impressive disease-free survival benefit at two years with the addition of osimertinib to provider-determined adjuvant therapy in stage II and IIIA patients (90% versus 44% for placebo; HR 0.17). Further, only 1% of patients receiving osimertinib developed CNS recurrence versus 10% of the placebo arm at two years. The adjuvant use of osimertinib was FDA approved on 18 December 2020 and extended to stage IB-IIIA NSCLC (non-squamous) patients whose tumors harbored EGFR exon 19 deletions or exon 21 L858R mutations [215]. This approval represents a paradigm shift, as increasing numbers of non-metastatic NSCLC patients will now receive molecular profiling whereas testing was previously relegated to the advanced setting. The additional genomic information received and potential uncovering of targetable molecular targets in the early-stage space provides a clinical challenge and opportunity for further study. Upon resistance to osimertinib, it is important to re-biopsy, if possible, and obtain tissue or liquid molecular profiling both to assess for small cell transformation, as well as potential targetable resistance mechanisms including *MET* amplifications, additional *EGFR* mutations or rare fusion events [245].

Finally, it should be noted that exon 20 insertion mutations represent the third most common alteration of *EGFR* and are generally not sensitive to TKIs. At this time, two agents selective to exon 20 insertions have received FDA Breakthrough Therapy Designation, amivantamab-vmjw [246] and mobocertinib [247]. On May 21, 2021, amivantamab, a bispecific antibody to EGFR and MET, was FDA approved for advanced NSCLC patients with *EGFR* exon 20 mutations after progression with chemotherapy. The approval was based upon the phase 1 CHRYSALIS study, which showed a 40% ORR with a median duration exceeding 11 months in 81 evaluated patients [246].

4.2. ALK, ROS1

Anaplastic lymphoma kinase (*ALK*; 2–5% of NSCLC) and *ROS1* (1–3%) rearrangements represent another subset of oncogenic drivers in NSCLC for which there are multiple effective targeted agents. Three precision drugs target both *ALK* and *ROS1* (crizotinib (which also has activity against *MET*) [248–252], ceritinib [253] and lorlatinib [254,255]. *ALK* can also be inhibited by alectinib (which also has activity against *RET*) [256–258] and brigatinib [259–262], while *ROS1* is also inhibited by entrectinib (previously discussed for *NTRK* fusions) [263]. In the first-line setting for *ALK*-rearranged disease, current preference should be given to alectinib, brigatinib or lorlatinib over crizotinib, as all three agents showed improved efficacy in randomized phase 3 trials compared to the first-generation *ALK* inhibitor [255–258,261,262]. For example, updated data from the ALEX trial recently established an advantage of alectinib over crizotinib for mature PFS (median 34.8 vs. 10.9 months; HR 0.43) and median OS (not reached vs. 57.4 months; HR 0.67), which was also seen for patients with brain metastases [258]. While ceritinib remains an FDA-approved frontline option based on the ASCEND-4 trial [253], a direct comparison to crizotinib or another TKI has not been published to date.

The toxicity profile should be considered before the use of any TKI in the management of *ALK*-rearranged NSCLC, such as myalgia, edema, hepatotoxicity, interstitial lung disease/pneumonitis and bradycardia with alectinib and respiratory symptoms [264,265], vision change, amylase and lipase elevation, hypertension and similarly bradycardia with brigatinib. Although associated with undesirable toxicities including cognitive effects, mood changes, peripheral neuropathy and elevated triglycerides or cholesterol, lorlatinib is a third-generation TKI that has ample CNS penetration and has emerged as an effective agent with not only front-line activity, but efficacy at progression for multiple *ALK* resistance mutations from early-generation inhibitors [255,266–268]. As with *EGFR*, the mechanism of resistance to *ALK*-inhibition should be sought with repeat tissue or liquid biopsy as targetable resistance mechanisms aside from *ALK* mutations may be identified [269].

Of the three available agents that target *ROS1*, entrectinib and crizotinib are FDA approved in advanced ROS1-rearranged NSCLC and should be prioritized over ceritinib in the first-line setting. Further, in addition to pulmonary toxicity seen with almost all TKIs utilized in NSCLC, ceritinib use includes heightened gastrointestinal toxicities such as diarrhea, nausea and vomiting, hepatotoxicity and pancreatitis that may make it less tolerable than other agents [253]. Both entrectinib and crizotinib provide ORR of approximately 70–80%, a significant portion of which are durable [252,263]; further, intracranial response of entrectinib is reported as 55%.

Upon progression, lorlatinib has likewise emerged as a preferred agent subsequent to either crizotinib or entrectinib [270,271]. Next-generation TKIs such as repotrectinib, which has impressive CNS penetration and activity against ROS1, ALK and NTRK, are currently being evaluated for first-line or subsequent-line use [272].

4.3. MET

Alterations in oncogenic driver MET occur in at least 3–5% of NSCLC and classically are affiliated with poor prognosis. While not all mutations are susceptible to targeted therapy, tumors with MET exon 14 lesions or a significantly elevated gene copy number may predict efficacy to TKIs [273]. In particular, MET exon 14 alterations are sensitive to inhibition with multi-kinase inhibitors crizotinib [274], cabozantinib [275], as well as recently FDA-approved selective inhibitors capmatinib [276,277] and tepotinib [277]. The GEOMETRY mono-1 trial reported a 68% response rate with capmatinib for untreated patients whose NSCLC contained MET exon 14 skipping mutations with a 12.6-month median duration of response. The authors reported a 40% response rate first-line for those harboring MET amplifications with a gene copy number of at least 10 [278]. Toxicity from this next-generation TKI is relatively modest and most frequently includes peripheral edema and nausea. Likewise, the efficacy of tepotinib was evaluated in the VISION trial, where 152 advanced NSCLC patients with exon 14 skipping mutations showed a 43% ORR (the same ORR was seen for treatment-naïve or those previously treated), with a median response duration of approximately 11 months. Combined with reports of effective CNS activity, capmatinib [278] or tepotinib [279,280] should be considered as the first-line options utilized for MET-directed therapy.

In addition to FDA-approved agents targeting sensitive alterations in EGFR, ALK, ROS1, BRAF, MET, RET and NTRK, the precision therapeutic arsenal in NSCLC may soon expand to other oncogenic drivers, including previously-cited KRAS G12C (13% of all NSCLC) [196] and HER2 exon 20 mutations [146] lending further credence to the necessity of molecular profiling in this target-rich disease.

5. Conclusions

As we have attempted to show, advances in molecular profiling have enabled genomic classification of a patient's tumor, leading to the development, approval and availability of precision therapies including TKIs, ADCs and ICIs. With this ever-expanding arsenal of treatment options and increasing availability of next-generation sequencing, the utilization of molecular profiling is primed to expand to most advanced solid tumors into early-stage disease and include combinatorial precision regimens based on complex molecular findings [281]. It is incumbent for the modern oncologist to be well-versed regarding the range of potentially targetable aberrations available, be comfortable with a molecular profiling platform he or she trusts and be able to effectively interpret resultant data to help patients make informed decisions with regards to treatment.

Author Contributions: Conceptualization, M.K.S. and A.V.; methodology, not applicable; software, not applicable; validation, not applicable; formal analysis, not applicable; investigation, M.K.S., O.O., K.P. and A.V.; resources, not applicable; data curation, M.K.S., O.O., K.P. and A.V.; writing—original draft preparation, M.K.S., O.O., K.P. and A.V.; writing—review and editing, M.K.S., O.O., K.P. and A.V.; visualization, A.V.; supervision, A.V.; project administration, A.V.; funding acquisition, not applicable. All authors have read and agreed to the published version of the manuscript.

Funding: This research received no external funding.

Data Availability Statement: All data reported in this paper is available in the cited references, available either at pubmed.gov or at the websites within the citations.

Conflicts of Interest: M.S.K., O.O. and K.P. declare no conflict of interest. A.V. has received research support from Amgen, is a consultant for Bristol-Myers Squibb and Elsevier, and participates in advisory boards for Roche/Genentech, Mirati, and Bristol-Myers Squibb.

References

1. Schwartzberg, L.; Kim, E.S.; Liu, D.; Schrag, D. Precision Oncology: Who, How, What, When, and When Not? *Am. Soc. Clin. Oncol. Educ. Book* **2017**, *37*, 160–169. [CrossRef] [PubMed]
2. Venter, J.C.; Adams, M.D.; Myers, E.W.; Li, P.W.; Mural, R.J.; Sutton, G.G.; Smith, H.O.; Yandell, M.; Evans, C.A.; Holt, R.A.; et al. The sequence of the human genome. *Science* **2001**, *291*, 1304–1351. [CrossRef]
3. Tao, J.J.; Schram, A.M.; Hyman, D.M. Basket Studies: Redefining Clinical Trials in the Era of Genome-Driven Oncology. *Annu. Rev. Med.* **2018**, *69*, 319–331. [CrossRef] [PubMed]
4. Verma, M. Personalized medicine and cancer. *J. Pers Med.* **2012**, *2*, 1–14. [CrossRef]
5. Druker, B.J.; Talpaz, M.; Resta, D.J.; Peng, B.; Buchdunger, E.; Ford, J.M.; Lydon, N.B.; Kantarjian, H.; Capdeville, R.; Ohno-Jones, S.; et al. Efficacy and safety of a specific inhibitor of the BCR-ABL tyrosine kinase in chronic myeloid leukemia. *N. Engl. J. Med.* **2001**, *344*, 1031–1037. [CrossRef] [PubMed]
6. Vogel, C.L.; Cobleigh, M.A.; Tripathy, D.; Gutheil, J.C.; Harris, L.N.; Fehrenbacher, L.; Slamon, D.J.; Murphy, M.; Novotny, W.F.; Burchmore, M.; et al. Efficacy and safety of trastuzumab as a single agent in first-line treatment of HER2-overexpressing metastatic breast cancer. *J. Clin. Oncol.* **2002**, *20*, 719–726. [CrossRef]
7. Slamon, D.J.; Leyland-Jones, B.; Shak, S.; Fuchs, H.; Paton, V.; Bajamonde, A.; Fleming, T.; Eiermann, W.; Wolter, J.; Pegram, M.; et al. Use of chemotherapy plus a monoclonal antibody against HER2 for metastatic breast cancer that overexpresses HER2. *N. Engl. J. Med.* **2001**, *344*, 783–792. [CrossRef]
8. VanderWalde, A.; Grothey, A.; Vaena, D.; Vidal, G.; ElNaggar, A.; Bufalino, G.; Schwartzberg, L. Establishment of a Molecular Tumor Board (MTB) and Uptake of Recommendations in a Community Setting. *J. Pers. Med.* **2020**, *10*, 252. [CrossRef]
9. FDA Grants Accelerated Approval to Pembrolizumab for First Tissue/Site Agnostic Indication. Available online: https://www.fda.gov/drugs/resources-information-approved-drugs/fda-grants-accelerated-approval-pembrolizumab-first-tissuesite-agnostic-indication (accessed on 21 April 2021).
10. FDA Grants Nivolumab Accelerated Approval for MSI-H or dMMR Colorectal Cancer. Content Current as of: 08/01/2017. Available online: https://www.fda.gov/drugs/resources-information-approved-drugs/fda-grants-nivolumab-accelerated-approval-msi-h-or-dmmr-colorectal-cancer (accessed on 28 April 2021).
11. FDA Grants Accelerated Approval to Ipilimumab for MSI-H or dMMR Metastatic Colorectal Cancer. Content Current as of: 07/11/2018. Available online: https://www.fda.gov/drugs/resources-information-approved-drugs/fda-grants-accelerated-approval-ipilimumab-msi-h-or-dmmr-metastatic-colorectal-cancer (accessed on 28 April 2021).
12. FDA Approves Pembrolizumab for First-Line Treatment of MSI-H/dMMR Colorectal Cancer. Content Current as of: 06/30/2020. Available online: https://www.fda.gov/drugs/drug-approvals-and-databases/fda-approves-pembrolizumab-first-line-treatment-msi-hdmmr-colorectal-cancer (accessed on 28 April 2021).
13. FDA News Release. FDA Approves Immunotherapy for Endometrial Cancer with Specific Biomarker. For Immediate Release: April 22, 2021. Available online: https://www.fda.gov/news-events/press-announcements/fda-approves-immunotherapy-endometrial-cancer-specific-biomarker (accessed on 24 April 2021).
14. FDA Approves Pembrolizumab for Adults and Children with TMB-H Solid Tumors. Available online: https://www.fda.gov/drugs/drug-approvals-and-databases/fda-approves-pembrolizumab-adults-and-children-tmb-h-solid-tumors (accessed on 22 April 2021).
15. FDA Approves Larotrectinib for Solid Tumors with NTRK Gene Fusions. Available online: https://www.fda.gov/drugs/fda-approves-larotrectinib-solid-tumors-ntrk-gene-fusions (accessed on 21 April 2021).
16. FDA Approves Entrectinib for NTRK Solid Tumors and ROS-1 NSCLC. Available online: https://www.fda.gov/drugs/resources-information-approved-drugs/fda-approves-entrectinib-ntrk-solid-tumors-and-ros-1-nsclc (accessed on 21 April 2021).
17. Kim, G.; McKee, A.E.; Ning, Y.M.; Hazarika, M.; Theoret, M.; Johnson, J.R.; Xu, Q.C.; Tang, S.; Sridhara, R.; Jiang, X.; et al. FDA approval summary: Vemurafenib for treatment of unresectable or metastatic melanoma with the BRAFV600E mutation. *Clin. Cancer Res.* **2014**, *20*, 4994–5000. [CrossRef]
18. Thompson, C.A. FDA approves two new drugs against advanced melanoma. *Am. J. Health Syst. Pharm.* **2013**, *70*, 1094. [CrossRef]
19. Novel Drug Approvals for 2015. Content Current as of: 11/15/2019. Available online: https://www.fda.gov/drugs/new-drugs-fda-cders-new-molecular-entities-and-new-therapeutic-biological-products/novel-drug-approvals-2015 (accessed on 29 April 2021).
20. Combination therapy approved for melanoma. *Cancer Discov.* **2014**, *4*, 262.
21. FDA Approves Encorafenib and Binimetinib in Combination for Unresectable or Metastatic Melanoma with BRAF Mutations. Content Current as of: 06/27/18. Available online: https://www.fda.gov/drugs/resources-information-approved-drugs/fda-approves-encorafenib-and-binimetinib-combination-unresectable-or-metastatic-melanoma-braf (accessed on 28 April 2021).

22. FDA Approves Dabrafenib Plus Trametinib for Adjuvant Treatment of Melanoma with BRAF V600E or V600K Mutations. Content Current as of: 05/01/2018. Available online: https://www.fda.gov/drugs/resources-information-approved-drugs/fda-approves-dabrafenib-plus-trametinib-adjuvant-treatment-melanoma-braf-v600e-or-v600k-mutations (accessed on 28 April 2021).
23. FDA Approves Atezolizumab for BRAF V600 Unresectable or Metastatic Melanoma. Content Current as of: 07/31/2020. Available online: https://www.fda.gov/drugs/resources-information-approved-drugs/fda-approves-atezolizumab-braf-v600-unresectable-or-metastatic-melanoma (accessed on 28 April 2021).
24. Odogwu, L.; Mathieu, L.; Blumenthal, G.; Larkins, E.; Goldberg, K.B.; Griffin, N.; Bijwaard, K.; Lee, E.Y.; Philip, R.; Jiang, X.; et al. FDA Approval Summary: Dabrafenib and Trametinib for the Treatment of Metastatic Non-Small Cell Lung Cancers Harboring BRAF V600E Mutations. *Oncologist* **2018**, *23*, 740–745. [CrossRef]
25. FDA NEWS RELEASE: FDA Approves New Uses for Two Drugs Administered Together for the Treatment of BRAF-Positive Anaplastic Thyroid Cancer. Content Current as of: 05/04/2018. Available online: https://www.fda.gov/news-events/press-announcements/fda-approves-new-uses-two-drugs-administered-together-treatment-braf-positive-anaplastic-thyroid (accessed on 28 April 2021).
26. FDA Approves Encorafenib in Combination with Cetuximab for Metastatic Colorectal Cancer with a BRAF V600E Mutation. Content Current as of: 04/09/2020. Available online: https://www.fda.gov/drugs/resources-information-approved-drugs/fda-approves-encorafenib-combination-cetuximab-metastatic-colorectal-cancer-braf-v600e-mutation (accessed on 28 April 2021).
27. Monoclonal antibody approved for metastatic breast cancer. *Oncology* **1998**, *12*, 1727.
28. Blumenthal, G.M.; Scher, N.S.; Cortazar, P.; Chattopadhyay, S.; Tang, S.; Song, P.; Li, Q.; Ringgold, K.; Pilaro, A.M.; Tilley, A.; et al. First FDA approval of dual anti-HER2 regimen: Pertuzumab in combination with trastuzumab and docetaxel for HER2-positive metastatic breast cancer. *Clin. Cancer Res.* **2013**, *19*, 4911–4916. [CrossRef]
29. Amiri-Kordestani, L.; Blumenthal, G.M.; Xu, Q.C.; Zhang, L.; Tang, S.W.; Ha, L.; Weinberg, W.C.; Chi, B.; Candau-Chacon, R.; Hughes, P.; et al. FDA approval: Ado-trastuzumab emtansine for the treatment of patients with HER2-positive metastatic breast cancer. *Clin. Cancer Res.* **2014**, *20*, 4436–4441. [CrossRef]
30. Singh, H.; Walker, A.J.; Amiri-Kordestani, L.; Cheng, J.; Tang, S.; Balcazar, P.; Barnett-Ringgold, K.; Palmby, T.R.; Cao, X.; Zehng, N.; et al. U.S. Food and Drug Administration Approval: Neratinib for the Extended Adjuvant Treatment of Early-Stage HER2-Positive Breast Cancer. *Clin. Cancer Res.* **2018**, *24*, 3486–3491. [CrossRef] [PubMed]
31. FDA Approves Fam-Trastuzumab Deruxtecan-Nxki for Unresectable or Metastatic HER2-Positive Breast Cancer. Content Current as of: 12/20/2019. Available online: https://www.fda.gov/drugs/resources-information-approved-drugs/fda-approves-fam-trastuzumab-deruxtecan-nxki-unresectable-or-metastatic-her2-positive-breast-cancer (accessed on 26 April 2021).
32. Ryan, Q.; Ibrahim, A.; Cohen, M.H.; Johnson, J.; Ko, C.W.; Sridhara, R.; Justice, R.; Pazdur, R. FDA drug approval summary: Lapatinib in combination with capecitabine for previously treated metastatic breast cancer that overexpresses HER-2. *Oncologist* **2008**, *13*, 1114–1119. [CrossRef] [PubMed]
33. FDA Approves Tucatinib for Patients with HER2-Positive Metastatic Breast Cancer. Content Current as of: 04/20/2020. Available online: https://www.fda.gov/drugs/resources-information-approved-drugs/fda-approves-tucatinib-patients-her2-positive-metastatic-breast-cancer (accessed on 26 April 2021).
34. 2010 Notifications. Content Current as of: 02/13/2018. Available online: https://www.fda.gov/drugs/resources-information-approved-drugs/2010-notifications (accessed on 27 April 2021).
35. FDA Approves Fam-Trastuzumab Deruxtecan-Nxki for HER2-Positive Gastric Adenocarcinomas. Content Current as of: 01/15/2021. Available online: https://www.fda.gov/drugs/drug-approvals-and-databases/fda-approves-fam-trastuzumab-deruxtecan-nxki-her2-positive-gastric-adenocarcinomas (accessed on 27 April 2021).
36. FDA Approves Selpercatinib for Lung and Thyroid Cancers with RET Gene Mutations or Fusions. Content Current as of: 05/11/2020. Available online: https://www.fda.gov/drugs/drug-approvals-and-databases/fda-approves-selpercatinib-lung-and-thyroid-cancers-ret-gene-mutations-or-fusions (accessed on 26 April 2021).
37. FDA Approves Pralsetinib for Lung Cancer with RET Gene Fusions. Available online: https://www.fda.gov/drugs/resources-information-approved-drugs/fda-approves-pralsetinib-lung-cancer-ret-gene-fusions (accessed on 22 April 2021).
38. Arora, S.; Balasubramaniam, S.; Zhang, H.; Berman, T.; Narayan, P.; Suzman, D.; Bloomquist, E.; Tang, S.; Gong, Y.; Sridhara, R.; et al. FDA Approval Summary: Olaparib Monotherapy or in Combination with Bevacizumab for the Maintenance Treatment of Patients with Advanced Ovarian Cancer. *Oncologist* **2021**, *26*, e164–e172. [CrossRef]
39. Balasubramaniam, S.; Beaver, J.A.; Horton, S.; Fernandes, L.L.; Tang, S.; Horne, H.N.; Liu, J.; Liu, C.; Schrieber, S.J.; Yu, J.; et al. FDA Approval Summary: Rucaparib for the Treatment of Patients with Deleterious BRCA Mutation-Associated Advanced Ovarian Cancer. *Clin. Cancer Res.* **2017**, *23*, 7165–7170. [CrossRef] [PubMed]
40. FDA Approves Rucaparib for Maintenance Treatment of Recurrent Ovarian, Fallopian Tube, or Primary Peritoneal Cancer. Content Current as of: 04/06/2018. Available online: https://www.fda.gov/drugs/resources-information-approved-drugs/fda-approves-rucaparib-maintenance-treatment-recurrent-ovarian-fallopian-tube-or-primary-peritoneal (accessed on 27 April 2021).
41. Ison, G.; Howie, L.J.; Amiri-Kordestani, L.; Zhang, L.; Tang, S.; Sridhara, R.; Pierre, V.; Charlab, R.; Ramamoorthy, A.; Song, P.; et al. FDA Approval Summary: Niraparib for the Maintenance Treatment of Patients with Recurrent Ovarian Cancer in Response to Platinum-Based Chemotherapy. *Clin. Cancer Res.* **2018**, *24*, 4066–4071. [CrossRef]

42. FDA Approves Niraparib for HRD-Positive Advanced Ovarian Cancer. Content Current as of: 10/23/2019. Available online: https://www.fda.gov/drugs/resources-information-approved-drugs/fda-approves-niraparib-hrd-positive-advanced-ovarian-cancer (accessed on 27 April 2021).
43. FDA Approves Olaparib for Germline BRCA-Mutated Metastatic Breast Cancer. Content Current as of: 01/12/2018. Available online: https://www.fda.gov/drugs/resources-information-approved-drugs/fda-approves-olaparib-germline-brca-mutated-metastatic-breast-cancer (accessed on 27 April 2021).
44. FDA Approves Talazoparib for gBRCAm HER2-Negative Locally Advanced or Metastatic Breast Cancer. Content Current as of: 12/14/2018. Available online: https://www.fda.gov/drugs/drug-approvals-and-databases/fda-approves-talazoparib-gbrcam-her2-negative-locally-advanced-or-metastatic-breast-cancer (accessed on 27 April 2021).
45. FDA Approves Olaparib for gBRCAm Metastatic Pancreatic Adenocarcinoma. Content Current as of: 12/30/2019. Available online: https://www.fda.gov/drugs/resources-information-approved-drugs/fda-approves-olaparib-gbrcam-metastatic-pancreatic-adenocarcinoma (accessed on 27 April 2021).
46. Anscher, M.S.; Chang, E.; Gao, X.; Gong, Y.; Weinstock, C.; Bloomquist, E.; Adeniyi, O.; Charlab, R.; Zimmerman, S.; Serlemitsos-Day, M.; et al. FDA Approval Summary: Rucaparib for the Treatment of Patients with Deleterious BRCA-Mutated Metastatic Castrate-Resistant Prostate Cancer. *Oncologist* **2021**, *26*, 139–146. [CrossRef]
47. FDA Approves Olaparib for HRR Gene-Mutated Metastatic Castration-Resistant Prostate Cancer. Content Current as of: 05/20/2020. Available online: https://www.fda.gov/drugs/drug-approvals-and-databases/fda-approves-olaparib-hrr-gene-mutated-metastatic-castration-resistant-prostate-cancer (accessed on 27 April 2021).
48. Marcus, L.; Lemery, S.J.; Keegan, P.; Pazdur, R. FDA Approval Summary: Pembrolizumab for the Treatment of Microsatellite Instability-High Solid Tumors. *Clin. Cancer Res.* **2019**, *25*, 3753–3758. [CrossRef]
49. Le, D.T.; Uram, J.N.; Wang, H.; Bartlett, B.R.; Kemberling, H.; Eyring, A.D.; Slora, A.D.; Luber, B.S.; Azad, N.S.; Laheru, D.; et al. PD-1 Blockade in Tumors with Mismatch-Repair Deficiency. *N. Engl. J. Med.* **2015**, *372*, 2509–2520. [CrossRef] [PubMed]
50. Le, D.T.; Kim, T.W.; van Cutsem, E.; Geva, R.; Jäger, D.; Hara, H.; Burge, M.; O'Neil, B.; Kavan, P.; Yoshino, T.; et al. Phase II Open-Label Study of Pembrolizumab in Treatment-Refractory, Microsatellite Instability-High/Mismatch Repair-Deficient Metastatic Colorectal Cancer: KEYNOTE-164. *J. Clin. Oncol.* **2020**, *38*, 11–19. [CrossRef] [PubMed]
51. Marabelle, A.; Le, D.T.; Ascierto, P.A.; Di Giacomo, A.M.; de Jesus-Acosta, A.; Delord, J.P.; Geva, R.; Gottfried, M.; Penel, N.; Hansen, A.R.; et al. Efficacy of Pembrolizumab in Patients with Noncolorectal High Microsatellite Instability/Mismatch Repair-Deficient Cancer: Results From the Phase II KEYNOTE-158 Study. *J. Clin. Oncol.* **2020**, *38*, 1–10. [CrossRef] [PubMed]
52. Overman, M.J.; McDermott, R.; Leach, J.L.; Lonardi, S.; Lenz, H.J.; Morse, M.A.; Desai, J.; Hill, A.; Axelson, M.; Moss, R.A.; et al. Nivolumab in patients with metastatic DNA mismatch repair-deficient or microsatellite instability-high colorectal cancer (CheckMate 142): An open-label, multicentre, phase 2 study. *Lancet Oncol.* **2017**, *18*, 1182–1191. [CrossRef]
53. Overman, M.J.; Lonardi, S.; Wong, K.Y.M.; Lenz, H.J.; Gelsomino, F.; Aglietta, M.; Morse, M.A.; Van Cutsem, E.; McDermott, R.; Hill, A.; et al. Durable Clinical Benefit with Nivolumab Plus Ipilimumab in DNA Mismatch Repair-Deficient/Microsatellite Instability-High Metastatic Colorectal Cancer. *J. Clin. Oncol.* **2018**, *36*, 773–779. [CrossRef]
54. André, T.; Shiu, K.K.; Kim, T.W.; Jensen, B.V.; Jensen, L.H.; Punt, C.; Smith, D.; Garcia-Carbonero, R.; Benavides, M.; Gibbs, P.; et al. Pembrolizumab in Microsatellite-Instability-High Advanced Colorectal Cancer. *N. Engl. J. Med.* **2020**, *383*, 2207–2218. [CrossRef]
55. Mandal, R.; Samstein, R.M.; Lee, K.W.; Havel, J.J.; Wang, H.; Krishna, C.; Sabio, E.Y.; Makarov, V.; Kuo, F.; Blecua, P.; et al. Genetic diversity of tumors with mismatch repair deficiency influences anti-PD-1 immunotherapy response. *Science* **2019**, *364*, 485–491. [CrossRef]
56. Sidaway, P. MSI-H: A truly agnostic biomarker? *Nat. Rev. Clin. Oncol.* **2020**, *17*, 68. [CrossRef]
57. Rosen, E.Y.; Goldman, D.A.; Hechtman, J.F.; Benayed, R.; Schram, A.M.; Cocco, E.; Shifman, S.; Gong, Y.; Kundra, R.; Solomon, J.P.; et al. TRK Fusions Are Enriched in Cancers with Uncommon Histologies and the Absence of Canonical Driver Mutations. *Clin. Cancer Res.* **2020**, *26*, 1624–1632. [CrossRef] [PubMed]
58. Drilon, A.; Laetsch, T.W.; Kummar, S.; DuBois, S.G.; Lassen, U.N.; Demetri, G.D.; Nathenson, M.; Doebele, R.C.; Farago, A.F.; Pappo, A.S.; et al. Efficacy of Larotrectinib in TRK Fusion-Positive Cancers in Adults and Children. *N. Engl. J. Med.* **2018**, *378*, 731–739. [CrossRef]
59. Hong, D.S.; DuBois, S.G.; Kummar, S.; Farago, A.F.; Albert, C.M.; Rohrberg, K.S.; van Tilburg, C.M.; Nagasubramanian, R.; Berlin, J.D.; Federman, N.; et al. Larotrectinib in patients with TRK fusion-positive solid tumours: A pooled analysis of three phase 1/2 clinical trials. *Lancet Oncol.* **2020**, *21*, 531–540. [CrossRef]
60. Doebele, R.C.; Drilon, A.; Paz-Ares, L.; Siena, S.; Shaw, A.T.; Farago, A.F.; Blakely, C.M.; Seto, T.; Cho, B.C.; Tosi, D.; et al. Entrectinib in patients with advanced or metastatic NTRK fusion-positive solid tumours: Integrated analysis of three phase 1-2 trials. *Lancet Oncol.* **2020**, *21*, 271–282. [CrossRef]
61. Drilon, A. TRK inhibitors in TRK fusion-positive cancers. *Ann. Oncol.* **2019**, *30* (Suppl. 8), viii23–viii30. [CrossRef]
62. Drilon, A.; Ou, S.I.; Cho, B.C.; Kim, D.W.; Lee, J.; Lin, J.J.; Zhu, V.W.; Ahn, M.J.; Camidge, D.R.; Nguyen, J.; et al. Repotrectinib (TPX-0005) Is a Next-Generation ROS1/TRK/ALK Inhibitor That Potently Inhibits ROS1/TRK/ALK Solvent-Front Mutations. *Cancer Discov.* **2018**, *8*, 1227–1236. [CrossRef]
63. Drilon, A.; Zhai, D.; Deng, W.; Zhang, J.; Lee, D.; Rogers, E.; Whitten, J.; Huang, Z.; Graber, A.; Liu, J.; et al. Abstract 442: Repotrectinib, a next generation TRK inhibitor, overcomes TRK resistance mutations including solvent front, gatekeeper and compound mutations. *Cancer Res.* **2019**, *79* (Suppl. 13), 442.

64. Drilon, A.; Nagasubramanian, R.; Blake, J.F.; Ku, N.; Touch, B.B.; Ebata, K.; Smith, S.; Lauriault, V.; Kolakowsky, G.R.; Brandhuber, B.J.; et al. A Next-Generation TRK Kinase Inhibitor Overcomes Acquired Resistance to Prior TRK Kinase Inhibition in Patients with TRK Fusion-Positive Solid Tumors. *Cancer Discov.* **2017**, *7*, 963–972. [CrossRef]
65. Marabelle, A.; Fakih, M.; Lopez, J.; Shah, M.; Shapira-Frommer, R.; Nakagawa, K.; Chung, H.C.; Kindler, H.L.; Lopez-Martin, J.A.; Miller, J.H., Jr.; et al. Association of tumour mutational burden with outcomes in patients with advanced solid tumours treated with pembrolizumab: Prospective biomarker analysis of the multicohort, open-label, phase 2 KEYNOTE-158 study. *Lancet Oncol.* **2020**, *21*, 1353–1365. [CrossRef]
66. Prasad, V.; Addeo, A. The FDA approval of pembrolizumab for patients with TMB >10 mut/Mb: Was it a wise decision? No. *Ann. Oncol.* **2020**, *31*, 1112–1114. [CrossRef]
67. McGrail, D.J.; Pilié, P.G.; Rashid, N.U.; Voorwerk, L.; Slagter, M.; Kok, M.; Jonasch, E.; Khasraw, M.; Heimberger, A.B.; Lim, B.; et al. High tumor mutation burden fails to predict immune checkpoint blockade response across all cancer types. *Ann. Oncol.* **2021**, *32*, 661–672. [CrossRef]
68. Subbiah, V.; Solit, D.B.; Chan, T.A.; Kurzrock, R. The FDA approval of pembrolizumab for adult and pediatric patients with tumor mutational burden (TMB) ≥10: A decision centered on empowering patients and their physicians. *Ann. Oncol.* **2020**, *31*, 1115–1118. [CrossRef]
69. Wang, F.; Zhao, Q.; Wang, Y.N.; Jin, Y.; He, M.M.; Liu, Z.X.; Xu, R.H. Evaluation of POLE and POLD1 Mutations as Biomarkers for Immunotherapy Outcomes Across Multiple Cancer Types. *JAMA Oncol.* **2019**, *5*, 1504–1506. [CrossRef]
70. Goodman, A.M.; Piccioni, D.; Kato, S.; Boichard, A.; Wang, H.Y.; Frampton, G.; Lippman, S.M.; Connelly, C.; Fabrizio, D.; Miller, V.; et al. Prevalence of PDL1 Amplification and Preliminary Response to Immune Checkpoint Blockade in Solid Tumors. *JAMA Oncol.* **2018**, *4*, 1237–1244. [CrossRef] [PubMed]
71. Straub, M.; Drecoll, E.; Pfarr, N.; Weichert, W.; Langer, R.; Hapfelmeier, A.; Gotz, C.; Wolff, K.D.; Kolk, A.; Specht, K. CD274/PD-L1 gene amplification and PD-L1 protein expression are common events in squamous cell carcinoma of the oral cavity. *Oncotarget* **2016**, *7*, 12024–12034. [CrossRef] [PubMed]
72. Sorscher, S.; Resnick, J.; Goodman, M. First Case Report of a Dramatic Radiographic Response to a Checkpoint Inhibitor in a Patient with Proficient Mismatch Repair Gene Expressing Metastatic Colorectal Cancer. *JCO Precis. Oncol.* **2017**, *1*, 1–4. [CrossRef]
73. Ikeda, S.; Goodman, A.M.; Cohen, P.R.; Jensen, T.J.; Ellison, C.K.; Frampton, G.; Miller, V.; Patel, S.P.; Kurzrock, R. Metastatic basal cell carcinoma with amplification of PD-L1: Exceptional response to anti-PD1 therapy. *NPJ Genom. Med.* **2016**, *1*, 16037. [CrossRef] [PubMed]
74. Flaherty, K.T.; Puzanov, I.; Kim, K.B.; Ribas, A.; McArthur, G.A.; Sosman, J.A.; O'Dwyer, P.J.; Lee, R.J.; Grippo, J.F.; Nolop, K.; et al. Inhibition of mutated, activated BRAF in metastatic melanoma. *N. Engl. J. Med.* **2010**, *363*, 809–819. [CrossRef]
75. Hauschild, A.; Grob, J.J.; Demidov, L.V.; Jouary, T.; Gutzmer, R.; Millward, M.; Rutkowski, P.; Blank, C.U.; Miller, W.H., Jr.; Kaempgen, E.; et al. Dabrafenib in BRAF-mutated metastatic melanoma: A multicentre, open-label, phase 3 randomised controlled trial. *Lancet* **2012**, *380*, 358–365. [CrossRef]
76. Flaherty, K.T.; Robert, C.; Hersey, P.; Nathan, P.; Garbe, C.; Milhem, M.; Demidov, L.V.; Hassel, J.C.; Rutkowski, P.; Mohr, P.; et al. Improved survival with MEK inhibition in BRAF-mutated melanoma. *N. Engl. J. Med.* **2012**, *367*, 107–114. [CrossRef] [PubMed]
77. Long, G.V.; Trefzer, U.; Davies, M.A.; Kefford, R.F.; Ascierto, P.A.; Chapman, P.B.; Puzanov, I.; Hauschild, A.; Robert, C.; Algazi, A.; et al. Dabrafenib in patients with Val600Glu or Val600Lys BRAF-mutant melanoma metastatic to the brain (BREAK-MB): A multicentre, open-label, phase 2 trial. *Lancet Oncol.* **2012**, *13*, 1087–1095. [CrossRef]
78. Bucheit, A.D.; Davies, M.A. Emerging insights into resistance to BRAF inhibitors in melanoma. *Biochem. Pharmacol.* **2014**, *87*, 381–389. [CrossRef] [PubMed]
79. Long, G.V.; Stroyakovskiy, D.; Gogas, H.; Levchenko, E.; de Braud, F.; Larkin, J.; Garbe, C.; Jouary, T.; Hauschild, A.; Grob, J.J.; et al. Combined BRAF and MEK inhibition versus BRAF inhibition alone in melanoma. *N. Engl. J. Med.* **2014**, *371*, 1877–1888. [CrossRef]
80. Long, G.V.; Stroyakovskiy, D.; Gogas, H.; Levchenko, E.; de Braud, F.; Larkin, J.; Garbe, C.; Jouary, T.; Hauschild, A.; Grob, J.J.; et al. Dabrafenib and trametinib versus dabrafenib and placebo for Val600 BRAF-mutant melanoma: A multicentre, double-blind, phase 3 randomised controlled trial. *Lancet* **2015**, *386*, 444–451. [CrossRef]
81. Long, G.V.; Flaherty, K.T.; Stroyakovskiy, D.; Gogas, H.; Levchenko, E.; de Braud, F.; Larkin, J.; Garbe, C.; Jouary, T.; Hauschild, A.; et al. Dabrafenib plus trametinib versus dabrafenib monotherapy in patients with metastatic BRAF V600E/K-mutant melanoma: Long-term survival and safety analysis of a phase 3 study. *Ann. Oncol.* **2017**, *28*, 1631–1639. [CrossRef]
82. Robert, C.; Karaszewska, B.; Schachter, J.; Rutkowski, P.; Mackiewicz, A.; Stroiakovski, D.; Lichinitser, M.; Dummer, R.; Grange, F.; Mortier, L.; et al. Improved overall survival in melanoma with combined dabrafenib and trametinib. *N. Engl. J. Med.* **2015**, *372*, 30–39. [CrossRef]
83. Robert, C.; Grob, J.J.; Stroyakovskiy, D.; Karaszewska, B.; Hauschild, A.; Levchenko, E.; Chiarion Sileni, V.; Schachter, J.; Garbe, C.; Bondarenko, I.; et al. Five-Year Outcomes with Dabrafenib plus Trametinib in Metastatic Melanoma. *N. Engl. J. Med.* **2019**, *381*, 626–636. [CrossRef]
84. Larkin, J.; Ascierto, P.A.; Dréno, B.; Atkinson, V.; Liszkay, G.; Maio, M.; Mandala, M.; Demidov, L.; Stroyakovskiy, D.; Thomas, L.; et al. Combined vemurafenib and cobimetinib in BRAF-mutated melanoma. *N. Engl. J. Med.* **2014**, *371*, 1867–1876. [CrossRef]

85. Ascierto, P.A.; McArthur, G.A.; Dréno, B.; Atkinson, V.; Liszkay, G.; Di Giacomo, A.M.; Mandala, M.; Demidov, L.; Stroyakovskiy, D.; Thomas, L.; et al. Cobimetinib combined with vemurafenib in advanced BRAF(V600)-mutant melanoma (coBRIM): Updated efficacy results from a randomised, double-blind, phase 3 trial. *Lancet Oncol.* **2016**, *17*, 1248–1260. [CrossRef]
86. Dummer, R.; Ascierto, P.A.; Gogas, H.J.; Arance, A.; Mandala, M.; Liszkay, G.; Garbe, C.; Schadendorf, D.; Krajsova, I.; Gutzmer, R.; et al. Encorafenib plus binimetinib versus vemurafenib or encorafenib in patients with BRAF-mutant melanoma (COLUMBUS): A multicentre, open-label, randomised phase 3 trial. *Lancet Oncol.* **2018**, *19*, 603–615. [CrossRef]
87. Dummer, R.; Ascierto, P.A.; Gogas, H.J.; Arance, A.; Mandala, M.; Liszkay, G.; Garbe, C.; Schadendorf, D.; Krajsova, I.; Gutzmer, R.; et al. Overall survival in patients with BRAF-mutant melanoma receiving encorafenib plus binimetinib versus vemurafenib or encorafenib (COLUMBUS): A multicentre, open-label, randomised, phase 3 trial. *Lancet Oncol.* **2018**, *19*, 1315–1327. [CrossRef]
88. Ascierto, P.A.; Dummer, R.; Gogas, H.J.; Flaherty, K.T.; Arance, A.; Mandala, M.; Liszkay, G.; Garbe, C.; Schadendorf, D.; Krajsova, I.; et al. Update on tolerability and overall survival in COLUMBUS: Landmark analysis of a randomised phase 3 trial of encorafenib plus binimetinib vs vemurafenib or encorafenib in patients with BRAF V600-mutant melanoma. *Eur. J. Cancer* **2020**, *126*, 33–44. [CrossRef]
89. Gogas, H.J.; Flaherty, K.T.; Dummer, R.; Ascierto, P.A.; Arance, A.; Mandala, M.; Liszkay, G.; Garbe, C.; Schadendorf, D.; Krajsova, I.; et al. Adverse events associated with encorafenib plus binimetinib in the COLUMBUS study: Incidence, course and management. *Eur. J. Cancer* **2020**, *119*, 97–106. [CrossRef] [PubMed]
90. Long, G.V.; Hauschild, A.; Santinami, M.; Atkinson, V.; Mandalà, M.; Chiarion-Sileni, V.; Larkin, J.; Nyakas, M.; Dutriaux, C.; Haydon, A.; et al. Adjuvant Dabrafenib plus Trametinib in Stage III BRAF-Mutated Melanoma. *N. Engl. J. Med.* **2017**, *377*, 1813–1823. [CrossRef]
91. Dummer, R.; Hauschild, A.; Santinami, M.; Atkinson, V.; Mandalà, M.; Kirkwood, J.M.; Chiarion Sileni, V.; Larkin, J.; Nyakas, M.; Dutriaux, C.; et al. Five-Year Analysis of Adjuvant Dabrafenib plus Trametinib in Stage III Melanoma. *N. Engl. J. Med.* **2020**, *383*, 1139–1148. [CrossRef]
92. Weber, J.; Mandala, M.; Del Vecchio, M.; Gogas, H.J.; Arance, A.M.; Cowey, C.L.; Dalle, S.; Schenker, M.; Chiarion-Sileni, V.; Marquez-Rodas, I.; et al. Adjuvant Nivolumab versus Ipilimumab in Resected Stage III or IV Melanoma. *N. Engl. J. Med.* **2017**, *377*, 1824–1835. [CrossRef]
93. Eggermont, A.M.M.; Blank, C.U.; Mandala, M.; Long, G.V.; Atkinson, V.; Dalle, S.; Haydon, A.; Lichinitser, M.; Khattak, A.; Carlino, M.S.; et al. Adjuvant Pembrolizumab versus Placebo in Resected Stage III Melanoma. *N. Engl. J. Med.* **2018**, *378*, 1789–1801. [CrossRef]
94. Ribas, A.; Puzanov, I.; Dummer, R.; Schadendorf, D.; Hamid, O.; Robert, C.; Hodi, F.S.; Schachter, J.; Pavlick, A.C.; Lewis, K.D.; et al. Pembrolizumab versus investigator-choice chemotherapy for ipilimumab-refractory melanoma (KEYNOTE-002): A randomised, controlled, phase 2 trial. *Lancet Oncol.* **2015**, *16*, 908–918. [CrossRef]
95. Robert, C.; Schachter, J.; Long, G.V.; Arance, A.; Grob, J.J.; Mortier, L.; Daud, A.; Carlino, M.S.; McNeil, C.; Lotem, M.; et al. Pembrolizumab versus Ipilimumab in Advanced Melanoma. *N. Engl. J. Med.* **2015**, *372*, 2521–2532. [CrossRef] [PubMed]
96. Larkin, J.; Chiarion-Sileni, V.; Gonzalez, R.; Grob, J.J.; Cowey, C.L.; Lao, C.D.; Schadendorf, D.; Dummer, R.; Smylie, M.; Rutkowski, P.; et al. Combined Nivolumab and Ipilimumab or Monotherapy in Untreated Melanoma. *N. Engl. J. Med.* **2015**, *373*, 23–34. [CrossRef]
97. Weber, J.S.; D'Angelo, S.P.; Minor, D.; Hodi, F.S.; Gutzmer, R.; Neyns, B.; Hoeller, C.; Khushalani, N.I.; Miller, W.H., Jr.; Lao, C.D.; et al. Nivolumab versus chemotherapy in patients with advanced melanoma who progressed after anti-CTLA-4 treatment (CheckMate 037): A randomised, controlled, open-label, phase 3 trial. *Lancet Oncol.* **2015**, *16*, 375–384. [CrossRef]
98. Postow, M.A.; Chesney, J.; Pavlick, A.C.; Robert, C.; Grossmann, K.; McDermott, D.; Linette, G.P.; Meyer, N.; Giguere, J.K.; Agarwala, S.S.; et al. Nivolumab and ipilimumab versus ipilimumab in untreated melanoma. *N. Engl. J. Med.* **2015**, *372*, 2006–2017. [CrossRef] [PubMed]
99. Gutzmer, R.; Stroyakovskiy, D.; Gogas, H.; Robert, C.; Lewis, K.; Protsenko, S.; Pereira, R.P.; Eigentler, T.; Rutkowski, P.; Demidov, L.; et al. Atezolizumab, vemurafenib, and cobimetinib as first-line treatment for unresectable advanced BRAFV600 mutation-positive melanoma (IMspire150): Primary analysis of the randomised, double-blind, placebo-controlled, phase 3 trial. *Lancet* **2020**, *395*, 1835–1844. [CrossRef]
100. Hatzivassiliou, G.; Song, K.; Yen, I.; Brandhuber, B.J.; Anderson, D.J.; Alvarado, R.; Ludlam, M.J.; Stokow, D.; Gloor, S.L.; Vigers, G.; et al. RAF inhibitors prime wild-type RAF to activate the MAPK pathway and enhance growth. *Nature* **2010**, *464*, 431–435. [CrossRef] [PubMed]
101. Menzer, C.; Menzies, A.M.; Carlino, M.S.; Reijers, I.; Groen, E.J.; Eigentler, T.; de Groot, J.W.B.; van der Veldt, A.A.M.; Johnson, D.B.; Meiss, F.; et al. Targeted Therapy in Advanced Melanoma with Rare BRAF Mutations. *J. Clin. Oncol* **2019**, *37*, 3142–3151. [CrossRef] [PubMed]
102. Owsley, J.; Stein, M.K.; Porter, J.; In, G.K.; Salem, M.; O'Day, S.; Elliott, A.; Poorman, K.; Gibney, G.; VanderWalde, A. Prevalence of class I-III BRAF mutations among 114,662 cancer patients in a large genomic database. *Exp. Biol Med.* **2021**, *246*, 31–39. [CrossRef] [PubMed]
103. Planchard, D.; Besse, B.; Groen, H.J.M.; Souquet, P.J.; Quoix, E.; Baik, C.S.; Barlesi, F.; Kim, T.M.; Mazieres, J.; Novello, S.; et al. Dabrafenib plus trametinib in patients with previously treated BRAF(V600E)-mutant metastatic non-small cell lung cancer: An open-label, multicentre phase 2 trial. *Lancet Oncol.* **2017**, *17*, 984–993. [CrossRef]

104. Planchard, D.; Kim, T.M.; Mazieres, J.; Quoix, E.; Riely, G.; Barlesi, F.; Souquet, P.J.; Smit, E.F.; Groen, H.J.; Kelly, R.J.; et al. Dabrafenib in patients with BRAF(V600E)-positive advanced non-small-cell lung cancer: A single-arm, multicentre, open-label, phase 2 trial. *Lancet Oncol.* **2016**, *17*, 642–650. [CrossRef]
105. Planchard, D.; Smit, E.F.; Groen, H.J.M.; Mazieres, J.; Besse, B.; Helland, Å.; Giannone, V.; D'Amilio, A.M., Jr.; Zhang, P.; Mookerjee, B.; et al. Dabrafenib plus trametinib in patients with previously untreated BRAFV600E-mutant metastatic non-small-cell lung cancer: An open-label, phase 2 trial. *Lancet Oncol.* **2017**, *18*, 1307–1316. [CrossRef]
106. Facchinetti, F.; Lacroix, L.; Mezquita, L.; Scoazec, J.Y.; Loriot, Y.; Tselikas, L.; Gazzah, A.; Rouleau, E.; Adam, J.; Michiels, S.; et al. Molecular mechanisms of resistance to BRAF and MEK inhibitors in BRAFV600E non-small cell lung cancer. *Eur. J. Cancer* **2020**, *132*, 211–223. [CrossRef] [PubMed]
107. Yarchoan, M.; LiVolsi, V.A.; Brose, M.S. BRAF mutation and thyroid cancer recurrence. *J. Clin. Oncol.* **2015**, *33*, 7–8. [CrossRef]
108. Liu, R.; Bishop, J.; Zhu, G.; Zhang, T.; Ladenson, P.W.; Xin, M. Mortality Risk Stratification by Combining BRAF V600E and TERT Promoter Mutations in Papillary Thyroid Cancer: Genetic Duet of BRAF and TERT Promoter Mutations in Thyroid Cancer Mortality. *JAMA Oncol.* **2017**, *3*, 202–208. [CrossRef]
109. Brose, M.S.; Cabanillas, M.E.; Cohen, E.E.; Wirth, L.J.; Riehl, T.; Yue, H.; Sherman, S.I.; Sherman, E.J. Vemurafenib in patients with BRAF(V600E)-positive metastatic or unresectable papillary thyroid cancer refractory to radioactive iodine: A non-randomised, multicentre, open-label, phase 2 trial. *Lancet Oncol.* **2016**, *17*, 1272–1282. [CrossRef]
110. Falchook, G.S.; Millward, M.; Hong, D.; Naing, A.; Piha-Paul, S.; Waguespack, S.G.; Cabanillas, M.E.; Sherman, S.I.; Ma, B.; Curtis, M.; et al. BRAF inhibitor dabrafenib in patients with metastatic BRAF-mutant thyroid cancer. *Thyroid* **2015**, *25*, 71–77. [CrossRef]
111. Untch, B.R.; Olson, J.A., Jr. Anaplastic thyroid carcinoma, thyroid lymphoma, and metastasis to thyroid. *Surg. Oncol. Clin. N. Am.* **2006**, *15*, 661–679. [CrossRef] [PubMed]
112. Guerra, A.; Di Crescenzo, V.; Garzi, A.; Cinelli, M.; Carlomagno, C.; Tonacchera, M.; Zeppa, P.; Vitale, M. Genetic mutations in the treatment of anaplastic thyroid cancer: A systematic review. *BMC Surg.* **2013**, *13* (Suppl. 2), S44. [CrossRef]
113. Subbiah, V.; Kreitman, R.J.; Wainberg, Z.A.; Cho, J.Y.; Schellens, J.H.M.; Soria, J.C.; Wen, P.Y.; Zielinski, C.; Cabanillas, M.E.; Urbanowitz, G.; et al. Dabrafenib and Trametinib Treatment in Patients with Locally Advanced or Metastatic BRAF V600-Mutant Anaplastic Thyroid Cancer. *J. Clin. Oncol.* **2018**, *36*, 7–13. [CrossRef] [PubMed]
114. Kopetz, S.; Grothey, A.; Yaeger, R.; van Cutsem, E.; Desai, J.; Yoshino, T.; Wasan, H.; Ciardiello, F.; Loupakis, F.; Hong, Y.S.; et al. Encorafenib, Binimetinib, and Cetuximab in BRAF V600E-Mutated Colorectal Cancer. *N. Engl. J. Med.* **2019**, *381*, 1632–1643. [CrossRef] [PubMed]
115. Tabernero, J.; Grothey, A.; van Cutsem, E.; Yaeger, R.; Wasan, H.; Yoshino, T.; Desai, J.; Ciardiello, F.; Loupakis, F.; Hong, Y.S.; et al. Encorafenib Plus Cetuximab as a New Standard of Care for Previously Treated BRAF V600E-Mutant Metastatic Colorectal Cancer: Updated Survival Results and Subgroup Analyses from the BEACON Study. *J. Clin. Oncol.* **2021**, *39*, 273–284. [CrossRef]
116. Cronin, K.A.; Harlan, L.C.; Dodd, K.W.; Abrams, J.S.; Ballard-Barbash, R. Population-based estimate of the prevalence of HER-2 positive breast cancer tumors for early stage patients in the US. *Cancer Invest.* **2010**, *28*, 963–968. [CrossRef]
117. Gordon, M.A.; Gundacker, H.M.; Benedetti, J.; Macdonald, J.S.; Baranda, J.C.; Levin, W.J.; Blanke, C.D.; Elatre, W.; Weng, P.; Zhou, J.Y.; et al. Assessment of HER2 gene amplification in adenocarcinomas of the stomach or gastroesophageal junction in the INT-0116/SWOG9008 clinical trial. *Ann. Oncol.* **2013**, *24*, 1754–1761. [CrossRef]
118. Slamon, D.J.; Clark, G.M.; Wong, S.G.; Levin, W.J.; Ullrich, A.; McGuire, W.L. Human breast cancer: Correlation of relapse and survival with amplification of the HER-2/neu oncogene. *Science* **1987**, *235*, 177–182. [CrossRef] [PubMed]
119. Lei, Y.Y.; Huang, J.Y.; Zhao, Q.R.; Jiang, N.; Xu, H.M.; Wang, Z.N.; Li, H.Q.; Zhang, S.B.; Sun, Z. The clinicopathological parameters and prognostic significance of HER2 expression in gastric cancer patients: A meta-analysis of literature. *World J. Surg Oncol.* **2017**, *15*, 68. [CrossRef] [PubMed]
120. Esteva, F.J.; Valero, V.; Booser, D.; Guerra, L.T.; Murray, J.L.; Pusztai, L.; Cristofanilli, M.; Arun, B.; Esmaeli, B.; Fritsche, H.A.; et al. Phase II study of weekly docetaxel and trastuzumab for patients with HER-2-overexpressing metastatic breast cancer. *J. Clin. Oncol.* **2002**, *20*, 1800–1808. [CrossRef]
121. Marty, M.; Cognetti, F.; Maraninchi, D.; Snyder, R.; Mauriac, L.; Tubiana-Hulin, M.; Chan, S.; Grimes, D.; Anton, A.; Lluch, A.; et al. Randomized phase II trial of the efficacy and safety of trastuzumab combined with docetaxel in patients with human epidermal growth factor receptor 2-positive metastatic breast cancer administered as first-line treatment: The M77001 study group. *J. Clin. Oncol.* **2005**, *23*, 4265–4274. [CrossRef]
122. Seidman, A.D.; Berry, D.; Cirrincione, C.; Harris, L.; Muss, H.; Marcom, P.K.; Gipson, G.; Burstein, H.; Lake, D.; Shapiro, C.; et al. Randomized phase III trial of weekly compared with every-3-weeks paclitaxel for metastatic breast cancer, with trastuzumab for all HER-2 overexpressors and random assignment to trastuzumab or not in HER-2 nonoverexpressors: Final results of Cancer and Leukemia Group B protocol 9840. *J. Clin. Oncol.* **2008**, *26*, 1642–1649. [PubMed]
123. Tolaney, S.M.; Barry, W.T.; Dang, C.T.; Yardley, D.A.; Moy, B.; Marcom, P.K.; Albain, K.S.; Rugo, H.S.; Ellis, M.; Shapira, I.; et al. Adjuvant paclitaxel and trastuzumab for node-negative, HER2-positive breast cancer. *N. Engl. J. Med.* **2015**, *372*, 134–141. [CrossRef] [PubMed]
124. Slamon, D.; Eiermann, W.; Robert, N.; Pienkowski, T.; Martin, M.; Press, M.; Mackey, J.; Glaspy, J.; Chan, A.; Pawlicki, M.; et al. Adjuvant trastuzumab in HER2-positive breast cancer. *N. Engl. J. Med.* **2011**, *365*, 1273–1283. [CrossRef] [PubMed]

125. Romond, E.H.; Perez, E.A.; Bryant, J.; Suman, V.J.; Geyer, C.E., Jr.; Davidson, N.E.; Tan-Chiu, E.; Martino, S.; Paik, S.; Kaufman, P.A.; et al. Trastuzumab plus adjuvant chemotherapy for operable HER2-positive breast cancer. *N. Engl. J. Med.* **2005**, *353*, 1673–1684. [CrossRef]
126. Geyer, C.E.; Forster, J.; Lindquist, D.; Chan, S.; Romieu, C.G.; Pienkowski, T.; Jagiello-Gruszfeld, A.; Crown, J.; Chan, A.; Kaufman, B.; et al. Lapatinib plus capecitabine for HER2-positive advanced breast cancer. *N. Engl. J. Med.* **2006**, *355*, 2733–2743. [CrossRef]
127. Blackwell, K.L.; Burstein, H.J.; Storniolo, A.M.; Rugo, H.; Sledge, G.; Koehler, M.; Ellis, C.; Casey, M.; Vukelja, S.; Bischoff, J.; et al. Randomized study of Lapatinib alone or in combination with trastuzumab in women with ErbB2-positive, trastuzumab-refractory metastatic breast cancer. *J. Clin. Oncol.* **2010**, *28*, 1124–1130. [CrossRef]
128. Baselga, J.; Cortés, J.; Kim, S.B.; Im, S.A.; Hegg, R.; Im, Y.H.; Roman, L.; Pedrini, J.L.; Pienkowski, T.; Knott, A.; et al. CLEOPATRA Study Group. Pertuzumab plus trastuzumab plus docetaxel for metastatic breast cancer. *N. Engl. J. Med.* **2012**, *366*, 109–119. [CrossRef] [PubMed]
129. Modi, S.; Saura, C.; Yamashita, T.; Park, Y.H.; Kim, S.B.; Tamura, K.; Andre, F.; Iwata, H.; Ito, Y.; Tsurutani, J.; et al. Trastuzumab Deruxtecan in Previously Treated HER2-Positive Breast Cancer. *N. Engl. J. Med.* **2020**, *382*, 610–621. [CrossRef] [PubMed]
130. Verma, S.; Miles, D.; Gianni, L.; Krop, I.E.; Welslau, M.; Baselga, J.; Pegram, M.; Oh, D.Y.; Dieras, V.; Guardino, E.; et al. Trastuzumab emtansine for HER2-positive advanced breast cancer. *N. Engl. J. Med.* **2012**, *367*, 1783–1791. [CrossRef]
131. Saura, C.; Oliveira, M.; Feng, Y.H.; Dai, M.S.; Chen, S.W.; Hurvitz, S.A.; Kim, S.B.; Moy, B.; Delaloge, S.; Gradishar, W.; et al. Neratinib Plus Capecitabine Versus Lapatinib Plus Capecitabine in HER2-Positive Metastatic Breast Cancer Previously Treated With ≥ 2 HER2-Directed Regimens: Phase III NALA Trial. *J. Clin. Oncol.* **2020**, *38*, 3138–3149. [CrossRef] [PubMed]
132. Murthy, R.K.; Loi, S.; Okines, A.; Paplomata, E.; Hamilton, E.; Hurvitz, S.A.; Lin, N.U.; Borges, V.; Abramson, V.; Anders, C.; et al. Tucatinib, Trastuzumab, and Capecitabine for HER2-Positive Metastatic Breast Cancer. *N. Engl. J. Med.* **2020**, *382*, 597–609. [CrossRef]
133. Schneeweiss, A.; Chia, S.; Hickish, T.; Harvey, V.; Eniu, A.; Hegg, R.; Tausch, C.; Seo, J.H.; Tsai, Y.F.; Ratnayake, J.; et al. Pertuzumab plus trastuzumab in combination with standard neoadjuvant anthracycline-containing and anthracycline-free chemotherapy regimens in patients with HER2-positive early breast cancer. *Ann. Oncol.* **2013**, *24*, 2278–2284. [CrossRef]
134. Swain, S.M.; Ewer, M.S.; Viale, G.; Delaloge, S.; Ferrero, J.M.; Verrill, M.; Colomer, R.; Vieira, C.; Werner, T.L.; Douthwaite, H.; et al. Pertuzumab, trastuzumab, and standard anthracycline- and taxane-based chemotherapy for the neoadjuvant treatment of patients with HER2-positive localized breast cancer (BERENICE): A phase II, open-label, multicenter, multinational cardiac safety study. *Ann. Oncol.* **2018**, *29*, 646–653. [CrossRef]
135. Lin, N.U.; Borges, V.; Anders, C.; Murthy, R.K.; Paplomata, E.; Hamilton, E.; Hurvitz, S.; Loi, S.; Okines, A.; Abramson, V.; et al. Intracranial Efficacy and Survival with Tucatinib Plus Trastuzumab and Capecitabine for Previously Treated HER2-Positive Breast Cancer With Brain Metastases in the HER2CLIMB Trial. *J. Clin. Oncol.* **2020**, *38*, 2610–2619. [CrossRef]
136. Bang, Y.J.; van Cutsem, E.; Feyereislova, A.; Chung, H.C.; Shen, L.; Sawaki, A.; Lordick, F.; Ohtsu, A.; Omuro, Y.; Satoh, T.; et al. Trastuzumab in combination with chemotherapy versus chemotherapy alone for treatment of HER2-positive advanced gastric or gastro-oesophageal junction cancer (ToGA): A phase 3, open-label, randomised controlled trial. *Lancet* **2010**, *376*, 687–697. [CrossRef]
137. Shitara, K.; Bang, Y.J.; Iwasa, S.; Sugimoto, N.; Ryu, M.H.; Sakai, D.; Chung, H.C.; Kawakami, H.; Yabusaki, H.; Lee, J.; et al. Trastuzumab Deruxtecan in Previously Treated HER2-Positive Gastric Cancer. *N. Engl. J. Med.* **2020**, *382*, 2419–2430. [CrossRef]
138. Meric-Bernstam, F.; Hurwitz, H.; Raghav, K.P.S.; McWilliams, R.R.; Fakih, M.; VanderWalde, A.; Swanton, C.; Kurzrock, R.; Burris, H.; Sweeney, C.; et al. Pertuzumab plus trastuzumab for HER2-amplified metastatic colorectal cancer (MyPathway): An updated report from a multicentre, open-label, phase 2a, multiple basket study. *Lancet Oncol.* **2019**, *20*, 518–530. [CrossRef]
139. Nakamura, Y.; Okamoto, W.; Kato, T.; Hasegawa, H.; Kato, K.; Iwasa, S.; Esaki, T.; Komatsu, Y.; Masuishi, T.; Nishina, T.; et al. TRIUMPH: Primary efficacy of a phase II trial of trastuzumab (T) and pertuzumab (P) in patients (pts) with metastatic colorectal cancer (mCRC) with HER2 (ERBB2) amplification (amp) in tumour tissue or circulating tumour DNA (ctDNA): A GOZILA sub-study. *Ann. Oncol.* **2019**, *30* (Suppl. 5), v199–v200. [CrossRef]
140. Sartore-Bianchi, A.; Trusolino, L.; Martino, C.; Bencardino, K.; Lonardi, S.; Bergamo, F.; Zagonel, V.; Leone, F.; Depetris, I.; Martinelli, E.; et al. Dual-targeted therapy with trastuzumab and lapatinib in treatment-refractory, KRAS codon 12/13 wild-type, HER2-positive metastatic colorectal cancer (HERACLES): A proof-of-concept, multicentre, open-label, phase 2 trial. *Lancet Oncol.* **2016**, *17*, 738–746. [CrossRef]
141. Strickler, J.H.; Zemla, T.; Ou, F.-S.; Cercek, A.; Wu, C.; Sanchez, F.A.; Hubbard, J.; Jaszewski, B.; Bandel, L.; Schweitzer, B.; et al. Trastuzumab and tucatinib for the treatment of HER2 amplified metastatic colorectal cancer (mCRC): Initial results from the MOUNTAINEER trial. *Ann. Oncol.* **2019**, *30* (Suppl. 5), v200. [CrossRef]
142. Sartore-Bianchi, A.; Lonardi, S.; Martino, C.; Fenocchio, E.; Tosi, F.; Ghezzi, S.; Leone, F.; Bergamo, F.; Zagonel, V.; Ciardiello, F.; et al. Pertuzumab and trastuzumab emtansine in patients with HER2-amplified metastatic colorectal cancer: The phase II HERACLES-B trial. *ESMO Open* **2020**, *5*, e000911. [CrossRef]
143. Siena, S.; Di Bartolomeo, M.; Raghav, K.; Masuishi, T.; Loupakis, F.; Kawakami, H.; Yamaguchi, K.; Nishina, T.; Faki, M.; Elez, E.; et al. Trastuzumab deruxtecan (DS-8201) in patients with HER2-expressing metastatic colorectal cancer (DESTINY-CRC01): A multicentre, open-label, phase 2 trial. *Lancet Oncol.* **2021**, *4*, S1470–S2045.
144. Hyman, D.M.; Piha-Paul, S.A.; Won, H.; Rodon, J.; Saura, C.; Shapiro, G.I.; Juric, D.; Quinn, D.I.; Moreno, V.; Doger, B.; et al. HER kinase inhibition in patients with HER2- and HER3-mutant cancers. *Nature* **2018**, *554*, 189–194. [CrossRef] [PubMed]

145. Li, B.T.; Shen, R.; Buonocore, D.; Olah, Z.T.; Ni, A.; Ginsberg, M.S.; Ulaner, G.A.; Offin, M.; Feldman, D.; Hembrough, T.; et al. Ado-Trastuzumab Emtansine for Patients with HER2-Mutant Lung Cancers: Results From a Phase II Basket Trial. *J. Clin. Oncol.* **2018**, *36*, 2532–2537. [CrossRef] [PubMed]
146. Smit, E.F.; Nakagawa, K.; Nagasaka, M.; Felip, E.; Goto, Y.; Li, B.T.; Pacheco, J.M.; Murakami, H.; Barlesi, F.; Saltos, A.N.; et al. Trastuzumab deruxtecan (T-DXd; DS-8201) in patients with HER2-mutated metastatic non-small cell lung cancer (NSCLC): Interim results of DESTINY-Lung01. *J. Clin. Oncol.* **2020**, *38* (Suppl.), 9504. [CrossRef]
147. Ciampi, R.; Romei, C.; Ramone, T.; Prete, A.; Tacito, A.; Cappagli, V.; Bottici, V.; Viola, D.; Torregrossa, L.; Ugolini, C.; et al. Genetic Landscape of Somatic Mutations in a Large Cohort of Sporadic Medullary Thyroid Carcinomas Studied by Next-Generation Targeted Sequencing. *iScience* **2019**, *20*, 324–336. [CrossRef] [PubMed]
148. Pozdeyev, N.; Gay, L.M.; Sokol, E.S.; Hartmaier, R.; Deaver, K.E.; Davis, S.; French, J.D.; Borre, P.V.; LaBarbera, D.V.; Tan, A.C.; et al. Genetic Analysis of 779 Advanced Differentiated and Anaplastic Thyroid Cancers. *Clin. Cancer Res.* **2018**, *24*, 3059–3068. [CrossRef] [PubMed]
149. Wang, R.; Hu, H.; Pan, Y.; Li, Y.; Ye, T.; Li, C.; Luo, X.; Wang, L.; Li, H.; Zhang, Y.; et al. RET fusions define a unique molecular and clinicopathologic subtype of non-small-cell lung cancer. *J. Clin. Oncol.* **2012**, *30*, 4352–4359. [CrossRef]
150. Drilon, A.; Oxnard, G.R.; Tan, D.S.W.; Loong, H.H.F.; Johnson, M.; Gainor, J.; McCoach, C.E.; Gautschi, O.; Besse, B.; Cho, B.C.; et al. Efficacy of Selpercatinib in RET Fusion-Positive Non-Small-Cell Lung Cancer. *N. Engl. J. Med.* **2020**, *383*, 813–824. [CrossRef]
151. Wirth, L.J.; Sherman, E.; Robinson, B.; Solomon, B.; Kang, H.; Lorch, J.; Worden, F.; Brose, M.; Patel, J.; Leboulleux, S.; et al. Efficacy of Selpercatinib in RET-Altered Thyroid Cancers. *N. Engl. J. Med.* **2020**, *383*, 825–835. [CrossRef]
152. Hu, M.; Subbiah, V.; Wirth, L.J.; Schuler, M.; Mansfield, A.S.; Brose, M.S.; Curigliano, G.; Leboulleux, S.; Zhu, V.W.; Keam, B.; et al. Results from the registrational phase I/II ARROW trial of pralsetinib (BLU-667) in patients (pts) with advanced RET mutation-positive medullary thyroid cancer (RET + MTC). *Ann. Oncol.* **2020**, *31* (Suppl. 4), S1084. [CrossRef]
153. Gainor, J.F.; Curigliano, G.; Kim, D.-W.; Lee, D.H.; Besse, B.; Baik, C.S.; Doebele, R.C.; Cassier, P.A.; Lopez, G.; Tan, D.S.-W.; et al. Registrational dataset from the phase I/II ARROW trial of pralsetinib (BLU-667) in patients (pts) with advanced RET fusion+ non-small cell lung cancer (NSCLC). *J. Clin. Oncol.* **2020**, *38*, 9515. [CrossRef]
154. Zhu, V.W.; Madison, R.; Schrock, A.B.; Ou, S.I. Emergence of High Level of MET Amplification as Off-Target Resistance to Selpercatinib Treatment in KIF5B-RET NSCLC. *J. Thorac. Oncol.* **2020**, *15*, e124–e127. [CrossRef]
155. Lin, J.J.; Liu, S.V.; McCoach, C.E.; Zhu, V.W.; Tan, A.C.; Yoda, S.; Peterson, J.; Do, A.; Prutisto-Chang, K.; Dagogo-Jack, I.; et al. Mechanisms of resistance to selective RET tyrosine kinase inhibitors in RET fusion-positive non-small-cell lung cancer. *Ann. Oncol.* **2020**, *31*, 1725–1733. [CrossRef]
156. Moore, K.; Colombo, N.; Scambia, G.; Kim, B.G.; Oaknin, A.; Friedlander, M.; Lisyanskaya, A.; Floquet, A.; Leary, A.; Sonke, G.S.; et al. Maintenance Olaparib in Patients with Newly Diagnosed Advanced Ovarian Cancer. *N. Engl. J. Med.* **2018**, *379*, 2495–2505. [CrossRef]
157. Ray-Coquard, I.; Pautier, P.; Pignata, S.; Pérol, D.; González-Martín, A.; Berger, R.; Fujiwara, K.; Vergote, I.; Colombo, N.; Mäenpää, J.; et al. Olaparib plus Bevacizumab as First-Line Maintenance in Ovarian Cancer. *N. Engl. J. Med.* **2019**, *381*, 2416–2428. [CrossRef] [PubMed]
158. Coleman, R.L.; Oza, A.M.; Lorusso, D.; Aghajanian, C.; Oaknin, A.; Dean, A.; Colombo, N.; Weberpals, J.I.; Clamp, A.; Scambia, G.; et al. Rucaparib maintenance treatment for recurrent ovarian carcinoma after response to platinum therapy (ARIEL3): A randomised, double-blind, placebo-controlled, phase 3 trial. *Lancet* **2017**, *390*, 1949–1961. [CrossRef]
159. González-Martín, A.; Pothuri, B.; Vergote, I.; DePont Christensen, R.; Graybill, W.; Mirza, M.R.; McCormick, C.; Lorusso, D.; Hoskins, P.; Freyer, G.; et al. Niraparib in Patients with Newly Diagnosed Advanced Ovarian Cancer. *N. Engl. J. Med.* **2019**, *381*, 2391–2402. [CrossRef]
160. de Bono, J.; Mateo, J.; Fizazi, K.; Saad, F.; Shore, N.; Sandhu, S.; Chi, K.N.; Sartor, O.; Agarwal, N.; Olmos, D.; et al. Olaparib for Metastatic Castration-Resistant Prostate Cancer. *N. Engl. J. Med.* **2020**, *382*, 2091–2102. [CrossRef]
161. Abida, W.; Patnaik, A.; Campbell, D.; Shapiro, J.; Bryce, A.H.; McDermott, R.; Sautois, B.; Vogelzang, N.J.; Bambury, R.M.; Voog, E.; et al. Rucaparib in Men with Metastatic Castration-Resistant Prostate Cancer Harboring a BRCA1 or BRCA2 Gene Alteration. *J. Clin. Oncol.* **2020**, *38*, 3763–3772. [CrossRef] [PubMed]
162. Robson, M.; Im, S.A.; Senkus, E.; Xu, B.; Domchek, S.M.; Masuda, N.; Delaloge, S.; Li, W.; Tung, N.; Armstrong, A.; et al. Olaparib for Metastatic Breast Cancer in Patients with a Germline BRCA Mutation. *N. Engl. J. Med.* **2017**, *377*, 523–533. [CrossRef] [PubMed]
163. Litton, J.K.; Rugo, H.S.; Ettl, J.; Hurvitz, S.A.; Gonçalves, A.; Lee, K.H.; Fehrenbacher, L.; Yerushalmi, R.; Mina, L.A.; Martin, M.; et al. Talazoparib in Patients with Advanced Breast Cancer and a Germline BRCA Mutation. *N. Engl. J. Med.* **2018**, *379*, 753–763. [CrossRef] [PubMed]
164. Holter, S.; Borgida, A.; Dodd, A.; Grant, R.; Semotiuk, K.; Hedley, D.; Dhani, N.; Narod, S.; Akbari, M.; Moore, M.; et al. Germline BRCA Mutations in a Large Clinic-Based Cohort of Patients with Pancreatic Adenocarcinoma. *J. Clin. Oncol.* **2015**, *33*, 3124–3129. [CrossRef] [PubMed]
165. Golan, T.; Hammel, P.; Reni, M.; van Cutsem, E.; Macarulla, T.; Hall, M.J.; Park, J.O.; Hochhauser, D.; Arnold, D.; Oh, D.Y.; et al. Maintenance Olaparib for Germline BRCA-Mutated Metastatic Pancreatic Cancer. *N. Engl. J. Med.* **2019**, *381*, 317–327. [CrossRef]
166. Keytruda Prescribing Information, Revised 02/2021. Available online: https://www.merck.com/product/usa/pi_circulars/k/keytruda/keytruda_pi.pdf (accessed on 20 April 2021).

167. Opdivo Prescribing Information. Revised 4/2021. Available online: https://packageinserts.bms.com/pi/pi_opdivo.pdf (accessed on 20 April 2021).
168. Tecentriq Prescribing Information. Revised 04/21. Available online: https://www.gene.com/download/pdf/tecentriq_prescribing.pdf (accessed on 20 April 2021).
169. Imfinzi Prescribing Information. Revised 02/21. Available online: https://den8dhaj6zs0e.cloudfront.net/50fd68b9-106b-4550-b5d0-12b045f8b184/9496217c-08b3-432b-ab4f-538d795820bd/9496217c-08b3-432b-ab4f-538d795820bd_viewable_rendition__v.pdf (accessed on 20 April 2021).
170. Bavencio Prescribing Information. Revised 11/2020. Available online: https://www.emdserono.com/us-en/pi/bavencio-pi.pdf (accessed on 20 April 2021).
171. Libtayo Prescribing Information. Revised 02/2021. Available online: https://www.regeneron.com/downloads/libtayo_fpi.pdf (accessed on 20 April 2021).
172. Jemperli Prescribing Information. Revised 04/2021. Available online: https://www.accessdata.fda.gov/drugsatfda_docs/label/2021/761174s000lbl.pdf (accessed on 24 April 2021).
173. Patel, S.P.; Kurzrock, R. PD-L1 Expression as a Predictive Biomarker in Cancer Immunotherapy. *Mol. Cancer Ther.* **2015**, *14*, 847–856. [CrossRef]
174. Festino, L.; Botti, G.; Lorigan, P.; Masucci, G.V.; Hipp, J.D.; Horak, C.E.; Melero, I.; Ascierto, P.A. Cancer Treatment with Anti-PD-1/PD-L1 Agents: Is PD-L1 Expression a Biomarker for Patient Selection? *Drugs* **2016**, *76*, 925–945. [CrossRef] [PubMed]
175. Davis, A.A.; Patel, V.G. The role of PD-L1 expression as a predictive biomarker: An analysis of all US Food and Drug Administration (FDA) approvals of immune checkpoint inhibitors. *J. Immunther. Cancer* **2019**, *7*, 278. [CrossRef]
176. Update on Phase III DANUBE Trial for Imfinzi and Tremelimumab in Unresectable, Stage IV Bladder Cancer, Published 6 March 2020. Available online: https://www.astrazeneca.com/media-centre/press-releases/2020/update-on-phase-iii-danube-trial-for-imfinzi-and-tremelimumab-in-unresectable-stage-iv-bladder-cancer-06032020.html (accessed on 27 April 2021).
177. Powles, T.; van der Heijden, M.S.; Castellano, D.; Galsky, M.D.; Loriot, Y.; Petrylak, D.P.; Ogawa, O.; Park, S.H.; Lee, J.L.; De Giorgi, U.; et al. Durvalumab alone and durvalumab plus tremelimumab versus chemotherapy in previously untreated patients with unresectable, locally advanced or metastatic urothelial carcinoma (DANUBE): A randomised, open-label, multicentre, phase 3 trial. *Lancet Oncol.* **2020**, *21*, 1574–1588. [CrossRef]
178. FDA Expands Pembrolizumab Indication for First-Line Treatment of NSCLC (TPS $\geq$1%). Content Current as of: 04/11/2019. Available online: https://www.fda.gov/drugs/fda-expands-pembrolizumab-indication-first-line-treatment-nsclc-tps-1 (accessed on 27 April 2021).
179. FDA Approves Nivolumab Plus Ipilimumab for First-Line mNSCLC (PD-L1 Tumor Expression $\geq$1%). Content Current as of: 05/15/2020. Available online: https://www.fda.gov/drugs/drug-approvals-and-databases/fda-approves-nivolumab-plus-ipilimumab-first-line-mnsclc-pd-l1-tumor-expression-1 (accessed on 27 April 2021).
180. FDA Approves Atezolizumab for First-Line Treatment of Metastatic NSCLC with High PD-L1 Expression. Content Current as of: 05/18/2020. Available online: https://www.fda.gov/drugs/resources-information-approved-drugs/fda-approves-atezolizumab-first-line-treatment-metastatic-nsclc-high-pd-l1-expression (accessed on 27 April 2021).
181. FDA Approves Cemiplimab-Rwlc for Non-Small Cell Lung Cancer with High PD-L1 Expression. Content Current as of: 02/22/2021. Available online: https://www.fda.gov/drugs/drug-approvals-and-databases/fda-approves-cemiplimab-rwlc-non-small-cell-lung-cancer-high-pd-l1-expression (accessed on 27 April 2021).
182. FDA Approves Pembrolizumab for First-Line Treatment of Head and Neck Squamous Cell Carcinoma. Content Current as of: 06/11/2019. Available online: https://www.fda.gov/drugs/resources-information-approved-drugs/fda-approves-pembrolizumab-first-line-treatment-head-and-neck-squamous-cell-carcinoma (accessed on 27 April 2021).
183. FDA Limits the Use of Tecentriq and Keytruda for Some Urothelial Cancer Patients. Content Current as of: 07/05/2018. Available online: https://www.fda.gov/drugs/resources-information-approved-drugs/fda-limits-use-tecentriq-and-keytruda-some-urothelial-cancer-patients (accessed on 27 April 2021).
184. Fashoyin-Aje, L.; Donoghue, M.; Chen, H.; He, K.; Veeraraghavan, J.; Goldberg, K.B.; Keegan, P.; McKee, A.E.; Pazdur, R. FDA Approval Summary: Pembrolizumab for Recurrent Locally Advanced or Metastatic Gastric or Gastroesophageal Junction Adenocarcinoma Expressing PD-L1. *Oncologist* **2019**, *24*, 103–109. [CrossRef]
185. FDA Approves Pembrolizumab for Advanced Esophageal Squamous Cell Cancer. Content Current as of: 07/31/2019. Available online: https://www.fda.gov/drugs/resources-information-approved-drugs/fda-approves-pembrolizumab-advanced-esophageal-squamous-cell-cancer (accessed on 27 April 2021).
186. FDA Approves Pembrolizumab for Advanced Cervical Cancer with Disease Progression during or after Chemotherapy. Content Current as of: 06/13/2018. Available online: https://www.fda.gov/drugs/resources-information-approved-drugs/fda-approves-pembrolizumab-advanced-cervical-cancer-disease-progression-during-or-after-chemotherapy (accessed on 27 April 2021).
187. Narayan, P.; Wahby, S.; Gao, J.J.; Amiri-Kordestani, L.; Ibrahim, A.; Bloomquist, E.; Tang, S.; Xu, Y.; Liu, J.; Fu, W.; et al. FDA Approval Summary: Atezolizumab Plus Paclitaxel Protein-bound for the Treatment of Patients with Advanced or Metastatic TNBC Whose Tumors Express PD-L1. *Clin. Cancer Res.* **2020**, *26*, 2284–2289. [CrossRef]

188. FDA Grants Accelerated Approval to Pembrolizumab for Locally Recurrent Unresectable or Metastatic Triple Negative Breast Cancer. Content Current as of: 11/13/2020. Available online: https://www.fda.gov/drugs/drug-approvals-and-databases/fda-grants-accelerated-approval-pembrolizumab-locally-recurrent-unresectable-or-metastatic-triple (accessed on 27 April 2021).
189. Bar-Sagi, D.; Knelson, E.H.; Sequist, L.V. A bright future for KRAS inhibitors. *Nat. Cancer* **2020**, *1*, 25–27. [CrossRef]
190. Nadal, E.; Chen, G.; Prensner, J.R.; Shiratsuchi, H.; Sam, C.; Zhao, L.; Kalemkerian, G.P.; Brenner, D.; Lin, J.; Reddy, R.M.; et al. KRAS-G12C mutation is associated with poor outcome in surgically resected lung adenocarcinoma. *J. Thorac. Oncol.* **2014**, *9*, 1513–1522. [CrossRef] [PubMed]
191. Jones, R.P.; Sutton, P.A.; Evans, J.P.; Clifford, R.; McAvoy, A.; Lewis, J.; Rousseau, A.; Mountford, R.; McWhirter, D.; Malik, H.Z. Specific mutations in KRAS codon 12 are associated with worse overall survival in patients with advanced and recurrent colorectal cancer. *Br. J. Cancer* **2017**, *116*, 923–929. [CrossRef]
192. Del Re, M.; Rofi, E.; Restante, G.; Crucitta, S.; Arrigoni, E.; Fogli, S.; DiMaio, M.; Petrini, I.; Danesi, R. Implications of KRAS mutations in acquired resistance to treatment in NSCLC. *Oncotarget* **2017**, *9*, 6630–6643. [CrossRef]
193. Ostrem, J.M.; Peters, U.; Sos, M.L.; Wells, J.A.; Shokat, K.M. K-Ras(G12C) inhibitors allosterically control GTP affinity and effector interactions. *Nature* **2013**, *503*, 548–551. [CrossRef] [PubMed]
194. Canon, J.; Rex, K.; Saiki, A.Y.; Mohr, C.; Cooke, K.; Bagal, D.; Gaida, K.; Holt, T.; Knutson, C.G.; Koppada, N.; et al. The clinical KRAS(G12C) inhibitor AMG 510 drives anti-tumour immunity. *Nature* **2019**, *575*, 217–223. [CrossRef]
195. Hallin, J.; Engstrom, L.D.; Hargis, L.; Calinisan, A.; Aranda, R.; Briere, D.M.; Sudhakar, N.; Bowcut, V.; Baer, B.R.; Ballard, J.A.; et al. The KRASG12C Inhibitor MRTX849 Provides Insight toward Therapeutic Susceptibility of KRAS-Mutant Cancers in Mouse Models and Patients. *Cancer Discov.* **2020**, *10*, 54–71. [CrossRef] [PubMed]
196. Hong, D.S.; Fakih, M.G.; Strickler, J.H.; Desai, J.; Durm, G.A.; Shapiro, G.I.; Falchook, G.S.; Price, T.J.; Sacher, A.; Denlinger, C.S.; et al. KRASG12C Inhibition with Sotorasib in Advanced Solid Tumors. *N. Engl. J. Med.* **2020**, *383*, 1207–1217. [CrossRef] [PubMed]
197. LoRusso, P.M.; Sebolt-Leopold, J.S. One Step at a Time—Clinical Evidence That KRAS Is Indeed Druggable. *N. Engl. J. Med.* **2020**, *383*, 1277–1278. [CrossRef]
198. Amodio, V.; Yaeger, R.; Arcella, P.; Cancelliere, C.; Lamba, S.; Lorenzato, A.; Arena, S.; Montone, M.; Mussolin, B.; Bian, Y.; et al. EGFR Blockade Reverts Resistance to KRASG12C Inhibition in Colorectal Cancer. *Cancer Discov.* **2020**, *10*, 1129–1139. [CrossRef]
199. Misale, S.; Fatherree, J.P.; Cortez, E.; Li, C.; Bilton, S.; Timonina, D.; Myers, D.T.; Lee, D.; Gomez-Caraballo, M.; Greenberg, M.; et al. KRAS G12C NSCLC Models Are Sensitive to Direct Targeting of KRAS in Combination with PI3K Inhibition. *Clin. Cancer Res.* **2019**, *25*, 796–807. [CrossRef]
200. Riely, G.J.; Ou, S.-H.I.; Rybkin, I.; Spira, A.; Papadopoulos, K.; Sabari, J.K.; Johnson, M.; Heist, R.S.; Bazhenova, L.; Barve, M.; et al. KRYSTAL-1: Activity and preliminary pharmacodynamic (PD) analysis of adagrasib (MRTX849) in patients (Pts) with advanced non–small cell lung cancer (NSCLC) harboring KRASG12C mutation. *J. Thorac. Oncol.* **2021**, *16*, S751–S752. [CrossRef]
201. Siegel, R.L.; Miller, K.D.; Jemal, A. Cancer Statistics, 2020. *CA Cancer J. Clin.* **2020**, *70*, 7–30. [CrossRef]
202. Noone, A.M.; Cronin, K.A.; Altekruse, S.F.; Howlader, N.; Lewis, D.R.; Petkov, V.I.; Penberthy, L. Cancer Incidence and Survival Trends by Subtype Using Data from the Surveillance Epidemiology and End Results Program, 1992–2013. *Cancer Epidemiol. Biomark. Prev.* **2017**, *26*, 632–641. [CrossRef] [PubMed]
203. Howlader, N.; Forjaz, G.; Mooradian, M.J.; Meza, R.; Kong, C.Y.; Cronin, K.A.; Mariotto, A.B.; Lowy, D.R.; Feuer, E.J. The Effect of Advances in Lung-Cancer Treatment on Population Mortality. *N. Engl. J. Med.* **2020**, *383*, 640–649. [CrossRef]
204. National Comprehensive Cancer Network. Non-Small Cell Lung Cancer (Version 4.2021-March 3, 2021). Available online: https://www.nccn.org/professionals/physician_gls/pdf/nscl.pdf (accessed on 22 April 2021).
205. Lindeman, N.I.; Cagle, P.T.; Aisner, D.L.; Arcila, M.E.; Beasley, M.B.; Bernicker, E.H.; Colasacco, C.; Dacic, S.; Hirsch, F.R.; Kerr, K.; et al. Updated Molecular Testing Guideline for the Selection of Lung Cancer Patients for Treatment with Targeted Tyrosine Kinase Inhibitors: Guideline From the College of American Pathologists, the International Association for the Study of Lung Cancer, and the Association for Molecular Pathology. *J. Mol. Diagn.* **2018**, *20*, 129–159.
206. Rolfo, C.; Mack, P.C.; Scagliotti, G.V.; Baas, P.; Barlesi, F.; Bivona, T.G.; Herbst, R.S.; Mok, T.S.; Peled, N.; Pirker, R.; et al. Liquid Biopsy for Advanced Non-Small Cell Lung Cancer (NSCLC): A Statement Paper from the IASLC. *J. Thorac. Oncol.* **2018**, *13*, 1248–1268. [CrossRef]
207. Leighl, N.B.; Page, R.D.; Raymond, V.M.; Daniel, D.B.; Divers, S.G.; Reckamp, K.L.; Villalona-Calero, M.S.; Dix, D.; Odegaard, J.I.; Lanman, R.B.; et al. Clinical Utility of Comprehensive Cell-free DNA Analysis to Identify Genomic Biomarkers in Patients with Newly Diagnosed Metastatic Non-Small Cell Lung Cancer. *Clin. Cancer Res.* **2019**, *25*, 4691–4700. [CrossRef]
208. Schoenfeld, A.J.; Arbour, K.C.; Rizvi, H.; Iqbal, A.N.; Gadgeel, S.M.; Girshman, J.; Kris, M.G.; Riely, G.J.; Yu, H.A.; Hellmann, M.D. Severe immune-related adverse events are common with sequential PD-(L)1 blockade and osimertinib. *Ann. Oncol.* **2019**, *30*, 839–844. [CrossRef]
209. Spigel, D.R.; Reynolds, C.; Waterhouse, D.; Garon, E.B.; Chandler, J.; Babu, S.; Thurmes, P.; Spira, A.; Jotte, R.; Zhu, J.; et al. Phase 1/2 Study of the Safety and Tolerability of Nivolumab Plus Crizotinib for the First-Line Treatment of Anaplastic Lymphoma Kinase Translocation—Positive Advanced Non-Small Cell Lung Cancer (CheckMate 370). *J. Thorac. Oncol.* **2018**, *13*, 682–688. [CrossRef]
210. Khozin, S.; Blumenthal, G.M.; Jiang, X.; He, K.; Boyd, K.; Murgo, A.; Justice, R.; Keegan, P.; Pazdur, R.U.S. Food and Drug Administration Approval Summary: Erlotinib for the First-Line Treatment of Metastatic Non-Small Cell Lung Cancer with

Epidermal Growth Factor Receptor Exon 19 Deletions or Exon 21 (L858R) Substitution Mutations. *Oncologist* **2014**, *19*, 774–779. [CrossRef]
211. Kazandjian, D.; Blumenthal, G.M.; Yuan, W.; He, K.; Keegan, P.; Pazdur, R. FDA Approval of Gefitinib for the Treatment of Patients with Metastatic EGFR Mutation-Positive Non-Small Cell Lung Cancer. *Clin. Cancer Res.* **2016**, *22*, 1307–1312. [CrossRef]
212. FDA Broadens Afatinib Indication to Previously Untreated, Metastatic NSCLC with Other Non-Resistant EGFR Mutations. Content Current as of: 01/16/2018. Available online: https://www.fda.gov/drugs/resources-information-approved-drugs/fda-broadens-afatinib-indication-previously-untreated-metastatic-nsclc-other-non-resistant-egfr (accessed on 26 April 2021).
213. FDA Approves Dacomitinib for Metastatic Non-Small Cell Lung Cancer. Content Current as of: 11/26/2018. Available online: https://www.fda.gov/drugs/drug-approvals-and-databases/fda-approves-dacomitinib-metastatic-non-small-cell-lung-cancer (accessed on 26 April 2021).
214. FDA Approves Osimertinib for First-Line Treatment of Metastatic NSCLC with Most Common EGFR Mutations. Content current as of: 04/19/2018. Available online: https://www.fda.gov/drugs/resources-information-approved-drugs/fda-approves-osimertinib-first-line-treatment-metastatic-nsclc-most-common-egfr-mutations (accessed on 26 April 2021).
215. FDA Approves Osimertinib as Adjuvant Therapy for Non-Small Cell Lung Cancer with EGFR Mutations. Available online: https://www.fda.gov/drugs/drug-approvals-and-databases/fda-approves-osimertinib-adjuvant-therapy-non-small-cell-lung-cancer-egfr-mutations (accessed on 23 April 2021).
216. FDA Grants Accelerated Approval to Amivantamab-Vmjw for Metastatic Non-Small Cell Lung Cancer. Content Current as of 05/21/2021. Available online: https://www.fda.gov/drugs/drug-approvals-and-databases/fda-grants-accelerated-approval-amivantamab-vmjw-metastatic-non-small-cell-lung-cancer (accessed on 26 May 2021).
217. Kazandjian, D.; Blumenthal, G.M.; Chen, H.Y.; He, K.; Patel, M.; Justice, R.; Keegan, P.; Pazdur, R. FDA approval summary: Crizotinib for the treatment of metastatic non-small cell lung cancer with anaplastic lymphoma kinase rearrangements. *Oncologist* **2014**, *19*, e5–e11. [CrossRef] [PubMed]
218. Khozin, S.; Blumenthal, G.M.; Zhang, L.; Tang, S.; Brower, M.; Fox, E.; Helms, W.; Leong, R.; Song, P.; Pan, Y.; et al. FDA approval: Ceritinib for the treatment of metastatic anaplastic lymphoma kinase-positive non-small cell lung cancer. *Clin. Cancer Res.* **2015**, *21*, 2436–2439. [CrossRef] [PubMed]
219. FDA Approves Lorlatinib for Second- or Third-Line Treatment of ALK-Positive Metastatic NSCLC. Content Current as of: 12/14/2018. Available online: https://www.fda.gov/drugs/fda-approves-lorlatinib-second-or-third-line-treatment-alk-positive-metastatic-nsclc (accessed on 26 April 2021).
220. Larkins, E.; Blumenthal, G.M.; Chen, H.; He, K.; Agarwal, R.; Gieser, G.; Stephens, O.; Zahalka, E.; Ringgold, K.; Helms, W.; et al. FDA Approval: Alectinib for the Treatment of Metastatic, ALK-Positive Non-Small Cell Lung Cancer Following Crizotinib. *Clin. Cancer Res.* **2016**, *22*, 5171–5176. [CrossRef] [PubMed]
221. Brigatinib. Content Current as of: 07/25/2017. Available online: https://www.fda.gov/drugs/resources-information-approved-drugs/brigatinib (accessed on 26 April 2021).
222. Kazandjian, D.; Blumenthal, G.M.; Luo, L.; He, K.; Fran, I.; Lemery, S.; Pazdur, R. Benefit-Risk Summary of Crizotinib for the Treatment of Patients with ROS1 Alteration-Positive, Metastatic Non-Small Cell Lung Cancer. *Oncologist* **2016**, *21*, 974–980. [CrossRef] [PubMed]
223. FDA Grants Accelerated Approval to Capmatinib for Metastatic Non-Small Cell Lung Cancer. Content Current as of: 05/06/2020. Available online: https://www.fda.gov/drugs/drug-approvals-and-databases/fda-grants-accelerated-approval-capmatinib-metastatic-non-small-cell-lung-cancer (accessed on 26 April 2021).
224. FDA Grants Accelerated Approval to Tepotinib for Metastatic Non-Small Cell Lung Cancer. Content Current as of: 02/03/2021. Available online: https://www.fda.gov/drugs/drug-approvals-and-databases/fda-grants-accelerated-approval-tepotinib-metastatic-non-small-cell-lung-cancer (accessed on 26 April 2021).
225. Hirsch, F.R.; Bunn, P.A., Jr. EGFR testing in lung cancer is ready for prime time. *Lancet Oncol.* **2009**, *10*, 432–433. [CrossRef]
226. O'Kane, G.M.; Bradbury, P.A.; Feld, R.; Leighl, N.B.; Liu, G.; Pisters, K.M.; Kamel-Reid, S.; Tsao, M.S.; Shepherd, F.A. Uncommon EGFR mutations in advanced non-small cell lung cancer. *Lung Cancer* **2017**, *109*, 137–144. [CrossRef]
227. Mok, T.S.; Wu, Y.L.; Thongprasert, S.; Yang, C.H.; Chu, D.T.; Saijo, N.; Sunpaweravong, P.; Han, B.; Margono, B.; Ichinose, Y.; et al. Gefitinib or carboplatin-paclitaxel in pulmonary adenocarcinoma. *N. Engl. J. Med.* **2009**, *361*, 947–957. [CrossRef]
228. Fukuoka, M.; Wu, Y.L.; Thongprasert, S.; Sunpaweravong, P.; Leong, S.S.; Sriuranpong, V.; Chao, T.Y.; Nakagawa, K.; Chu, D.T.; Saijo, N.; et al. Biomarker analyses and final overall survival results from a phase III, randomized, open-label, first-line study of gefitinib versus carboplatin/paclitaxel in clinically selected patients with advanced non-small-cell lung cancer in Asia (IPASS). *J. Clin. Oncol.* **2011**, *29*, 2866–2874. [CrossRef]
229. Douillard, J.Y.; Ostoros, G.; Cobo, M.; Ciuleanu, T.; McCormack, R.; Webster, A.; Milenkova, T. First-line gefitinib in Caucasian EGFR mutation-positive NSCLC patients: A phase-IV, open-label, single-arm study. *Br. J. Cancer* **2014**, *110*, 55–62. [CrossRef]
230. Rosell, R.; Carcereny, E.; Gervais, R.; Vergnenegre, A.; Massuti, B.; Felip, E.; Palmero, R.; Garcia-Gomez, R.; Pallares, C.; Sanchez, J.M.; et al. Erlotinib versus standard chemotherapy as first-line treatment for European patients with advanced EGFR mutation-positive non-small-cell lung cancer (EURTAC): A multicentre, open-label, randomised phase 3 trial. *Lancet Oncol.* **2012**, *13*, 239–246. [CrossRef]

231. Nakagawa, K.; Garon, E.B.; Seto, T.; Nishio, M.; Ponce Aix, S.; Paz-Ares, L.; Chiu, C.H.; Park, K.; Novello, S.; Nadal, E.; et al. Ramucirumab plus erlotinib in patients with untreated, EGFR-mutated, advanced non-small-cell lung cancer (RELAY): A randomised, double-blind, placebo-controlled, phase 3 trial. *Lancet Oncol.* **2019**, *20*, 1655–1669. [CrossRef]
232. Saito, H.; Fukuhara, T.; Furuya, N.; Watanabe, K.; Sugawara, S.; Iwasawa, S.; Tsunezuka, Y.; Yamaguchi, O.; Okada, M.; Yoshimori, K.; et al. Erlotinib plus bevacizumab versus erlotinib alone in patients with EGFR-positive advanced non-squamous non-small-cell lung cancer (NEJ026): Interim analysis of an open-label, randomised, multicentre, phase 3 trial. *Lancet Oncol.* **2019**, *20*, 625–635. [CrossRef]
233. Yang, J.C.; Sequist, L.V.; Geater, S.L.; Tsai, C.M.; Mok, T.S.; Schuler, M.; Yamamoto, N.; Yu, C.J.; Ou, S.H.; Zhou, C.; et al. Clinical activity of afatinib in patients with advanced non-small-cell lung cancer harbouring uncommon EGFR mutations: A combined post-hoc analysis of LUX-Lung 2, LUX-Lung 3, and LUX-Lung 6. *Lancet Oncol.* **2015**, *16*, 830–838. [CrossRef]
234. Yang, J.C.; Schuler, M.; Popat, S.; Miura, S.; Heeke, S.; Park, K.; Märten, A.; Kim, E.S. Afatinib for the Treatment of NSCLC Harboring Uncommon EGFR Mutations: A Database of 693 Cases. *J. Thorac. Oncol.* **2020**, *15*, 803–815. [CrossRef]
235. Wu, Y.L.; Cheng, Y.; Zhou, X.; Lee, K.H.; Nakagawa, K.; Niho, S.; Tsuji, F.; Linke, R.; Rosell, R.; Corral, J.; et al. Dacomitinib versus gefitinib as first-line treatment for patients with EGFR-mutation-positive non-small-cell lung cancer (ARCHER 1050): A randomised, open-label, phase 3 trial. *Lancet Oncol.* **2017**, *18*, 1454–1466. [CrossRef]
236. Mok, T.S.; Cheng, Y.; Zhou, X.; Lee, K.H.; Nakagawa, K.; Niho, S.; Lee, M.; Linke, R.; Rosell, R.; Corral, J.; et al. Improvement in Overall Survival in a Randomized Study That Compared Dacomitinib With Gefitinib in Patients with Advanced Non-Small-Cell Lung Cancer and EGFR-Activating Mutations. *J. Clin. Oncol.* **2018**, *36*, 2244–2250. [CrossRef] [PubMed]
237. Mok, T.S.; Wu, Y.-L.; Ahn, M.-J.; Garassino, M.C.; Kim, H.R.; Ramalingam, S.S.; Shepherd, F.A.; He, Y.; Akamatsu, H.; Theelen, W.S.; et al. Osimertinib or Platinum-Pemetrexed in EGFR T790M-Positive Lung Cancer. *N. Engl. J. Med.* **2017**, *376*, 629–640. [CrossRef]
238. Soria, J.C.; Ohe, Y.; Vansteenkiste, J.; Reungwetwattana, T.; Chewaskulyong, B.; Lee, K.H.; Dechaphunkul, A.; Imamura, F.; Nogami, N.; Kurata, T.; et al. Osimertinib in Untreated EGFR-Mutated Advanced Non-Small-Cell Lung Cancer. *N. Engl. J. Med.* **2018**, *378*, 113–125. [CrossRef] [PubMed]
239. Ramalingam, S.S.; Vansteenkiste, J.; Planchard, D.; Cho, B.C.; Gray, J.E.; Ohe, Y.; Zhou, C.; Reungwetwattana, T.; Cheng, Y.; Chewaskulyong, B.; et al. Overall Survival with Osimertinib in Untreated, EGFR-Mutated Advanced NSCLC. *N. Engl. J. Med.* **2020**, *382*, 41–50. [CrossRef] [PubMed]
240. Reungwetwattana, T.; Nakagawa, K.; Cho, B.C.; Cobo, M.; Cho, E.K.; Bertolini, A.; Bohnet, S.; Zhou, C.; Lee, K.H.; Nogami, N.; et al. CNS Response to Osimertinib Versus Standard Epidermal Growth Factor Receptor Tyrosine Kinase Inhibitors in Patients with Untreated EGFR-Mutated Advanced Non-Small-Cell Lung Cancer. *J. Clin. Oncol.* **2018**, *36*, 3290–3297. [CrossRef]
241. Yang, J.C.H.; Kim, S.W.; Kim, D.W.; Lee, J.S.; Cho, B.C.; Ahn, J.S.; Lee, D.H.; Kim, T.M.; Goldman, J.W.; Natale, R.B.; et al. Osimertinib in Patients with Epidermal Growth Factor Receptor Mutation-Positive Non-Small-Cell Lung Cancer and Leptomeningeal Metastases: The BLOOM Study. *J. Clin. Oncol.* **2020**, *38*, 538–547. [CrossRef]
242. Coleman, N.; Woolf, D.; Welsh, L.; McDonald, F.; MacMahon, S.; Yousaf, N.; Popat, S. EGFR Exon 20 Insertion (A763_Y764insFQEA) Mutant NSCLC Is Not Identified by Roche Cobas Version 2 Tissue Testing but Has Durable Intracranial and Extracranial Response to Osimertinib. *J. Thorac. Oncol.* **2020**, *15*, e162–e165. [CrossRef] [PubMed]
243. Sehgal, K.; Rangachari, D.; VanderLaan, P.A.; Kobayashi, S.S.; Costa, D.B. Clinical Benefit of Tyrosine Kinase Inhibitors in Advanced Lung Cancer with EGFR-G719A and Other Uncommon EGFR Mutations. *Oncologist* **2021**, *26*, 281–287. [CrossRef]
244. Wu, Y.L.; Tsuboi, M.; He, J.; John, T.; Grohe, C.; Majem, M.; Goldman, J.W.; Laktionov, K.; Kim, S.W.; Kato, T.; et al. Osimertinib in Resected EGFR-Mutated Non-Small-Cell Lung Cancer. *N. Engl. J. Med.* **2020**, *383*, 1711–1723. [CrossRef]
245. Piper-Vallillo, A.J.; Sequist, L.V.; Piotrowska, Z. Emerging Treatment Paradigms for EGFR-Mutant Lung Cancers Progressing on Osimertinib: A Review. *J. Clin. Oncol.* **2020**, *38*, 2926–2936. [CrossRef]
246. Sabari, J.K.; Shu, C.A.; Park, K.; Leighl, N.; Mitchell, P.; Kim, S.; Lee, J.; Kim, D.; Viteri, S.; Spira, A.; et al. Amivantamab in Post-platinum EGFR Exon 20 Insertion Mutant Non-Small Cell Lung Cancer. *J. Thorac. Oncol.* **2021**, *16*, S108–S109. [CrossRef]
247. Zhou, C.; Ramalingam, S.; Li, B.; Fang, J.; Kim, T.M.; Kim, S.; Yang, J.C.; Riely, J.; Mekhail, T.; Nguyen, D.; et al. Mobocertinib in NSCLC With EGFR Exon 20 Insertions: Results from EXCLAIM and Pooled Platinum-Pretreated Patient Populations. *J. Thorac. Oncol.* **2021**, *16*, S108. [CrossRef]
248. Kwak, E.L.; Bang, Y.J.; Camidge, D.R.; Shaw, A.T.; Solomon, B.; Maki, R.G.; Ou, S.H.; Dezube, B.J.; Jänne, P.A.; Costa, D.B.; et al. Anaplastic lymphoma kinase inhibition in non-small-cell lung cancer. *N. Engl. J. Med.* **2010**, *363*, 1693–1703. [CrossRef] [PubMed]
249. Camidge, D.R.; Bang, Y.J.; Kwak, E.L.; Iafrate, A.J.; Varella-Garcia, M.; Fox, S.B.; Riely, G.J.; Solomon, B.; Ou, S.H.; Kim, D.W.; et al. Activity and safety of crizotinib in patients with ALK-positive non-small-cell lung cancer: Updated results from a phase 1 study. *Lancet Oncol.* **2012**, *13*, 1011–1019. [CrossRef]
250. Kim, D.-W.; Ahn, M.-J.; Shi, Y.; de Pas, T.M.; Yang, P.-C.; Riely, G.J.; Crino, L.; Evans, T.L.; Liu, X.; Han, J.-Y.; et al. Results of a global phase II study with crizotinib in advanced ALK-positive non-small cell lung cancer (NSCLC). *J. Clin. Oncol.* **2012**, *30* (Suppl.), 7533. [CrossRef]
251. Shaw, A.T.; Ou, S.H.; Bang, Y.J.; Camidge, D.R.; Solomon, B.J.; Salgia, R.; Riely, G.J.; Varella-Garcia, M.; Shapiro, G.I.; Costa, D.B.; et al. Crizotinib in ROS1-rearranged non-small-cell lung cancer. *N. Engl. J. Med.* **2014**, *371*, 1963–1971. [CrossRef] [PubMed]

252. Shaw, A.T.; Riely, G.J.; Bang, Y.J.; Kim, D.W.; Camidge, D.R.; Solomon, B.J.; Varella-Garcia, M.; Iafrate, A.J.; Shapiro, G.I.; Usari, T.; et al. Crizotinib in ROS1-rearranged advanced non-small-cell lung cancer (NSCLC): Updated results, including overall survival, from PROFILE 1001. *Ann. Oncol.* **2019**, *30*, 1121–1126. [CrossRef] [PubMed]
253. Soria, J.C.; Tan, D.S.W.; Chiari, R.; Wu, Y.L.; Paz-Ares, L.; Wolf, J.; Geater, S.L.; Orlov, S.; Cortinovis, D.; Yu, C.J.; et al. First-line ceritinib versus platinum-based chemotherapy in advanced ALK-rearranged non-small-cell lung cancer (ASCEND-4): A randomised, open-label, phase 3 study. *Lancet* **2017**, *389*, 917–929. [CrossRef]
254. Shaw, A.T.; Felip, E.; Bauer, T.M.; Besse, B.; Navarro, A.; Postel-Vinay, S.; Gainor, J.F.; Johnson, M.; Dietrich, J.; James, L.P.; et al. Lorlatinib in non-small-cell lung cancer with ALK or ROS1 rearrangement: An international, multicentre, open-label, single-arm first-in-man phase 1 trial. *Lancet Oncol.* **2017**, *18*, 1590–1599. [CrossRef]
255. Shaw, A.T.; Bauer, T.M.; de Marinis, F.; Felip, E.; Goto, Y.; Liu, G.; Mazieres, J.; Kim, D.W.; Mok, T.; Polli, A.; et al. First-Line Lorlatinib or Crizotinib in Advanced ALK-Positive Lung Cancer. *N. Engl. J. Med.* **2020**, *383*, 2018–2029. [CrossRef] [PubMed]
256. Camidge, D.R.; Dziadziuszko, R.; Peters, S.; Mok, T.; Noe, J.; Nowicka, M.; Gadgeel, S.M.; Cheema, P.; Pavlakis, N.; de Marinis, F.; et al. Updated Efficacy and Safety Data and Impact of the EML4-ALK Fusion Variant on the Efficacy of Alectinib in Untreated ALK-Positive Advanced Non-Small Cell Lung Cancer in the Global Phase III ALEX Study. *J. Thorac. Oncol.* **2019**, *14*, 1233–1243. [CrossRef] [PubMed]
257. Mok, T.; Camidge, D.R.; Gadgeel, S.M.; Rosell, R.; Dziadziuszko, R.; Kim, D.W.; Perol, M.; Ou, S.I.; Ahn, J.S.; Shaw, A.T.; et al. Updated overall survival and final progression-free survival data for patients with treatment-naive advanced ALK-positive non-small-cell lung cancer in the ALEX study. *Ann. Oncol.* **2020**, *31*, 1056–1064. [CrossRef]
258. Kim, D.W.; Tiseo, M.; Ahn, M.J.; Reckamp, K.L.; Hansen, K.H.; Kim, S.W.; Huber, R.M.; West, H.L.; Groen, H.J.M.; Hochmair, M.J.; et al. Brigatinib in Patients with Crizotinib-Refractory Anaplastic Lymphoma Kinase-Positive Non-Small-Cell Lung Cancer: A Randomized, Multicenter Phase II Trial. *J. Clin. Oncol.* **2017**, *35*, 2490–2498. [CrossRef] [PubMed]
259. Huber, R.M.; Hansen, K.H.; Paz-Ares Rodríguez, L.; West, H.L.; Reckamp, K.L.; Leighl, N.B.; Tiseo, M.; Smit, E.F.; Kim, D.W.; Gettinger, S.N.; et al. Brigatinib in Crizotinib-Refractory ALK+ NSCLC: 2-Year Follow-up on Systemic and Intracranial Outcomes in the Phase 2 ALTA Trial. *J. Thorac. Oncol.* **2020**, *15*, 404–415. [CrossRef] [PubMed]
260. Camidge, D.R.; Kim, H.R.; Ahn, M.J.; Yang, J.C.; Han, J.Y.; Lee, J.S.; Hochmair, M.J.; Li, J.Y.; Gridelli, C.; Delmonte, A.; et al. Brigatinib versus Crizotinib in ALK-Positive Non-Small-Cell Lung Cancer. *N. Engl. J. Med.* **2018**, *379*, 2027–2039. [CrossRef]
261. Camidge, D.R.; Kim, H.R.; Ahn, M.J.; Yang, J.C.H.; Han, J.Y.; Hochmair, M.J.; Lee, K.H.; Delmonte, A.; Garcia Campelo, M.R.; Kim, D.W.; et al. Brigatinib Versus Crizotinib in Advanced ALK Inhibitor-Naive ALK-Positive Non-Small Cell Lung Cancer: Second Interim Analysis of the Phase III ALTA-1L Trial. *J. Clin. Oncol.* **2020**, *38*, 3592–3603. [CrossRef] [PubMed]
262. Drilon, A.; Siena, S.; Dziadziuszko, R.; Barlesi, F.; Krebs, M.G.; Shaw, A.T.; de Braud, F.; Rolfo, C.; Ahn, M.J.; Wolf, J.; et al. Entrectinib in ROS1 fusion-positive non-small-cell lung cancer: Integrated analysis of three phase 1-2 trials. *Lancet Oncol.* **2020**, *21*, 261–270. [CrossRef]
263. Camidge, D.R.; Pabani, A.; Miller, R.M.; Rizvi, N.A.; Bazhenova, L. Management Strategies for Early-Onset Pulmonary Events Associated with Brigatinib. *J. Thorac. Oncol.* **2019**, *14*, 1547–1555. [CrossRef]
264. Ng, T.L.; Narasimhan, N.; Gupta, N.; Venkatakrishnan, K.; Kerstein, D.; Camidge, D.R. Early-Onset Pulmonary Events Associated with Brigatinib Use in Advanced NSCLC. *J. Thorac. Oncol.* **2020**, *15*, 1190–1199. [CrossRef]
265. Shaw, A.T.; Friboulet, L.; Leshchiner, I.; Gainor, J.F.; Bergqvist, S.; Brooun, A.; Burke, B.J.; Deng, Y.L.; Liu, W.; Dardaei, L.; et al. Resensitization to Crizotinib by the Lorlatinib ALK Resistance Mutation L1198F. *N. Engl. J. Med.* **2016**, *374*, 54–61. [CrossRef]
266. Sakamoto, M.R.; Honce, J.M.; Lindquist, D.L.; Camidge, D.R. Lorlatinib Salvages CNS Relapse in an ALK-Positive Non-Small-Cell Lung Cancer Patient Previously Treated with Crizotinib and High-Dose Brigatinib. *Clin. Lung Cancer* **2019**, *20*, e133–e136. [CrossRef]
267. Shaw, A.T.; Solomon, B.J.; Besse, B.; Bauer, T.M.; Lin, C.C.; Soo, R.A.; Riely, G.J.; Ou, S.I.; Clancy, J.S.; Li, S.; et al. ALK Resistance Mutations and Efficacy of Lorlatinib in Advanced Anaplastic Lymphoma Kinase-Positive Non-Small Cell Lung Cancer. *J. Clin. Oncol.* **2019**, *37*, 1370–1379. [CrossRef] [PubMed]
268. Shi, R.; Filho, S.N.M.; Li, M.; Fares, A.; Weiss, J.; Pham, N.A.; Ludkovski, O.; Raghavan, V.; Li, Q.; Ravi, D.; et al. BRAF V600E mutation and MET amplification as resistance pathways of the second-generation anaplastic lymphoma kinase (ALK) inhibitor alectinib in lung cancer. *Lung Cancer* **2020**, *146*, 78–85. [CrossRef]
269. Coleman, N.; Yousaf, N.; Arkenau, H.T.; Welsh, L.; Popat, S. Lorlatinib Salvages Central Nervous System-Only Relapse on Entrectinib in ROS1-Positive NSCLC. *J. Thorac. Oncol.* **2020**, *15*, e142–e144. [CrossRef] [PubMed]
270. Peters, S.; Camidge, D.R.; Shaw, A.T.; Gadgeel, S.; Ahn, J.S.; Kim, D.W.; Ou, S.I.; Perol, M.; Dziadziuszko, R.; Rosell, R.; et al. Alectinib versus Crizotinib in Untreated ALK-Positive Non-Small-Cell Lung Cancer. *N. Engl. J. Med.* **2017**, *377*, 829–838. [CrossRef]
271. Yun, M.R.; Kim, D.H.; Kim, S.Y.; Joo, H.S.; Lee, Y.W.; Choi, H.M.; Park, C.W.; Heo, S.G.; Kang, H.N.; Lee, S.S.; et al. Repotrectinib Exhibits Potent Antitumor Activity in Treatment-Naïve and Solvent-Front-Mutant ROS1-Rearranged Non-Small Cell Lung Cancer. *Clin. Cancer Res.* **2020**, *26*, 3287–3295. [CrossRef]
272. Schuler, M.; Berardi, R.; Lim, W.T.; de Jonge, M.; Bauer, T.M.; Azaro, A.; Gottfried, M.; Han, J.Y.; Lee, D.H.; Wollner, M.; et al. Molecular correlates of response to capmatinib in advanced non-small-cell lung cancer: Clinical and biomarker results from a phase I trial. *Ann. Oncol.* **2020**, *31*, 789–797. [CrossRef] [PubMed]

273. Drilon, A.; Clark, J.W.; Weiss, J.; Ou, S.I.; Camidge, D.R.; Solomon, B.J.; Otterson, G.A.; Villaruz, L.C.; Riely, G.J.; Heist, R.S.; et al. Antitumor activity of crizotinib in lung cancers harboring a MET exon 14 alteration. *Nat. Med.* **2020**, *26*, 47–51. [CrossRef]
274. Paik, P.K.; Drilon, A.; Fan, P.D.; Yu, H.; Rekhtman, N.; Ginsberg, M.S.; Borsu, L.; Schultz, N.; Berger, M.F.; Rudin, C.M.; et al. Response to MET inhibitors in patients with stage IV lung adenocarcinomas harboring MET mutations causing exon 14 skipping. *Cancer Discov.* **2015**, *5*, 842–849. [CrossRef] [PubMed]
275. Klempner, S.J.; Borghei, A.; Hakimian, B.; Ali, S.M.; Ou, S.I. Intracranial Activity of Cabozantinib in MET Exon 14-Positive NSCLC with Brain Metastases. *J. Thorac. Oncol.* **2017**, *12*, 152–156. [CrossRef]
276. Wolf, J.; Seto, T.; Han, J.Y.; Reguart, N.; Garon, E.B.; Groen, H.J.M.; Tan, D.S.W.; Hida, T.; de Jonge, M.; Orlov, S.V.; et al. Capmatinib in MET Exon 14-Mutated or MET-Amplified Non-Small-Cell Lung Cancer. *N. Engl. J. Med.* **2020**, *383*, 944–957. [CrossRef] [PubMed]
277. Paik, P.K.; Felip, E.; Veillon, R.; Sakai, H.; Cortot, A.B.; Garassino, M.C.; Mazieres, J.; Viteri, S.; Senellart, H.; Van Meerbeeck, J.; et al. Tepotinib in Non-Small-Cell Lung Cancer with MET Exon 14 Skipping Mutations. *N. Engl. J. Med.* **2020**, *383*, 931–941. [CrossRef]
278. Garon, E.B.; Heist, R.S.; Seto, T.; Han, J.-Y.; Reguart, N.; Groen, H.J.M.; Tan, D.S.W.; Hida, T.; De Jonge, M.J.A.; Orlov, S.V.; et al. Capmatinib in METex14-mutated (mut) advanced non-small cell lung cancer (NSCLC): Results from the phase II GEOMETRY mono-1 study, including efficacy in patients (pts) with brain metastases (BM). In Proceedings of the 111th Annual Meeting of the American Association for Cancer Research 2020 Virtual Meeting, Philadelphia, PA, USA, 27–28 April and 22–24 June 2020. Abstract nr CT2082.
279. Roth, K.G.; Mambetsariev, I.; Salgia, R. Prolonged survival and response to tepotinib in a non-small-cell lung cancer patient with brain metastases harboring MET exon 14 mutation: A research report. *Cold Spring Harb. Mol. Case Stud.* **2020**, *6*, a005785. [CrossRef]
280. Takamori, S.; Matsubara, T.; Fujishita, T.; Ito, K.; Toyozawa, R.; Seto, T.; Yamaguchi, M.; Okamoto, T. Dramatic intracranial response to tepotinib in a patient with lung adenocarcinoma harboring MET exon 14 skipping mutation. Thorac Cancer. *Thorac. Cancer* **2021**, *12*, 978–980. [CrossRef] [PubMed]
281. Sicklick, J.K.; Kato, S.; Okamura, R.; Schwaederle, M.; Hahn, M.E.; Williams, C.B.; De, P.; Krie, A.; Piccioni, D.E.; Miller, V.A.; et al. Molecular profiling of cancer patients enables personalized combination therapy: The I-PREDICT study. *Nat. Med.* **2019**, *25*, 744–750. [CrossRef]

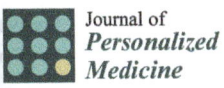

Article

Endothelin-1 as a Mediator of Heme Oxygenase-1-Induced Stemness in Colorectal Cancer: Influence of p53

Sandra Ríos-Arrabal [1,†], Jose D. Puentes-Pardo [1,2,†], Sara Moreno-SanJuan [1,3,†], Ágata Szuba [4,†], Jorge Casado [1], María García-Costela [1], Julia Escudero-Feliu [1], Michela Verbeni [5], Carlos Cano [5], Cristina González-Puga [1,6], Alicia Martín-Lagos Maldonado [1,7], Ángel Carazo [1,‡] and Josefa León [1,7,*,‡]

1. Instituto de Investigación Biosanitaria de Granada, ibs.GRANADA, 18012 Granada, Spain; sandrariosarrabal@hotmail.com (S.R.-A.); josedavidpupa@correo.ugr.es (J.D.P.-P.); sara.moreno@ibsgranada.es (S.M.-S.); jorgecasado@ugr.es (J.C.); gmaria92@correo.ugr.es (M.G.-C.); juliaescuderofeliu@gmail.com (J.E.-F.); crisgona2@hotmail.com (C.G.-P.); aliciamartin-lagos@hotmail.com (A.M.-L.M.); angelcarazogallego@gmail.com (Á.C.)
2. Departamento de Farmacología, Facultad de Farmacia, Universidad de Granada, 18071 Granada, Spain
3. Cytometry and Microscopy Research Service, Instituto de Investigación Biosanitaria de Granada, ibs.GRANADA, 18012 Granada, Spain
4. Unidad de Gestión Clínica de Cirugía, Complejo Hospitalario de Jaén, 23007 Jaén, Spain; agata_szuba@wp.pl
5. Departamento de Ciencias de la Computación e Inteligencia Artificial, E.T.S. de Ingenierías Informática y de Telecomunicación, Universidad de Granada, 18014 Granada, Spain; michelav@decsai.ugr.es (M.V.); ccano@decsai.ugr.es (C.C.)
6. Unidad de Gestión Clínica de Cirugía, Hospital Universitario San Cecilio de Granada, 18016 Granada, Spain
7. Unidad de Gestión Clínica de Aparato Digestivo, Hospital Universitario San Cecilio de Granada, 18016 Granada, Spain
* Correspondence: pepileon@ugr.es; Tel.: +34-958023199
† These authors contributed equally to this work.
‡ These authors contributed equally to this work.

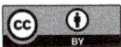

Abstract: Heme oxygenase-1 (HO-1) is an antioxidant protein implicated in tumor progression, metastasis, and resistance to therapy. Elevated HO-1 expression is associated with stemness in several types of cancer, although this aspect has not yet been studied in colorectal cancer (CRC). Using an in vitro model, we demonstrated that HO-1 overexpression regulates stemness and resistance to 5-FU treatment, regardless of p53. In samples from CRC patients, HO-1 and endothelin converting enzyme-1 (ECE-1) expression correlated significantly, and p53 had no influence on this result. Carbon monoxide (CO) activated the ECE-1/endothelin-1 (ET-1) pathway, which could account for the protumoral effects of HO-1 in p53 wild-type cells, as demonstrated after treatment with bosentan (an antagonist of both ETRA and ETRB endothelin-1 receptors). Surprisingly, in cells with a non-active p53 or a mutated p53 with gain-of-function, ECE-1-produced ET-1 acted as a protective molecule, since treatment with bosentan led to increased efficiency for spheres formation and percentage of cancer stem cells (CSCs) markers. In these cells, HO-1 could activate or inactivate certain unknown routes that could induce these contrary responses after treatment with bosentan in our cell model. However more research is warranted to confirm these results. Patients carrying tumors with a high expression of both HO-1 and ECE-1 and a non-wild-type p53 should be considered for HO-1 based-therapies instead of ET-1 antagonists-based ones.

Keywords: colorectal cancer; cancer stem cells; heme oxygenase-1; endothelin-1; endothelin converting enzyme-1; bosentan

1. Introduction

Worldwide, colorectal cancer (CRC) annually affects more than one million men and women and causes more than half a million deaths [1]. Drug-resistance remains one of the challenges for the low survival rates of patients in advanced stages of the disease [2].

Tumor heterogeneity associated with changes in gene expression or in epigenetics supports the existence of therapy-resistant cancer cells. These cells, usually called cancer stem cells (CSCs) or tumor-initiating cells (TICs), represent a small fraction within the cancer and are also responsible for initiating, maintaining, and developing cancer growth [3]. Therefore, current research has been focused on the discovery of molecular targets involved in the appearance and maintenance of CSCs [3].

The enzyme heme oxygenase-1 (HO-1) or heat shock protein 32 (Hsp32) is the inducible isoform of HO, which catalyzes the limiting step in the oxidation of the heme group in equimolar quantities of CO, ferrous iron, and biliverdin [4]. HO-1 is a protein sensitive to oxidative stress, growth factors, pathogen-associated molecular patterns (PAMPs), cytokines, metalloporphyrins, heme, and heavy metals. It has been widely accepted that HO-1 is a cytoprotective protein in several pathological conditions, acting as an anti-inflammatory, antioxidant, and antiapoptotic agent through several mechanisms [5–8]. On the contrary, in some cell types and under certain circumstances, it may amplify intracellular oxidative stress and exacerbate the disease process [9].

Overexpression of HO-1 has been observed in preneoplastic and neoplastic tissues [4]. It has been implicated in tumor progression, invasiveness, angiogenesis, metastasis, and immune scape, acting at both microenvironment and tumor levels [10,11]. These effects are highly dependent on the intracellular localization of HO-1 (nuclear, mitochondrial, or cytoplasmic) [12,13] and the type of cancer studied [10]. Recent reports showed that at low levels of expression, HO-1 induces cancer progression, while excessive activation of HO-1 leads to cell death by activating ferroptosis [14], which could explain the contradictory effects found in several types of cancer, including CRC [10]. Specifically, in this type of cancer, HO-1 overexpression is associated with long-term survival in patients [15], reducing cell viability through induction of cell cycle arrest and apoptosis in tumor cells, although a functional p53 protein is required for these effects [16]. However, and contrary to this, other reports showed that overexpression of HO-1 mediates EGF-induced colon cancer cell proliferation [17] and promotes tumor progression and metastasis of colorectal carcinoma cells by inhibiting antitumor immunity [18] and increasing angiogenesis [19,20].

HO-1 has also been implicated in therapy resistance in a variety of cancers, including CRC [21,22]. As mentioned before, this ability of cancers to escape therapy has been attributed to the existence of subpopulations of CSCs, which activate DNA repair, increase drug efflux, and their quiescent state [23]. Elevated HO-1 expression is associated with stemness and cell self-renewal in glioblastoma [24], breast cancer [25], and in leukemia [26]. However, this aspect remains to be studied in CRC.

Endothelins (ETs) are a family of three 21 amino-acid peptides (ET-1, 2 and 3). Prepro-ET-1 peptide is the primary translation product of the ET-1 gene (EDN-1), which is finally cleaved by an endothelin-converting enzyme (ECE-1) to form the biologically active ET-1. This peptide mediates physiological functions such as vasoconstriction and cell proliferation in vascular and non-vascular tissues through two cell-surface receptors, ETRA and ETRB [27,28]. In tumor cells, ET-1 promotes angiogenesis in addition to cell proliferation, metastasis, and suppression of apoptosis [28]. It was proposed that CSCs from CRC secrete ET-1 and that the activation of the ETRA receptor/β-arrestin1 axis induces the cross-talk with β-catenin signaling to sustain stemness, the epithelial-to-mesenchymal transition (EMT) phenotype, and regulates the response to chemotherapy [29].

Previous studies unrelated to cancer have reported a relationship between HO-1 and the ECE-1/ET-1 pathway. HO-1-produced CO regulates ET-1 production by smooth muscle cells under normal and hypoxic conditions [30] and in several models of disease [31–33]. In addition, chemical inhibition of ECE-1 lead to HO-1 overexpression on ischemic-reperfusion spinal cord injury in rats [34].

Taking into account all the above, in this study, we aimed to investigate the role of HO-1 in regulating stemness in CRC and the mediating effects of the ECE-1/ET-1 system in this process.

2. Materials and Methods

2.1. Cell Culture and Reagents

Three CRC cell lines with different p53 statuses were used in this study: HCT-116 (p53 wild-type), HCT-116 p53 -/- (p53 null), and HT-29 (p53 mutated). HCT-116 and HCT-116 p53 null were obtained from Horizon Discovery (Cambridge, UK). HT-29 cells were obtained from American Type Culture Collection (ATCC, Rockville, MD, USA). All cell types were cultivated in RPMI-1640 medium (Gibco, Carlsbad, CA, USA) supplemented with 2 mM L-glutamine, 10% FBS, and a 1% antibiotic-antimycotic cocktail containing penicillin (100 U/mL), streptomycin (100 µg/mL), and amphotericin B (250 ng/mL) (Gibco, Carlsbad, CA, USA) at 37 °C with 5% CO_2.

CORM3, biliverdin, hemin, and CoPPIX were purchased from Sigma-Aldric Co. (St. Luis, MO, USA). Bosentan was purchased from Selleckchem (Houston, TX, USA).

2.2. Patients

This research work was part of a larger, ongoing prospective study that aimed to investigate CSCs regulatory pathways in CRC. Initially, 183 patients were recruited, of which 150 were included in this study [35]. Samples were obtained from patients who underwent surgery for primary sporadic CRC and were provided by the Andalusian Tumor Bank Network (RBTA) (Table S1). Viable tumor tissues and adjacent normal mucosa were dissected immediately and fresh-frozen in Tissue-Tek1 (Optimal Cutting Temperature Compound, Sakura Finetek Europe B.V., Zoeterwoude, The Netherlands). The inclusion criteria included people over 18 years, without hereditary burden, not treated with neoadjuvant therapy, and not previously diagnosed or treated for cancer. The Ethical Committee of Clinical Research of Granada (project code: PI-067/2013; date of approval: 24 January 2014) approved the study. All patients gave written informed consent for the use of samples in biomedical research.

2.3. Transient Transfection of HO-1

Cells at 60–70% of confluence were transiently transfected with lipofectamine 2000 transfection reagent (Thermo Fisher Scientific, Waltham, MA, USA) according to the manufacturer's instructions. Transfected cells were then collected 24–96 h after transfection. Plasmid expression vector pCMV6 containing the human *HMOX1* gene and the corresponding empty vector were purchased from Origene Technologies (Rockville, MA, USA).

2.4. Western Blotting

After treatments, cells were washed in ice-cold DPBS and incubated in RIPA buffer containing protease inhibitors. Then, proteins were separated by SDS-PAGE and transferred to PVDF filters. Finally, blots were probed with appropriate antibodies raised against HO-1 (Abcam, Cambridge, UK), ECE-1 (Abcam, Cambridge, UK), NF-κB (p65; Santa Cruz Biotechnology, Inc., Dallas, TX, USA), pNF-κB at Ser^{529} (phospho-p65; Becton Dickinson, Franklin Lakes, NJ, USA), AP-1 (c-jun; Santa Cruz Biotechnology, Inc., Dallas, TX, USA), pAP-1 at Ser^{243} (phosphor-c-jun; Santa Cruz Biotechnology, Inc., Dallas, TX, USA), and β-actin (Santa Cruz Biotechnology, Inc., Dallas, TX, USA). Proteins were visualized by enhanced chemiluminescence using appropriate HRP-conjugated secondary antibodies (Santa Cruz Biotechnology, Inc., Dallas, TX, USA). The intensity of the bands was estimated using Quantity One 4.6.8 (Bio-Rad Laboratories, Inc., Hercules, CA, USA) for Windows analytic software.

2.5. ET-1 ELISA

ET-1 was analyzed in 100 µL of conditioned media using a colorimetric ELISA kit (R & D Systems, Minneapolis, MN, USA) in accordance with the manufacturer's protocol using a microplate reader TRIAD Multimode Reader series (Dynex Technologies, Chantilly, VA, USA) at 450 nm. Results were determined by comparison with standard curves and normalized to the number of cells in each well.

2.6. RNA Isolation and cDNA Synthesis

Total RNA from tissue samples was isolated using the RNeasy Mini Kit (Qiagen, Hilden, Germany). The amount of total RNA was determined by UV spectrophotometry, and RNA integrity was assessed by agarose gel electrophoresis. First-strand cDNA was prepared by a reverse transcription cDNA synthesis kit (qScript cDNA Synthesis, Quantabio, Beverly, MA, USA).

2.7. Real Time PCR

Quantitative analysis of mRNA expression was performed using the PerfeCTa SYBR Green SuperMix Kit (Quantabio, Beverly, MA, USA) on a CFX96 Dx Real-Time PCR Detection System (Bio-Rad, Hercules, CA, USA) following manufacturer's instructions. Expression of mRNA was evaluated through standard curves generated for each target gene by plotting Ct values versus log cDNA dilution. UBC was used to normalize mRNA levels. PCR products were verified by a melting profile and agarose gel electrophoresis to rule out nonspecific PCR products and primer dimers.

2.8. DNA Extraction and p53 Mutations Analysis

DNA was extracted from tissues using the QIAamp ADN mini Kit (Qiagen, Hilden, Germany) and quantified on a NanoDrop ND-1000 spectrophotometer (Implen GmbH, Munich, Germany). Mutations were analyzed in 2–10 exons using specific primers (Table S3) in two independent amplifications. IARC p53 database (http://www.p53.iarc.fr/) was consulted (15 January 2021) for p53 activity of mutants. A transcriptional activity < 75% was considered partially functional and classified as mutant [35].

2.9. ALDEFLUOR Assay

An ALDEFLUOR™ Kit (Stem Cell Technologies, Vancouver, BC, Canada) was used to detect enzyme ALDH1 activity in cultured cells according to the manufacturer's instructions. After treatments, cells were incubated with BODIPY-aminoacetaldehyde (BAAA), a fluorescent non-toxic substrate for ALDH, which was converted into BODIPY-aminoacate (BAA) and retained inside the cells. Viable ALDH1+ cells were quantified by flow cytometry on a FACS Aria IIIu (BD Biosciences, San Jose, CA, USA). The specific inhibitor of ALDH, diethylaminobenzaldehyde (DEAB), was used to control for background fluorescence.

2.10. Isolation and Characterization of CSCs

Enrichment of CSCs was achieved via serial trypsin treatment, as previously described [36,37]. Briefly, cells at 60–80% of confluence were washed with PBS and treated with 0.05% trypsin for 2 min at 37 °C. Detached cells were plated and allowed to attach for 24 h. Then, the above procedure was repeated, and the cells obtained were considered CSCs. After the first trypsin treatment, remaining cells attached to the dishes were washed twice with PBS and incubated with 0.05% trypsin for 4 min at 37 °C. Cells detached from this trypsinization were discarded. Dishes with remaining trypsin-resistant cells were considered non-CSCs

Once isolated, cell surface marker levels of CSCs were determined with human anti-CD44-PE, anti-CD326-FITC, and anti-CD133-APC antibodies (Biolegend, San Diego, CA, USA). Samples were measured and analyzed by flow cytometry on a FACS Aria IIIu (BD Biosciences, San Jose, CA, USA).

2.11. Sphere Forming Assay

For self-renewal analysis, 24 h after transfection with either pCMV6-HMOX1 or an empty vector, CSCs and non-CSCs cells were collected and quantified. Then, 3000 cells were resuspended in sphere culture medium (DMEM:F12, 1% penicilin/streptomycin, B27, 10 µg/mL ITS, 1 µg/mL Hydrocortisone, 4 ng/mL Heparin, 10 ng/mL EGF, and 20 ng/mL FGF) in ultra-low attachment 24-well plates (Corning). Spheres >75 µM diameter were counted after 4 days by light microscopy.

2.12. MTT Assay

Cells were seeded in 96 well-plates at a concentration of 40,000 cells/mL, allowed to attach overnight, and transfected with either pCMV6-HMOX1 or an empty vector. Then, the cells were treated with the vehicle or the corresponding drug, 24 h after transfection. After 72 h, 10 µL of 5 mg/mL MTT were added to each well. Four hours later, cells were lysed with 100 µL buffer (20% SDS in 50% formamide at pH 4.7) at 37 °C overnight. Absorbance was measured in a TRIAD Multimode Reader series, (Dynex Technologies, Chantilly, VA, USA) at 570 nm. Means were estimated from the results of four samples in each experimental group. All experiments were performed two times.

2.13. Statistical Analysis

For each patient, mRNA levels of genes in tumor samples were normalized to mRNA levels in normal mucosa. Descriptive statistics were reported as medians with interquartile ranges (IQR) for continuous variables and as whole numbers and percentages for categorical variables. Low and high levels of CSCs markers were obtained through the median of the mRNA expression levels in our cohort of patients. Associations between clinicopathological features of CRC patients and gene expression were analyzed with the Kruskal–Wallis and Mann–Whitney non-parametric tests. For the correlation analysis, the Pearson test was used after transforming the variables applying natural logarithms. All confidence intervals (CIs) were stated at the 95% level. Statistical significance was defined as $p < 0.05$. All statistical calculations were performed using SPSS software version 15.0 for Windows (IBM, Chicago, IL, USA).

3. Results

3.1. HO-1 Overexpression Induces Stemness in CRC In Vitro Regardless of p53 Status

In order to investigate whether HO-1 conferred stem cell properties on CRC cells, we used the pCMV6-*HMOX1* plasmid to transiently overexpress HO-1 in HCT-116, HCT-116 p53 null, and HT-29 cells. Overexpression of HO-1 increased aldehyde dehydrogenase 1 positive (ALDH1+) subpopulation, representing the subpopulation of CSCs, in HCT-116 and HCT-116 p53 null cells at 96 h after transfection (Figure 1a,b). In HT-29 cells, the percentage of ALDH1+ cells was lower in pCMV6-HMOX1 versus mock transfected cells at 72 h after transfection, whereas the percentage of this subpopulation was similar in control (mock) and HO-1 overexpressing cells at 96 h (Figure 1c).

The percentage of cells with high expression of CSCs markers in the total population (TP) of cells increased in pCMV6-*HMOX1* versus mock transfected cells at 96 h after transfection. At this time, the percentage of $CD133_{high}/CD44_{high}/CD326_{high}$ cells significantly increased in the TP of pCMV6-*HMOX1* versus mock HCT-116 and HT29 transfected cells at 96 h after transfection (Figure 1d). We did not find triple-labeled subpopulation cells in the HCT-116 p53 null line; however, the percentage of $CD44_{high}/CD326_{high}$ cells significantly increased in the TP of pCMV6-*HMOX1* versus mock HCT-116 p53 null transfected cells at 96 h after transfection (Figure 1e). Similarly, in HT-29 cells, the percentage of the $CD44_{high}/CD326_{high}$ subpopulation significantly increased in the TP of pCMV6-*HMOX1* versus mock transfected cells at 96 h after transfection (Figure 1e). In addition, the percentage of $CD44_{high}/CD326_{high}$ cells increased in the CSCs subpopulation of pCMV6-*HMOX1* versus mock transfected cells at 96 h after transfection in the three cell lines studied (Figure 1f). These results indicate that HO-1 overexpression increases the proportion of cancer cells with a CSC phenotype in the different subpopulations analyzed.

Next, we studied the anchorage-independent growth of CSCs and non-CSCs subpopulations extracted from HCT-116 and HCT-116 p53 null after transient overexpression of HO-1 under free-serum conditions. As shown in Figure 2, CSCs and non-CSCs from both cell lines formed spheres with similar efficiency in mock transfected cells; however, CSCs subpopulations formed spheres more efficiently than non-CSCs when parental cells were transfected with the pCMV6-*HMOX1* plasmid, indicating that HO-1 overexpression increases the self-renewal capacity of CSCs subpopulations, regardless of p53 status.

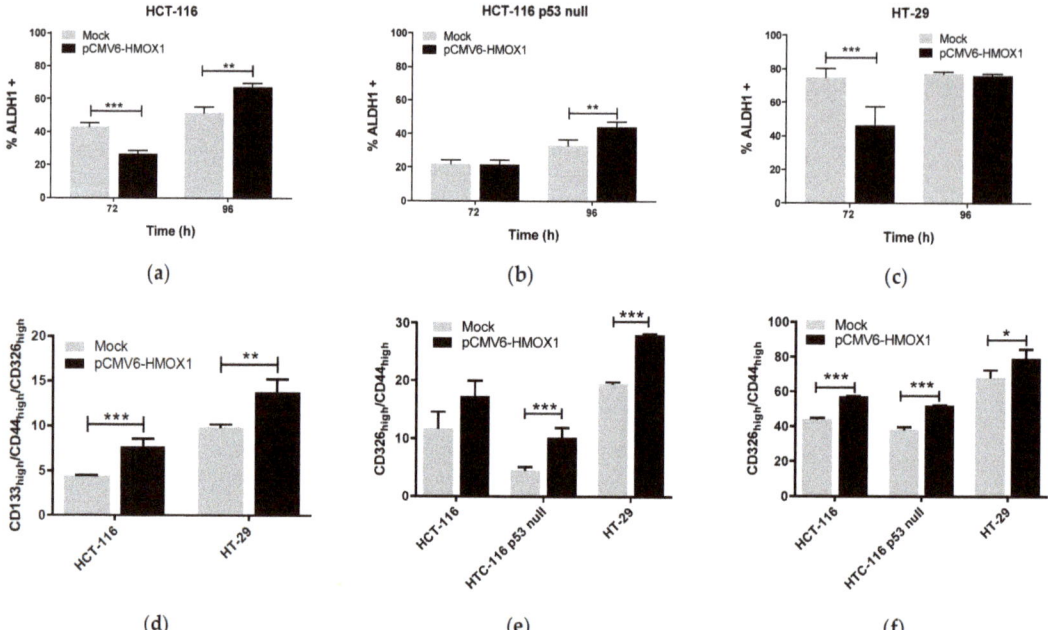

Figure 1. HO-1 overexpression increases stemness in CRC regardless of p53 status. Cells were pCMV6-*HMOX1* or mock transfected, collected at 72 and 96 hours after transfection, and used to characterize the percentage of ALDH1+ cells by flow cytometry in the total population (TP) of (**a**) HCT-116, (**b**) HCT-116 p53 null, and (**c**) HT-29 CRC cells. In other experiments, cells were collected at 96 h after pCMV6-*HMOX1* or empty vector (mock) transfections and used to quantify, in the TP, (**d**) the percentage of $CD133_{high}/CD44_{high}/CD326_{high}$ and (**e**) the percentage of $CD44_{high}/CD326_{high}$ cells or (**f**) the percentage of $CD44_{high}/CD326_{high}$ cells in CSCs subpopulations, obtained as described in the Materials and Methods section. Data represent the mean ± SD of two experiments performed in duplicate. *, $p < 0.05$; **, $p < 0.01$; ***, $p < 0.001$.

3.2. HO-1 Overexpression Induces ECE-1 Expression and ET-1 Production by CRC Cells

We next investigated the mechanism by which HO-1 could induce stemness in CRC. As mentioned before, HO-1 could modulate ET-1 production in several models of health and disease [37–41].

It was interesting to find high mRNA and protein content of both HO-1 and ECE-1 in the CSC versus the non-CSCs subpopulation in the three cell lines studied (Figure 3a–c). We also analyzed the mRNA expression of HO-1, ECE-1, and the CSCs markers CD44 and CD133 by quantitative RT-PCR in 150 cases of CRC patients. Tumors showing high expression of CSCs markers ($CD133_{high}CD44_{high}$) also exhibited higher expression of HO-1 (Figure 3d) and ECE-1 (Figure 3e) than tumors with low expression of these markers ($CD133_{low}CD44_{low}$). It was very interesting to find that HO-1 and ECE-1 expression highly correlated in both $CD133_{high}CD44_{high}$ and $CD133_{high}CD44_{high}$ tumors, while no correlations were found between HO-1 and END-1 (Table S3). The status of P53 did not influence any of the results mentioned above (Figure 3 and Table S3).

Next, we studied whether HO-1 could regulate ET-1 production in CRC. As shown in Figure 4a, HO-1 induced ECE-1 expression at 72 and 96 h after transfection with the pCMV6-*HMOX1* plasmid in HCT-116, HCT-116 p53 null, and HT-29 cells versus vector (mock) transfected cells. In addition, HO-1 overexpression induced ET-1 synthesis in HCT-116 and HCT-116 p53 null cells at 96 h after transfection (Figure 4b,c). In HT-29 cells, HO-1 overexpression induced inhibition of ET-1 at 72 h, whereas, at 96 h, its levels increased until reaching the levels of control (mock) cells (Figure 4d).

In the cohort of CRC patients, HO-1 and ECE-1 expressions positively correlated in all cases (Rp = 0.723, $p < 0.001$; Figure 4e) in tumors harboring a wild-type p53 (Rp = 0.699, $p < 0.001$; Figure 4f) and in tumors with mutations in this gene (Rp = 0.755, $p < 0.001$; Figure 4g). END-1, the first gene implicated in the synthesis of ET-1, did not correlate with HO-1 at any of the conditions mentioned above (Rp = 0.042, $p = 0.614$; Rp = 0.042, $p = 0.905$; Rp = 0.093, $p = 0.506$, for all cases, p53 wild-type tumors, and p53 mutated tumors, respectively). As shown in Table S2, none of these genes correlated with any of the clinicopathological features of the patients included in the study.

We next investigated which of the subproducts of the HO-1 reaction is responsible for ECE-1 activation after HO-1 overexpression in CRC cells. To assess this, we treated cells with 10 µM CORM3 (a CO donor) and 10 µM biliverdin. We also used 5 µM hemin and 1 µM CoPPIX treatments as positive controls. CORM3, hemin, and CoPPIX induced ECE-1 protein expression at the doses used in both HCT-116 and HCT-116 p53 null cells, whereas biliverdin was unable to induce it (Figure 5a). We also studied ET-1 production by cells after treatments at the doses specified above (Figure 5b,c). CORM3 induced a significant increase in ET-1 production at all times analyzed in both cell lines. Treatment with hemin induced increased ET-1 production in HCT-116 cells, although only after 24 h, while this effect appeared after 24, 48, and 72 h in HCT-116 p53 null cells. After showing that CO is responsible for the activation of ECE-1, we next investigated the mechanism by which it carries out this effect. As shown in Figure 5d, CO seemed to induce ECE-1 expression through the activation of pNF-kβ and pc-Jun in HCT-116 and HCT-116 p53 null cells, respectively.

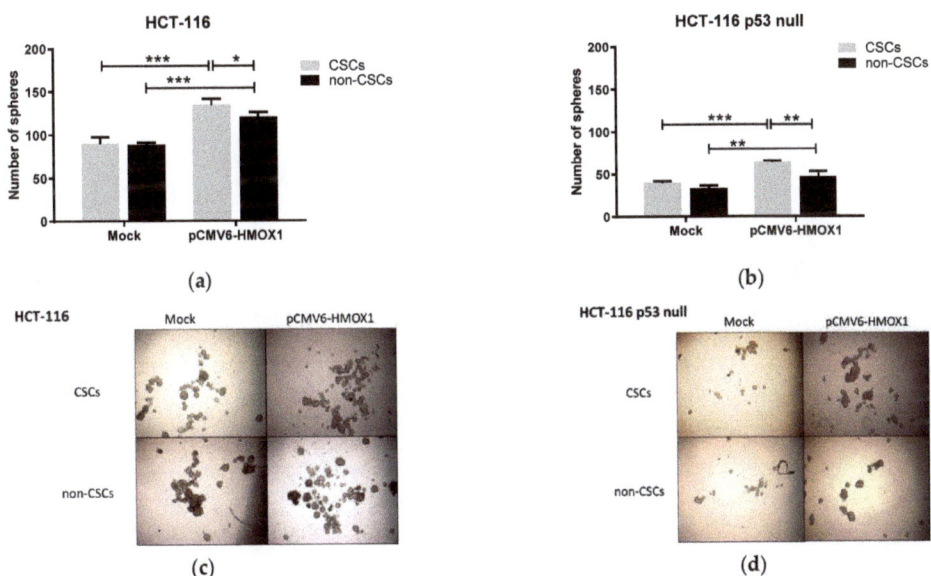

Figure 2. HO-1 overexpression increases self-renewal ability of isolated CRCssubpopulations in cultured cells, regardless of p53 status. The number of spheres formed by subpopulations obtained from mock and pCMV6-*HMOX1* (a) HCT-116 and (b) HCT-116 p53 null transiently transfected cells. Representative images of tumorospheres formed from different subpopulations of pCMV6-*HMOX1* (c) HCT-116 and (d) HCT-116 p53 null transiently transfected cells. TP: total population; CSCs: cancer stem cells subpopulation; non-CSCs: non-cancer stem cells subpopulation. *, $p < 0.05$; **, $p < 0.01$; ***, $p < 0.001$.

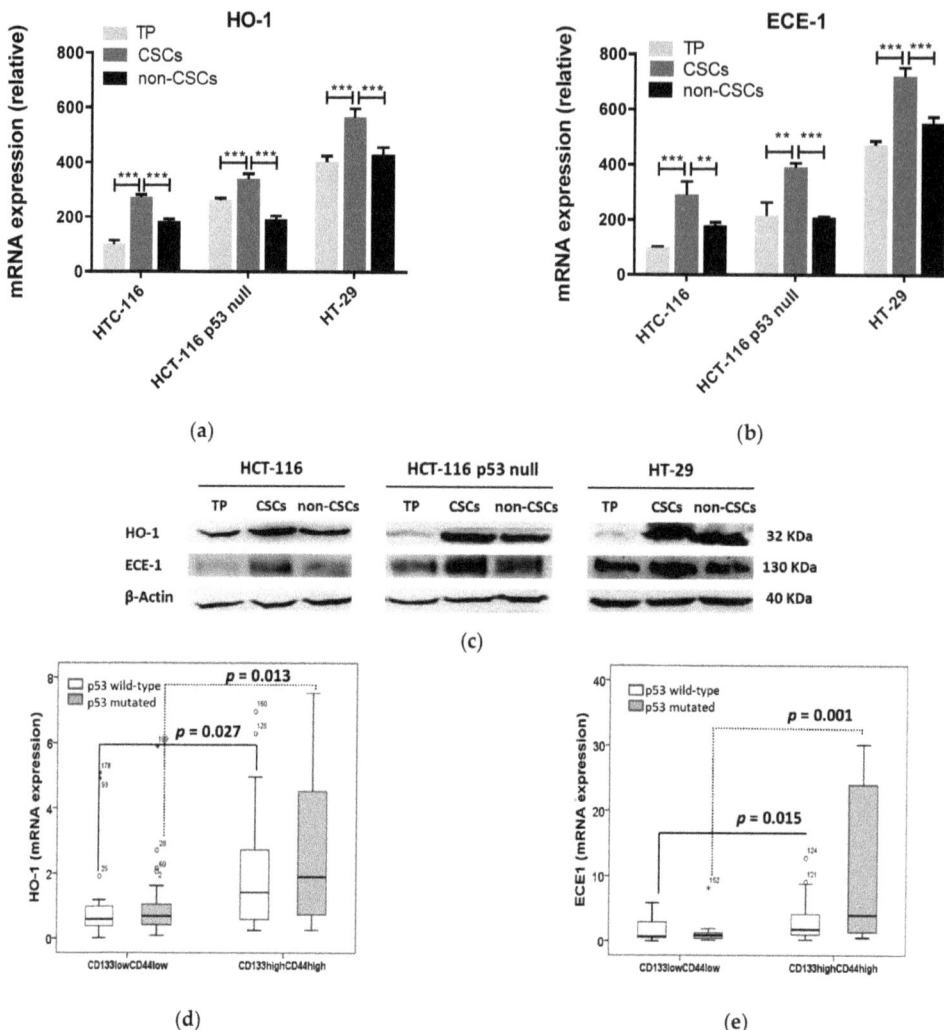

Figure 3. HO-1 and ECE-1 expression is higher in the CSCs vs. non-CSCs subpopulation in CRC regardless of p53 status. The CSCs and non-CSCs subpopulations from HCT-116, HT-116 p53 null, and HT-29 cells were obtained as described in the Materials and Methods section and used to measure mRNA expression of (**a**) HO-1 and (**b**) ECE-1. Data represent the relative expression of HO-1 and ECE-1 to the TP of HCT-116 and express the mean ± SD of two experiments performed in duplicate. **, $p < 0.01$; ***, $p < 0.001$. (**c**) Protein expression of HO-1 and ECE-1 in HCT-116, HT-116 p53 null, and HT-29 cells in the TP, CSCs, and non-CSCs subpopulations. β-actin was used as housekeeping. TP: total population; CSCs: cancer stem cells subpopulation; non-CSCs: non-cancer stem cells subpopulation. Box plots representing the relative mRNA expression of of (**d**) HO-1 and (**e**) ECE-1 in CRC samples from patients considering the levels of CSCs markers and the status of p53. Data represent the median and the interquartile range of the genes analyzed. *, distant values more than 3 box lengths from 75th percentile; °, distant values more than 1.5 box lengths from 75th percentile.

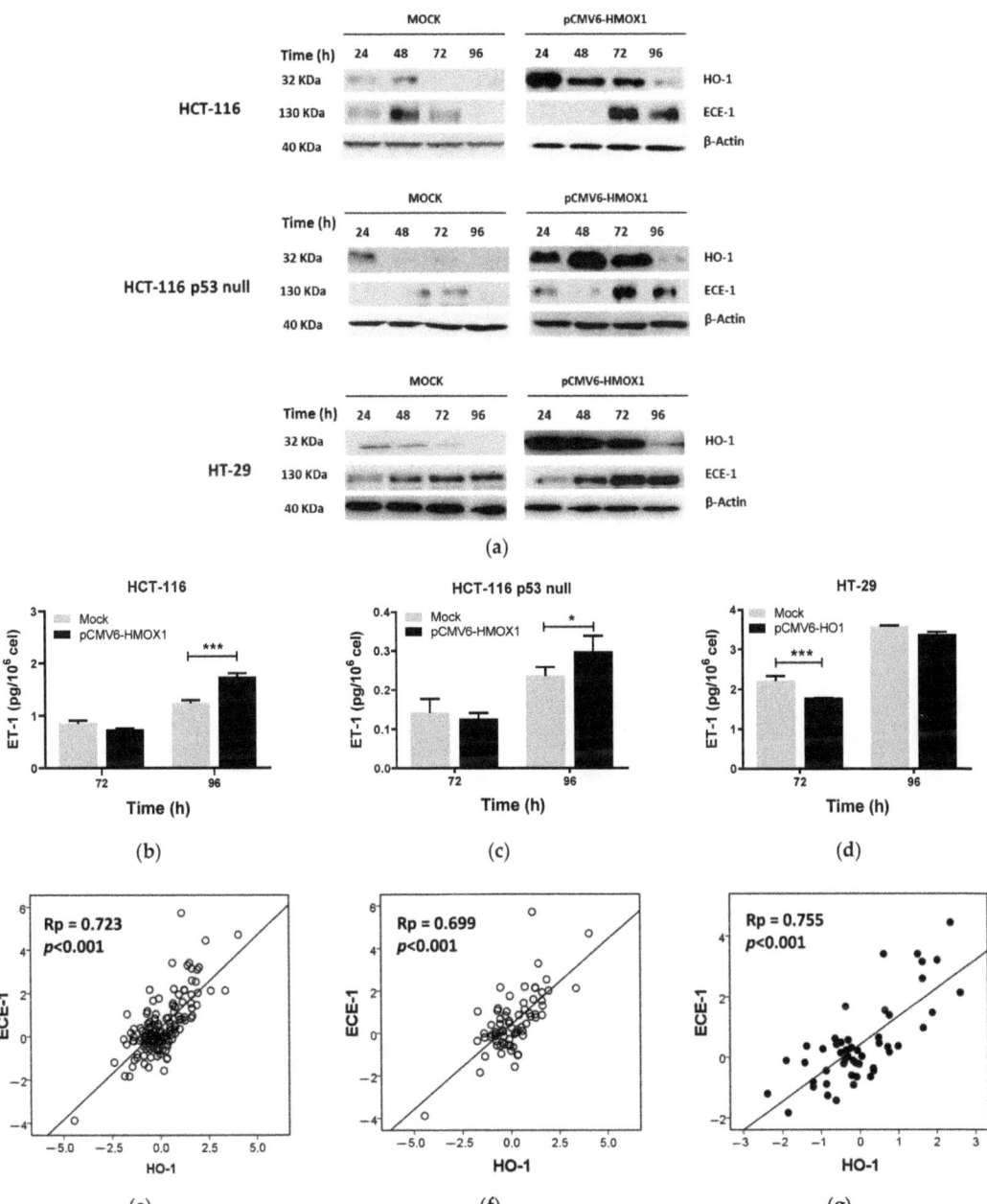

Figure 4. HO-1 overexpression induces ECE-1 expression and ET-1 production in CRC cells regardless of p53 status. Cells were transiently transfected with pCMV6-*HMOX1* or an empty vector and collected 24–96 h later for (**a**) HO-1 and ECE-1 protein expression by western blotting or ET-1 measurements in the supernatants of (**b**) HCT-116, (**c**) HCT-116 p53 null, (**d**) and HT-29 cells. Data represent the median ± SD of two experiments in duplicate. *, $p < 0.05$; ***, $p < 0.001$. Correlation of ECE-1 and HO-1 expression in tumors from CRC patients considering (**e**) all cases, (**f**) p53 wild-type tumors, and (**g**) p53 mutated tumors.

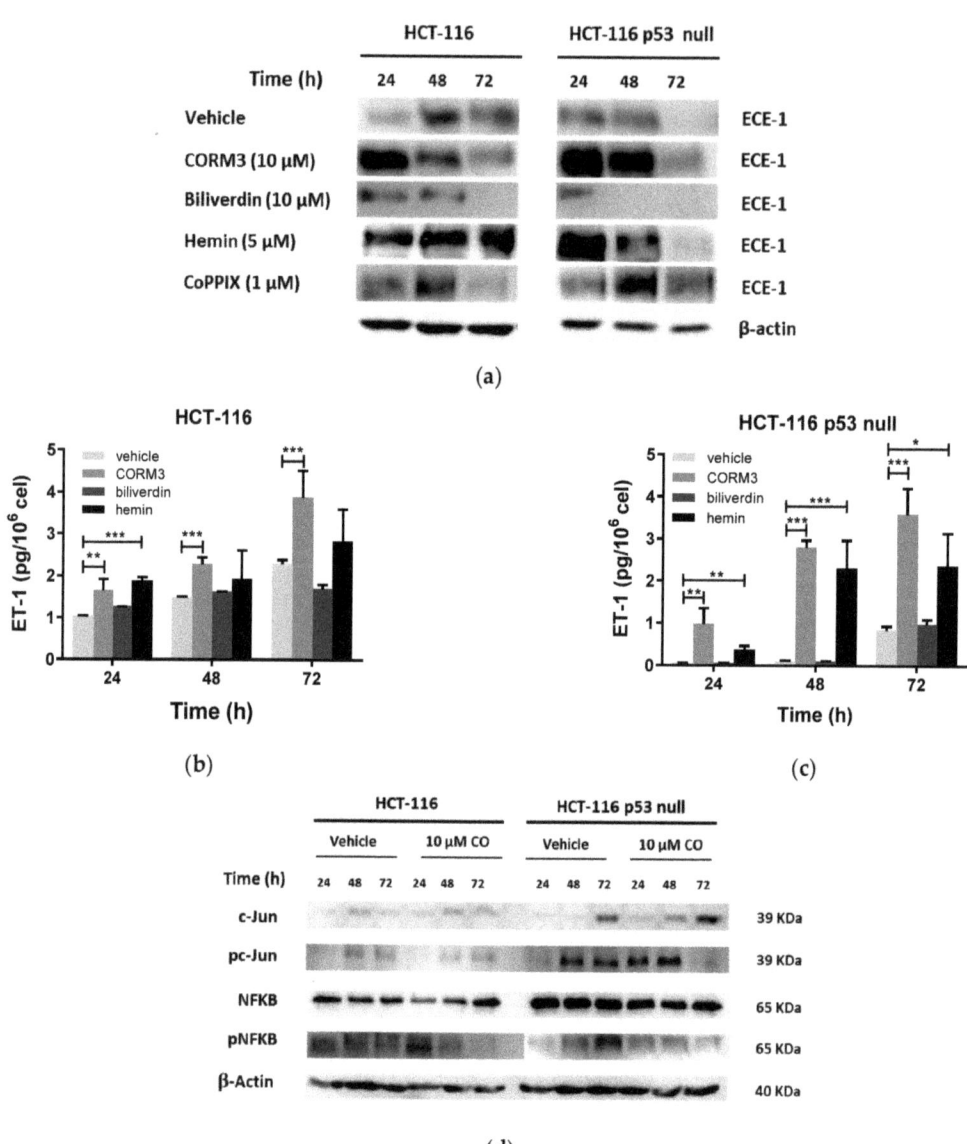

Figure 5. CO induces ECE-1 expression in CRC cells in vitro through the activation of NF-kβ and c-Jun in HCT-116 and HCT-116 p53 null cells, respectively. HCT-116 and HCT-116 p53 null cells were treated with 10 μM CORM3, 10 μM biliverdin, 5 μM hemin, and 1 μM CoPPIX during 24, 48, and 72 h. After treatments, we collected (**a**) cells for the analysis of ECE-1 protein expression by western blotting and supernatants for the analysis of ET-1 in (**b**) HCT-116 and (**c**) HCT-116 p53 null cells. Data represent the median ± SD of two experiments performed in duplicate. *, $p < 0.05$; **, $p < 0.01$; ***, $p < 0.001$. (**d**) The mechanism of CO-induced ECE-1 expression in CRC cells. Cells were treated with 10 μM CORM3 and collected for the analysis of c-Jun, pc-Jun, NF-kβ, and pNF-kβ proteins expression in whole cell lysates by western blotting. The expression of β-actin was used as housekeeping.

3.3. HO-1 Overexpression Induces Stemness in CRC Cell Lines through ECE-1/ET-1 Only in p53 Wild-Type Cells

To study whether HO-1 overexpression induces stemness in our model of CRC in vitro through ET-1 produced by ECE-1, we analyzed the percentage of ALDH1+ cells after HO-1 overexpression in the presence of bosentan, an antagonist of both ETRA and ETRB receptors. In this case, and contrary to what happened in the absence of bosentan, HO-1 overexpression was not able to induce an increase in the ALDH1+ subpopulation in HCT-116 cells (Figure 6a), and the percentage of $CD133_{high}/CD44_{high}/CD326_{high}$ cells in the TP was similar in pCMV6-HMOX1 versus mock transfected cells (Figure 6d). However, the percentage of $CD44_{high}/CD326_{high}$ cells increased in pCMV6-HMOX1 versus mock transfected cells (Figure 6e). Therefore, HO-1 induces stemness in CRC cells harboring a wild-type p53 trough ET-1.

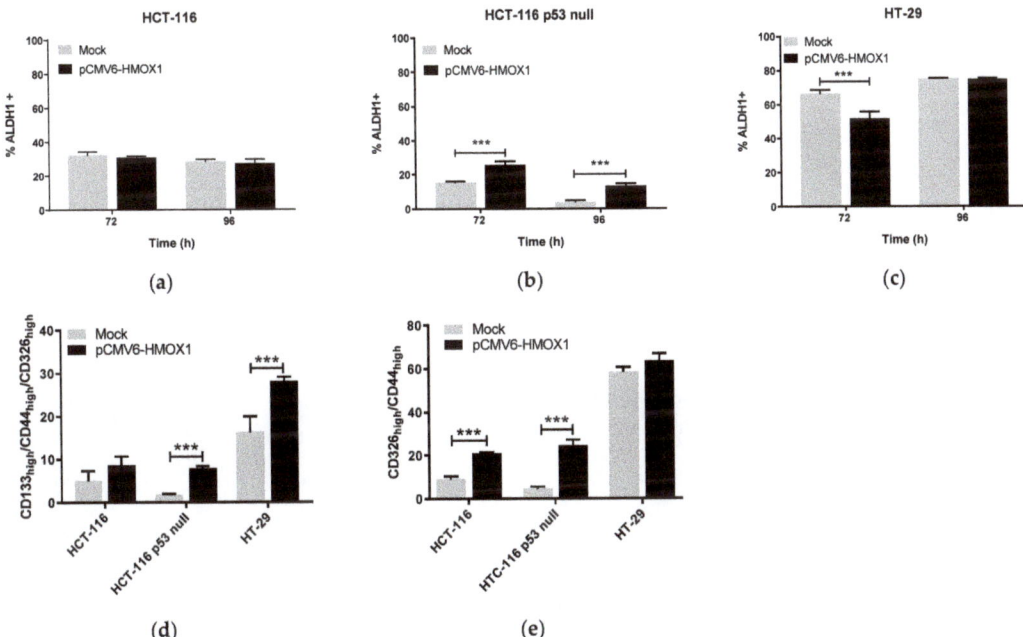

Figure 6. Blockade of endothelin-1 receptors eliminates the HO-1-induced stemness only in p53 wild-type CRC cells. Cells were pCMV6-HMOX1 or mock transfected, treated with 10 µM bosentan 24 h after, collected at 72 and 96 h after transfection, and used to characterize the percentage of ALDH1+ cells by flow cytometry in the TP of (**a**) HCT-116, (**b**) HCT-116 p53 null, and (**c**) HT-29 CRC cells. In other experiments, cells were collected at 96 h after pCMV6-HMOX1 or empty vector (mock) transfections and used to quantify, in the TP, (**d**) the percentage of $CD133_{high}/CD44_{high}/CD326_{high}$ and (**e**) $CD44_{high}/CD326_{high}$ cells. Data represent the mean ± SD of two experiments performed in duplicate. ***, $p < 0.001$.

On the contrary, the addition of bosentan after HO-1 overexpression led to an increase in the percentage of ALDH1+ cells at 72 and 96 h after transfection (Figure 6b) as well as to the appearance of the $CD133_{high}/CD44_{high}/CD326_{high}$ subpopulation in HCT-116 p53 null cells (Figure 6e). In HT-29 cells, the presence of bosentan after HO-1 overexpression did not modify the percentage of ALDH1+ cells, although the $CD44_{high}/CD326_{high}$ subpopulation seemed to decrease, while the difference in the percentage of the $CD133_{high}/CD44_{high}/CD326_{high}$ subpopulation increased in pCMV6-HMOX1 versus mock transfected cells (Figure 6d,e), when comparing this result in the absence of bosentan (Figure 1d). According to these results, the blockade of ET-1 receptors induces an increase in the CSCs subpopulation in cells without an active p53 or with a mutated p53 with a gain of function, and ET-1 seems to act as a protective agent in these cells after HO-1 overexpression.

The presence of bosentan in the cultured media also influenced the self-renewal capacity of CSCs and non-CSCs subpopulations extracted from transiently transfected HCT-116 and HCT-116 p53 null cells with empty vector (mock) and pCMV6-*HMOX1* plasmid. On these working conditions, the capacity of subpopulations to form spheres was similar in mock and pCMV6-*HMOX1* transfected HCT-116 cells (Figure 7a). However, CSCs and non-CSCs subpopulations from HCT-116 p53 null cells increased their ability to form spheres (Figure 7b). Considering these results, ET-1 increases the self-renewal capacity in cells with a wild-type p53 and decreases it in cells with an inactive p53 after HO-1 overexpression, and the presence of bosentan eliminates these effects.

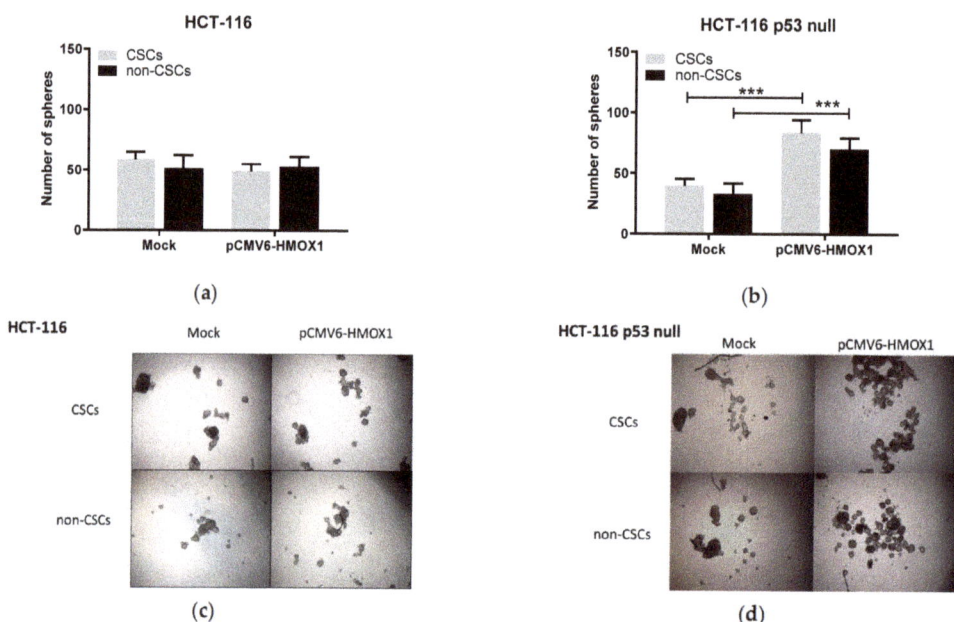

Figure 7. Blockade of endothelin-1 receptors eliminates the HO-1-induced self-renewal ability in p53 wild-type CRC cells and enhances it in p53 null cells. The number of spheres formed by subpopulations obtained from mock and pCMV6-*HMOX1* (**a**) HCT-116 and (**b**) HCT-116 p53 null transiently transfected cells. Representative images of tumorospheres formed from different subpopulations of pCMV6-*HMOX1* (**c**) HCT-116 and (**d**) HCT-116 p53 null transiently transfected cells. ***, $p < 0.001$.

3.4. HO-1 Overexpression Induces Resistance to 5-FU Treatment in CRC In Vitro

Given the implication of CSCs on therapy resistance in cancer, we analyzed whether HO-1 overexpression induced this effect on CRC in vitro and the mediation of the ECE-1/ET-1 system on it. The treatment of mock and pCMV6-*HMOX1* HCT-116, HCT-116 p53 null, and HT-29 transfected cells with 5-fluorouracil (5-FU) at different doses (0–4 µM) showed that HO-1 overexpression induced resistance to this treatment in HCT-116 cells (Figure 8a). We did not find different 5-FU sensitivity after HO-1 overexpression in HCT-116 p53 null nor in HT-29 cells (Figure 8b,c), at least at the doses of 5-FU used. The presence of bosentan in the culture media sensitized HCT-116 cells overexpressing HO-1 to 5-FU (Figure 8a); however, no effect was found in HCT-116 p53 null cells (Figure 8b). On the contrary, in HT-29 cells transfected with pCMV6-*HMOX1*, the presence of bosentan induced resistance to 5-FU (Figure 8c). We could conclude that HO-1 overexpression induces 5-FU resistance in cells with a wild-type p53 and that ET-1 is responsible, at least in part, for this effect. On the contrary, in cells with a non-wild-type p53, HO-1 overexpression seemed to not affect the response to 5-FU treatment at the doses used in this study. In addition, ET-1 increases the response to this treatment in cells with a mutated p53 with a gain of function.

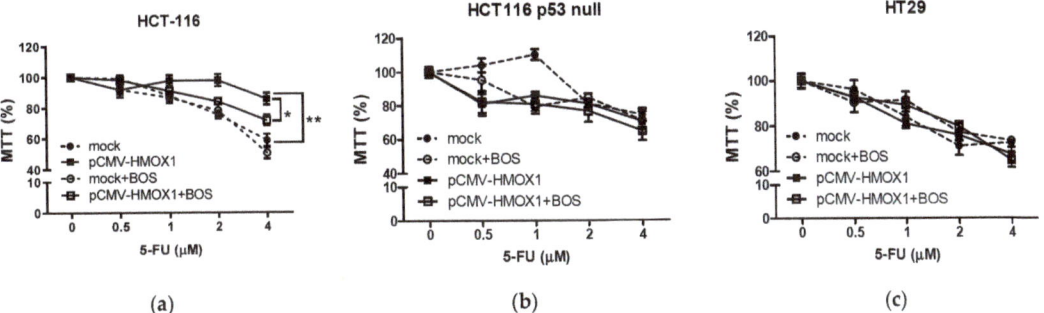

Figure 8. Influence of HO-1 overexpression on therapy resistance in CRC. As described in the Materials and Methods section, cells were seeded in 96 well-plates, transfected with vector or pCMV6-*HMOX1* plasmid, and treated with increasing doses of 5-FU (0–4 Mm) during 72 h in the presence or absence of 10 µM bosentan. The viability of cells was analyzed using the MTT assay in (**a**) HCT-116, (**b**) HCT-116 p53 null, and (**c**) HT-29 cells. Data represent the mean ± SD of two experiments performed in quadruplicate. *, $p < 0.05$; **, $p < 0.01$.

4. Discussion

In the recent years, numerous research works have tried to elucidate the role of HO-1 in colorectal cancer. This has not been an easy task, since this enzyme is found in both cancer and stromal cells, including immune cells [38–41]. In addition, HO-1 in CRC cells is able to regulate immune-mediated cytotoxicity against CRC cells [18]. In this complex scenario, the results from the scientific literature have shown contradictory effects of HO-1 in this type of cancer [15–20], which highlights the need to continue this field of research. The metabolic status of cancer cells influences how heme-degrading enzymes modulate tumor growth. Conversely, CO and biliverdin can modulate lipid and glucose metabolism [42]. Specifically, CO can promote increased mitochondrial biogenesis and induce an anti-Warburg effect [43], which has been linked to a lower rate of proliferation and cell differentiation [44]. In addition, the presence of HO-1 in cytosol or its translocation into the nucleus can also affect its activity and, therefore, its effects on tumors [42].

We used the CRC cell lines HCT-116, HCT-116 p53 null, and HT-29 to conduct our in vitro model. These cells have the ability to form tumorospheres within 3–5 days after being seeded in appropriate plates and medium [45–47], which allowed us to carry out our study even though the transformation of the parental cells was performed by transient transfection [48,49].

In this study, we found that HO-1 regulates the proportion and phenotype of CSCs in CRC, a result that is not surprising considering that we also found a higher expression of this protein in the CSCs subpopulation compared to non-CSCs in cell cultures. In tumors from CRC patients, samples with a higher expression of CSCs markers also showed a higher expression of HO-1. These results agree with previous works that reported a direct implication of HO-1 in regulating CSCs in leukemia, glioma, melanoma, breast, pancreatic, and lung cancers [24,49–51]. According to our results, HO-1 could regulate stemness in CRC independently of p53; however, previous reports have demonstrated an important relationship between them [16,52]. In fact, HO-1 is a p53-dependent target gene that is responsible for p53-dependent cellular survival after oxidative treatment [52]. Other works have suggested that HO activity is involved in the regulation of p53 expression in normal [53] and cancer cells [54].

In our in vitro model, CO produced after HO-1 overexpression led to increased expression of ECE-1 and ET-1 secretion by CRC cells through the activation of NF-κB and AP-1 in cells harboring a wild-type p53 and in cells with a mutated p53, respectively. These transcription factors are essential for ECE-1 activation in endothelial cells [55]. The CO releasing molecule CORM3 has been reported to activate AP-1 in vitro [56,57]. The regulation of NF-κB by CO has been previously described in several models of disease [58,59]. This molecule is also able to induce ROS production in vitro [60]. Interestingly, ROS production and NF-κB activation are critical events in CSCs appearance and CRC initiation [61]. Biliverdin was unable to activate the ECE-1/ET-1 pathway in our study. Biliverdin is converted to bilirubin by bilirubin reductase [62]. The ROS scavenging properties of both heme metabolites contribute to their antitumoral activities [11,63]. We did not test the possible role of ferrous ions on ECE/ET-1 induction by HO-1 overexpression. Similarly to bilirubin, literature to date has shown protective effects of ferrous iron against cancer, mainly due to the induction of ferroptosis and cell death [11,41,64,65].

The endothelin system regulates stem properties of cells in CRC. The END-1 gene is highly expressed in CSCs isolated from cultured CRC cells [66]. ET-1 regulates important pathways for the maintenance of the stemness phenotype, such as MAPK, PI3K/Akt, and Wnt/β-catenin [29]. However, given the short half-life of ET-1, its biological effects are totally dependent on the maintenance of a critical concentration by ECE-1 [67]. Of the four described isoforms of ECE-1 (a, b, c and d), ECE-1c has been implicated in CSCs generation in CRC [67]. In our study, we did not analyze which isoform of ECE-1 increased after HO-1 overexpression. However, ETRA and ETRB receptors blockaded with bosentan led to a decrease in the ALDH1+ population, in the percentage of $CD133_{high}/CD44_{high}/CD326_{high}$ cells, and in the resistance to 5-FU treatment in the total population and a decrease in the ability for self-renewal of the CSCs subpopulation of wild-type p53 cells. Previous studies have reported that ETRA receptors are responsible for ET-1-mediated stemness in CRC [29].

On the other hand, treatment with bosentan after HO-1 overexpression induced an increase in the ALDH1+ and the appearance of $CD133_{high}/CD44_{high}/CD326_{high}$ subpopulations in the total population, and it increased the ability to form spheres in the CSCs subpopulation of cells lacking p53. Similarly, in cells harboring a mutated p53, the ETR blockade induced a loss of $CD44_{high}/CD326_{high}$ cells and an increase in $CD133_{high}/CD44_{high}/CD326_{high}$ ones. These results could indicate that even though HO-1 overexpression induces increased expression of ECE-1 and ET-1 production regardless of p53, in cells without an active p53 or even a p53 with gain of function, like HT-29 cells, another mechanism that does not involve the ECE-1/ET-1 system is responsible for the increase in the stem subpopulation. More interestingly, the HO-1-induced ECE-1/ET-1 system seems to exert a protective effect in these p53 not-active or with gain of function CRC cells. Contrary to these results, previous reports have shown that treatment with bosentan is proapoptotic and antiproliferative in HT-29 [68] cells and sensitizes them to Fas-L-induced cell death [69,70]. An ET-1-independent mechanism of ECE-1 in CRC and other cancers has also been described [67], but in these cases it acts as a protumoral protein [67]. On the contrary, clinical trials with approved endothelin receptor antagonists, including bosentan, were not so promising, with no statistically significant results, even though the drugs were well-tolerated [71]. Although more research is warranted to confirm our results, HO-1 overexpression probably activates or inactivates certain unknown pathways that could induce these contrary results after treatment with bosentan in our cell model.

5. Conclusions

HO-1 regulates stemness and resistance to 5-FU treatment in CRC in vitro. CO produced after HO-1 overexpression seemed to activate the ECE-1/ET-1 pathway, which could be the final effectors of HO-1 protumoral events in p53 wild-type cells. Surprisingly, in cells with a non-active p53 or a gain-of-function mutated p53, ECE-1-produced ET-1 seems to act as a protective molecule. These results could implicate that patients carrying tumors with high expression of both HO-1 and ECE-1 and a non-wild-type p53 should be considered for HO-1 based-therapies instead of ET-1 antagonists-based ones.

Supplementary Materials: The following are available online at https://www.mdpi.com/article/10.3390/jpm11060509/s1, Table S1: Characteristics of the patients included in the study; Table S2: Relationship between HO-1 and ECE-1 expression with the clinicopathological characteristics of the patients included in the study; Table S3: Correlations between HO-1 and genes related to ET-1 synthesis, according to p53 status and levels of CSC markers.

Author Contributions: Conceptualization, J.L. and Á.C.; methodology, S.R.-A., J.D.P.-P., S.M.-S., J.C. and Á.S.; formal analysis, M.V. and C.C.; investigation, J.L.; data curation, J.L., S.R.-A., J.D.P.-P., S.M.-S. and Á.S.; writing—original draft preparation, J.L., S.R.-A., J.D.P.-P., S.M.-S. and Á.S.; writing—review and editing, J.L., S.R.-A., J.D.P.-P., S.M.-S., J.C., Á.S., A.M.-L.M., C.G.-P., C.C., M.V., M.G.-C., J.E.-F., Á.C.; supervision, J.L. and Á.C.; project administration, J.L.; funding acquisition, J.L. and Á.C. All authors have read and agreed to the published version of the manuscript.

Funding: This work was supported by a research grant from the Instituto de Salud Carlos III-FEDER (PI18/01947) and MINECO grant (DPI2017-84439-R). J.L. was supported by the Nicolás Monardes Program from the Andalusian Health Service (C-0033-2015). J.D.P.-P. is funded by a FPU2019 fellowship (FPU19/02269) from the Ministerio de Ciencia, Innovación y Universidades (Spain).

Institutional Review Board Statement: The study was conducted according to the guidelines of the Declaration of Helsinki and approved by the Institutional Review Board (or Ethics Committee) of Granada (project code: PI-067/2013; date of approval: 24 January 2014).

Informed Consent Statement: Informed consent was obtained from all subjects involved in the study.

Conflicts of Interest: The authors declare no conflict of interest.

References

1. Bray, F.; Ferlay, J.; Soerjomataram, I.; Siegel, R.L.; Torre, L.A.; Jemal, A. Global cancer statistics 2018: GLOBOCAN estimates of incidence and mortality worldwide for 36 cancers in 185 countries. *CA Cancer J. Clin.* **2018**, *68*, 394–424. [CrossRef]
2. Van der Jeught, K.; Xu, H.C.; Li, Y.J.; Lu, X.B.; Ji, G. Drug resistance and new therapies in colorectal cancer. *World J. Gastroenterol.* **2018**, *24*, 3834–3848. [CrossRef]
3. Zeuner, A.; Todaro, M.; Stassi, G.; De Maria, R. Colorectal cancer stem cells: From the crypt to the clinic. *Cell Stem Cell* **2014**, *15*, 692–705. [CrossRef]
4. Jozkowicz, A.; Was, H.; Dulak, J. Heme oxygenase-1 in tumors: Is it a false friend? *Antioxid. Redox Signal.* **2007**, *9*, 2099–2117. [CrossRef]
5. Loboda, A.; Damulewicz, M.; Pyza, E.; Jozkowicz, A.; Dulak, J. Role of Nrf2/HO-1 system in development, oxidative stress response and diseases: An evolutionarily conserved mechanism. *Cell. Mol. Life Sci.* **2016**, *73*, 3221–3247. [CrossRef]
6. Vijayan, V.; Wagener, F.; Immenschuh, S. The macrophage heme-heme oxygenase-1 system and its role in inflammation. *Biochem. Pharmacol.* **2018**, *153*, 159–167. [CrossRef]
7. Rochette, L.; Zeller, M.; Cottin, Y.; Vergely, C. Redox Functions of Heme Oxygenase-1 and Biliverdin Reductase in Diabetes. *Trends Endocrinol. Metab.* **2018**, *29*, 74–85. [CrossRef] [PubMed]
8. Liu, Y.T.; Lin, Z.M.; He, S.J.; Zuo, J.P. Heme oxygenase-1 as a potential therapeutic target in rheumatic diseases. *Life Sci.* **2018**. [CrossRef] [PubMed]
9. Yang, C.M.; Lin, C.C.; Hsieh, H.L. High-Glucose-Derived Oxidative Stress-Dependent Heme Oxygenase-1 Expression from Astrocytes Contributes to the Neuronal Apoptosis. *Mol. Neurobiol.* **2017**, *54*, 470–483. [CrossRef]
10. Nitti, M.; Piras, S.; Marinari, U.M.; Moretta, L.; Pronzato, M.A.; Furfaro, A.L. HO-1 Induction in Cancer Progression: A Matter of Cell Adaptation. *Antioxidants.* **2017**, *6*, 29. [CrossRef] [PubMed]
11. Chiang, S.K.; Chen, S.E.; Chang, L.C. A Dual Role of Heme Oxygenase-1 in Cancer Cells. *Int. J. Mol. Sci.* **2018**, *20*, 39. [CrossRef] [PubMed]
12. Biswas, C.; Shah, N.; Muthu, M.; La, P.; Fernando, A.P.; Sengupta, S.; Yang, G.; Dennery, P.A. Nuclear heme oxygenase-1 (HO-1) modulates subcellular distribution and activation of Nrf2, impacting metabolic and anti-oxidant defenses. *J. Biol. Chem.* **2014**, *289*, 26882–26894. [CrossRef]
13. Lin, P.L.; Chang, J.T.; Wu, D.W.; Huang, C.C.; Lee, H. Cytoplasmic localization of Nrf2 promotes colorectal cancer with more aggressive tumors via upregulation of PSMD4. *Free Radic. Biol. Med.* **2016**, *95*, 121–132. [CrossRef] [PubMed]
14. Chang, L.C.; Chiang, S.K.; Chen, S.E.; Yu, Y.L.; Chou, R.H.; Chang, W.C. Heme oxygenase-1 mediates BAY 11-7085 induced ferroptosis. *Cancer Lett.* **2018**, *416*, 124–137. [CrossRef]

15. Becker, J.C.; Fukui, H.; Imai, Y.; Sekikawa, A.; Kimura, T.; Yamagishi, H.; Yoshitake, N.; Pohle, T.; Domschke, W.; Fujimori, T. Colonic expression of heme oxygenase-1 is associated with a better long-term survival in patients with colorectal cancer. *Scand. J. Gastroenterol.* **2007**, *42*, 852–858. [CrossRef]
16. Andrés, N.C.; Fermento, M.E.; Gandini, N.A.; Romero, A.L.; Ferro, A.; Donna, L.G.; Curino, A.C.; Facchinetti, M.M. Heme oxygenase-1 has antitumoral effects in colorectal cancer: Involvement of p53. *Exp. Mol. Pathol.* **2014**, *97*, 321–331. [CrossRef]
17. Lien, G.S.; Wu, M.S.; Bien, M.Y.; Chen, C.H.; Lin, C.H.; Chen, B.C. Epidermal growth factor stimulates nuclear factor-kappaB activation and heme oxygenase-1 expression via c-Src, NADPH oxidase, PI3K, and Akt in human colon cancer cells. *PLoS ONE* **2014**, *9*, e104891. [CrossRef]
18. Seo, G.S.; Jiang, W.Y.; Chi, J.H.; Jin, H.; Park, W.C.; Sohn, D.H.; Park, P.H.; Lee, S.H. Heme oxygenase-1 promotes tumor progression and metastasis of colorectal carcinoma cells by inhibiting antitumor immunity. *Oncotarget* **2015**, *6*, 19792–19806. [CrossRef]
19. Hellmuth, M.; Wetzler, C.; Nold, M.; Chang, J.H.; Frank, S.; Pfeilschifter, J.; Muhl, H. Expression of interleukin-8, heme oxygenase-1 and vascular endothelial growth factor in DLD-1 colon carcinoma cells exposed to pyrrolidine dithiocarbamate. *Carcinogenesis* **2002**, *23*, 1273–1279. [CrossRef]
20. Kim, T.H.; Hur, E.G.; Kang, S.J.; Kim, J.A.; Thapa, D.; Lee, Y.M.; Ku, S.K.; Jung, Y.; Kwak, M.K. NRF2 blockade suppresses colon tumor angiogenesis by inhibiting hypoxia-induced activation of HIF-1alpha. *Cancer Res.* **2011**, *71*, 2260–2275. [CrossRef] [PubMed]
21. Waghela, B.N.; Vaidya, F.U.; Pathak, C. Upregulation of NOX-2 and Nrf-2 Promotes 5-Fluorouracil Resistance of Human Colon Carcinoma (HCT-116) Cells. *Biochemistry* **2021**, *86*, 262–274. [PubMed]
22. Yin, H.; Fang, J.; Liao, L.; Maeda, H.; Su, Q. Upregulation of heme oxygenase-1 in colorectal cancer patients with increased circulation carbon monoxide levels, potentially affects chemotherapeutic sensitivity. *BMC Cancer* **2014**, *14*, 1471–2407. [CrossRef] [PubMed]
23. Shibue, T.; Weinberg, R.A. EMT, CSCs, and drug resistance: The mechanistic link and clinical implications. *Nat. Rev. Clin. Oncol.* **2017**, *14*, 611–629. [CrossRef] [PubMed]
24. Ghosh, D.; Ulasov, I.V.; Chen, L.; Harkins, L.E.; Wallenborg, K.; Hothi, P.; Rostad, S.; Hood, L.; Cobbs, C.S. TGFbeta-Responsive HMOX1 Expression Is Associated with Stemness and Invasion in Glioblastoma Multiforme. *Stem Cells* **2016**, *34*, 2276–2289. [CrossRef]
25. Kim, D.H.; Yoon, H.J.; Cha, Y.N.; Surh, Y.J. Role of heme oxygenase-1 and its reaction product, carbon monoxide, in manifestation of breast cancer stem cell-like properties: Notch-1 as a putative target. *Free Radic. Res.* **2018**, *52*, 1336–1347. [CrossRef]
26. Jang, J.E.; Eom, J.I.; Jeung, H.K.; Chung, H.; Kim, Y.R.; Kim, J.S.; Cheong, J.W.; Min, Y.H. PERK/NRF2 and autophagy form a resistance mechanism against G9a inhibition in leukemia stem cells. *J. Exp. Clinical Cancer Res.* **2020**, *39*, 66. [CrossRef] [PubMed]
27. Horinouchi, T.; Terada, K.; Higashi, T.; Miwa, S. Endothelin receptor signaling: New insight into its regulatory mechanisms. *J. Pharmacol. Sci.* **2013**, *123*, 85–101. [CrossRef]
28. Rosano, L.; Bagnato, A. Endothelin therapeutics in cancer: Where are we? *Am. J. Physiol.-Regul. Integr. Comp. Physiol.* **2016**, *310*, R469–R475. [CrossRef]
29. Cianfrocca, R.; Rosano, L.; Tocci, P.; Sestito, R.; Caprara, V.; Di Castro, V.; De Maria, R.; Bagnato, A. Blocking endothelin-1-receptor/beta-catenin circuit sensitizes to chemotherapy in colorectal cancer. *Cell Death Differ.* **2017**, *24*, 1811–1820. [CrossRef] [PubMed]
30. Morita, T.; Kourembanas, S. Endothelial cell expression of vasoconstrictors and growth factors is regulated by smooth muscle cell-derived carbon monoxide. *J. Clin. Investig.* **1995**, *96*, 2676–2682. [CrossRef]
31. Zhang, F.; Kaide, J.I.; Yang, L.; Jiang, H.; Quan, S.; Kemp, R.; Gong, W.; Balazy, M.; Abraham, N.G.; Nasjletti, A. CO modulates pulmonary vascular response to acute hypoxia: Relation to endothelin. *Am. J. Physiol.-Heart Circ. Physiol.* **2004**, *286*, H137–H144. [CrossRef]
32. Liou, S.F.; Hsu, J.H.; Chen, Y.T.; Chen, I.J.; Yeh, J.L. KMUP-1 Attenuates Endothelin-1-Induced Cardiomyocyte Hypertrophy through Activation of Heme Oxygenase-1 and Suppression of the Akt/GSK-3beta, Calcineurin/NFATc4 and RhoA/ROCK Pathways. *Molecules* **2015**, *20*, 10435–10449. [CrossRef]
33. Lin, H.C.; Su, S.L.; Lu, C.Y.; Lin, A.H.; Lin, W.C.; Liu, C.S.; Yang, Y.C.; Wang, H.M.; Lii, C.K.; Chen, H.W. Andrographolide inhibits hypoxia-induced HIF-1alpha-driven endothelin 1 secretion by activating Nrf2/HO-1 and promoting the expression of prolyl hydroxylases 2/3 in human endothelial cells. *Environ. Toxicol.* **2017**, *32*, 918–930. [CrossRef]
34. Chou, A.K.; Chen, T.I.; Winardi, W.; Dai, M.H.; Chen, S.C.; Howng, S.L.; Yen, C.P.; Lin, T.K.; Jeng, A.Y.; Kwan, A.L. Functional neuroprotective effect of CGS 26303, a dual ECE inhibitor, on ischemic-reperfusion spinal cord injury in rats. *Exp. Biol. Med.* **2007**, *232*, 214–218.
35. Casado, J.; Iñigo-Chaves, A.; Jiménez-Ruiz, S.M.; Ríos-Arrabal, S.; Carazo-Gallego, Á.; González-Puga, C.; Núñez, M.I.; Ruíz-Extremera, Á.; Salmerón, J.; León, J. AA-NAT, MT1 and MT2 Correlates with Cancer Stem-Like Cell Markers in Colorectal Cancer: Study of the Influence of Stage and p53 Status of Tumors. *Int. J. Mol. Sci.* **2017**, *18*, 1251. [CrossRef] [PubMed]
36. Witte, K.E.; Hertel, O.; Windmöller, B.A.; Helweg, L.P.; Höving, A.L.; Knabbe, C.; Busche, T.; Greiner, J.F.W.; Kalinowski, J.; Noll, T.; et al. Nanopore Sequencing Reveals Global Transcriptome Signatures of Mitochondrial and Ribosomal Gene Expressions in Various Human Cancer Stem-like Cell Populations. *Cancers* **2021**, *13*, 1136. [CrossRef]

37. Morata-Tarifa, C.; Jiménez, G.; García, M.A.; Entrena, J.M.; Griñán-Lisón, C.; Aguilera, M.; Picon-Ruiz, M.; Marchal, J.A. Low adherent cancer cell subpopulations are enriched in tumorigenic and metastatic epithelial-to-mesenchymal transition-induced cancer stem-like cells. *Sci. Rep.* **2016**, *6*, 18772. [CrossRef] [PubMed]
38. Hemmati, M.; Yousefi, B.; Bahar, A.; Eslami, M. Importance of Heme Oxygenase-1 in Gastrointestinal Cancers: Functions, Inductions, Regulations, and Signaling. *J. Gastrointest. Cancer* **2021**, *52*, 454–461. [CrossRef] [PubMed]
39. Germanova, D.; Keirsse, J.; Köhler, A.; Hastir, J.F.; Demetter, P.; Delbauve, S.; Elkrim, Y.; Verset, L.; Larbanoix, L.; Preyat, N.; et al. Myeloid tumor necrosis factor and heme oxygenase-1 regulate the progression of colorectal liver metastases during hepatic ischemia-reperfusion. *Int. J. Cancer* **2021**, *148*, 1276–1288. [CrossRef]
40. Sebastián, V.P.; Salazar, G.A.; Coronado-Arrázola, I.; Schultz, B.M.; Vallejos, O.P.; Berkowitz, L.; Álvarez-Lobos, M.M.; Riedel, C.A.; Kalergis, A.M.; Bueno, S.M. Heme Oxygenase-1 as a Modulator of Intestinal Inflammation Development and Progression. *Front. Immunol.* **2018**, *9*, 1956. [CrossRef] [PubMed]
41. Puentes-Pardo, J.D.; Moreno-SanJuan, S.; Carazo, Á.; León, J. Heme Oxygenase-1 in Gastrointestinal Tract Health and Disease. *Antioxidants* **2020**, *9*, 214. [CrossRef]
42. Wegiel, B.; Nemeth, Z.; Correa-Costa, M.; Bulmer, A.C.; Otterbein, L.E. Heme oxygenase-1: A metabolic nike. *Antioxid. Redox Signal.* **2014**, *20*, 1709–1722. [CrossRef]
43. Wegiel, B.; Gallo, D.; Csizmadia, E.; Harris, C.; Belcher, J.; Vercellotti, G.M.; Penacho, N.; Seth, P.; Sukhatme, V.; Ahmed, A.; et al. Carbon monoxide expedites metabolic exhaustion to inhibit tumor growth. *Cancer Res.* **2013**, *73*, 7009–7021. [CrossRef] [PubMed]
44. Almeida, A.S.; Sonnewald, U.; Alves, P.M.; Vieira, H.L. Carbon monoxide improves neuronal differentiation and yield by increasing the functioning and number of mitochondria. *J. Neurochem.* **2016**, *138*, 423–435. [CrossRef] [PubMed]
45. Li, Y.; Rogoff, H.A.; Keates, S.; Gao, Y.; Murikipudi, S.; Mikule, K.; Leggett, D.; Li, W.; Pardee, A.B.; Li, C.J. Suppression of cancer relapse and metastasis by inhibiting cancer stemness. *Proc. Natl. Acad. Sci. USA* **2015**, *112*, 1839–1844. [CrossRef] [PubMed]
46. Ryoo, I.G.; Kim, G.; Choi, B.H.; Lee, S.H.; Kwak, M.K. Involvement of NRF2 Signaling in Doxorubicin Resistance of Cancer Stem Cell-Enriched Colonospheres. *Biomol. Ther.* **2016**, *24*, 482–488. [CrossRef]
47. Shiokawa, D.; Sakai, H.; Ohata, H.; Miyazaki, T.; Kanda, Y.; Sekine, S.; Narushima, D.; Hosokawa, M.; Kato, M.; Suzuki, Y.; et al. Slow-Cycling Cancer Stem Cells Regulate Progression and Chemoresistance in Colon Cancer. *Cancer Res.* **2020**, *80*, 4451–4464. [CrossRef] [PubMed]
48. Sharif, T.; Dai, C.; Martell, E.; Ghassemi-Rad, M.S.; Hanes, M.R.; Murphy, P.J.; Kennedy, B.E.; Venugopal, C.; Subapanditha, M.; Giacomantonio, C.A.; et al. TAp73 Modifies Metabolism and Positively Regulates Growth of Cancer Stem-Like Cells in a Redox-Sensitive Manner. *Clin. Cancer Res.* **2019**, *25*, 2001–2017. [CrossRef]
49. Leis, O.; Eguiara, A.; Lopez-Arribillaga, E.; Alberdi, M.J.; Hernandez-Garcia, S.; Elorriaga, K.; Pandiella, A.; Rezola, R.; Martin, A.G. Sox2 expression in breast tumours and activation in breast cancer stem cells. *Oncogene* **2012**, *31*, 1354–1365. [CrossRef]
50. Abdalla, M.Y.; Ahmad, I.M.; Rachagani, S.; Banerjee, K.; Thompson, C.M.; Maurer, H.C.; Olive, K.P.; Bailey, K.L.; Britigan, B.E.; Kumar, S. Enhancing responsiveness of pancreatic cancer cells to gemcitabine treatment under hypoxia by heme oxygenase-1 inhibition. *Transl. Res.* **2019**, *207*, 56–69. [CrossRef]
51. Zhan, L.; Zhang, H.; Zhang, Q.; Woods, C.G.; Chen, Y.; Xue, P.; Dong, J.; Tokar, E.J.; Xu, Y.; Hou, Y.; et al. Regulatory role of KEAP1 and NRF2 in PPARγ expression and chemoresistance in human non-small-cell lung carcinoma cells. *Free Radic. Biol. Med.* **2012**, *53*, 758–768. [CrossRef]
52. Nam, S.Y.; Sabapathy, K. p53 promotes cellular survival in a context-dependent manner by directly inducing the expression of haeme-oxygenase-1. *Oncogene* **2011**, *30*, 4476–4486. [CrossRef]
53. Lee, S.Y.; Jo, H.J.; Kim, K.M.; Song, J.D.; Chung, H.T.; Park, Y.C. Concurrent expression of heme oxygenase-1 and p53 in human retinal pigment epithelial cell line. *Biochem. Biophys. Res. Commun.* **2008**, *365*, 870–874. [CrossRef] [PubMed]
54. Kim, D.H.; Song, N.Y.; Kim, E.H.; Na, H.K.; Joe, Y.; Chung, H.T.; Surh, Y.J. 15-Deoxy-Δ12,14-prostaglandin J2 induces p53 expression through Nrf2-mediated upregulation of heme oxygenase-1 in human breast cancer cells. *Free Radical Res.* **2014**, *48*, 1018–1027. [CrossRef] [PubMed]
55. Martínez-Miguel, P.; Medrano-Andrés, D.; Griera-Merino, M.; Ortiz, A.; Rodríguez-Puyol, M.; Rodríguez-Puyol, D.; López-Ongil, S. Tweak up-regulates endothelin-1 system in mouse and human endothelial cells. *Cardiovasc. Res.* **2017**, *113*, 207–221. [CrossRef] [PubMed]
56. Serizawa, F.; Patterson, E.; Potter, R.F.; Fraser, D.D.; Cepinskas, G. Pretreatment of human cerebrovascular endothelial cells with CO-releasing molecule-3 interferes with JNK/AP-1 signaling and suppresses LPS-induced proadhesive phenotype. *Microcirculation* **2015**, *22*, 28–36. [CrossRef] [PubMed]
57. Lin, C.C.; Yang, C.C.; Hsiao, L.D.; Chen, S.Y.; Yang, C.M. Heme Oxygenase-1 Induction by Carbon Monoxide Releasing Molecule-3 Suppresses Interleukin-1β-Mediated Neuroinflammation. *Front. Mol. Neurosci.* **2017**, *10*, 387. [CrossRef] [PubMed]
58. Brouard, S.; Berberat, P.O.; Tobiasch, E.; Seldon, M.P.; Bach, F.H.; Soares, M.P. Heme Oxygenase-1-derived Carbon Monoxide Requires the Activation of Transcription Factor NF-κB to Protect Endothelial Cells from Tumor Necrosis Factor-α-mediated Apoptosis. *J. Biol. Chem.* **2002**, *277*, 17950–17961. [CrossRef] [PubMed]
59. Chhikara, M.; Wang, S.; Kern, S.J.; Ferreyra, G.A.; Barb, J.J.; Munson, P.J.; Danner, R.L. Carbon monoxide blocks lipopolysaccharide-induced gene expression by interfering with proximal TLR4 to NF-kappaB signal transduction in human monocytes. *PLoS ONE* **2009**, *4*, e8139. [CrossRef] [PubMed]

60. Mizuguchi, S.; Capretta, A.; Suehiro, S.; Nishiyama, N.; Luke, P.; Potter, R.F.; Fraser, D.D.; Cepinskas, G. Carbon monoxide-releasing molecule CORM-3 suppresses vascular endothelial cell SOD-1/SOD-2 activity while up-regulating the cell surface levels of SOD-3 in a heparin-dependent manner. *Free Radic. Biol. Med.* **2010**, *49*, 1534–1541. [CrossRef]
61. Myant, K.B.; Cammareri, P.; McGhee, E.J.; Ridgway, R.A.; Huels, D.J.; Cordero, J.B.; Schwitalla, S.; Kalna, G.; Ogg, E.L.; Athineos, D.; et al. ROS production and NF-κB activation triggered by RAC1 facilitate WNT-driven intestinal stem cell proliferation and colorectal cancer initiation. *Cell Stem Cell* **2013**, *12*, 761–773. [CrossRef]
62. Vítek, L.; Schwertner, H.A. The heme catabolic pathway and its protective effects on oxidative stress-mediated diseases. *Adv. Clin. Chem.* **2007**, *43*, 1–57. [PubMed]
63. Zheng, J.; Nagda, D.A.; Lajud, S.A.; Kumar, S.; Mouchli, A.; Bezpalko, O.; O'Malley, B.W., Jr.; Li, D. Biliverdin's regulation of reactive oxygen species signalling leads to potent inhibition of proliferative and angiogenic pathways in head and neck cancer. *Br. J. Cancer* **2014**, *110*, 2116–2122. [CrossRef] [PubMed]
64. Trachootham, D.; Alexandre, J.; Huang, P. Targeting cancer cells by ROS-mediated mechanisms: A radical therapeutic approach? *Nat. Rev. Drug Discov.* **2009**, *8*, 579–591. [CrossRef]
65. Kajarabille, N.; Latunde-Dada, G.O. Programmed Cell-Death by Ferroptosis: Antioxidants as Mitigators. *Int. J. Mol. Sci.* **2019**, *20*, 4968. [CrossRef]
66. Puglisi, M.A.; Barba, M.; Corbi, M.; Errico, M.F.; Giorda, E.; Saulnier, N.; Boninsegna, A.; Piscaglia, A.C.; Carsetti, R.; Cittadini, A.; et al. Identification of Endothelin-1 and NR4A2 as CD133-regulated genes in colon cancer cells. *J. Pathol.* **2011**, *225*, 305–314. [CrossRef]
67. Pérez-Moreno, P.; Indo, S.; Niechi, I.; Huerta, H.; Cabello, P.; Jara, L.; Aguayo, F.; Varas-Godoy, M.; Burzio, V.A.; Tapia, J.C. Endothelin-converting enzyme-1c promotes stem cell traits and aggressiveness in colorectal cancer cells. *Mol. Oncol.* **2020**, *14*, 347–362. [CrossRef] [PubMed]
68. Peduto Eberl, L.; Bovey, R.; Juillerat-Jeanneret, L. Endothelin-receptor antagonists are proapoptotic and antiproliferative in human colon cancer cells. *Br. J. Cancer* **2003**, *88*, 788–795. [CrossRef]
69. Eberl, L.P.; Valdenaire, O.; Saintgiorgio, V.; Jeannin, J.F.; Juillerat-Jeanneret, L. Endothelin receptor blockade potentiates FasL-induced apoptosis in rat colon carcinoma cells. *Int. J. Cancer* **2000**, *86*, 182–187. [CrossRef]
70. Eberl, L.P.; Egidy, G.; Pinet, F.; Juillerat-Jeanneret, L. Endothelin receptor blockade potentiates FasL-induced apoptosis in colon carcinoma cells via the protein kinase C-pathway. *J. Cardiovasc. Pharmacol.* **2000**, *36*, S354–S356. [CrossRef] [PubMed]
71. Enevoldsen, F.C.; Sahana, J.; Wehland, M.; Grimm, D.; Infanger, M.; Krüger, M. Endothelin Receptor Antagonists: Status Quo and Future Perspectives for Targeted Therapy. *J. Clin. Med.* **2020**, *9*, 824. [CrossRef] [PubMed]

Commentary

Germline Mutations in Other Homologous Recombination Repair-Related Genes Than *BRCA1/2*: Predictive or Prognostic Factors?

Laura Cortesi *, Claudia Piombino and Angela Toss

Genetic Oncology Unit, Department of Oncology and Haematology, University Hospital of Modena, 41125 Modena, Italy; claudia.piombino@outlook.com (C.P.); angela.toss@unimore.it (A.T.)
* Correspondence: hbc@unimore.it

Abstract: The homologous recombination repair (HRR) pathway repairs double-strand DNA breaks, mostly by BRCA1 and BRCA2, although other proteins such as ATM, CHEK2, and PALB2 are also involved. *BRCA1/2* germline mutations are targeted by PARP inhibitors. The aim of this commentary is to explore whether germline mutations in HRR-related genes other than *BRCA1/2* have to be considered as prognostic factors or predictive to therapies by discussing the results of two articles published in December 2020. The TBCRC 048 trial published by Tung et al. showed an impressive objective response rate to olaparib in metastatic breast cancer patients with germline *PALB2* mutation compared to germline *ATM* and *CHEK2* mutation carriers. Additionally, Yadav et al. observed a significantly longer overall survival in pancreatic adenocarcinoma patients with germline HRR mutations compared to non-carriers. In our opinion, assuming that *PALB2* is a high-penetrant gene with a key role in the HRR system, *PALB2* mutations are predictive factors for response to treatment. Moreover, germline mutations in the *ATM* gene provide a better outcome in pancreatic adenocarcinoma, being more often associated to wild-type *KRAS*. In conclusion, sequencing of HRR-related genes other than *BRCA1/2* should be routinely offered as part of a biological characterization of pancreatic and breast cancers.

Keywords: BRCA1; BRCA2; PALB2; homologous recombination repair

1. Introduction

1.1. DNA Repair Mechanisms

DNA damage and deficiencies of repair are central features of cancer pathology. Healthy cells defend themselves against DNA damage through different pathways. The DNA damage can induce a single-strand break or a double-strand break. The single-strand break can be repaired by different systems: base excision repair (BER), nucleotide excision repair (NER), or mismatch repair (MMR). The poly (ADP-ribose) polymerase (PARP) enzyme belongs to the BER system (Figure 1A), whereas ERCC excision repair 1, endonuclease non-catalytic subunit (ERCC1) enzyme repairs bulky adducts by the NER systems, and the MutL homolog 1 (MLH1), MutS homolog 6 (MSH6), and MutT homolog 1 (MTH1) proteins repair the single nucleotide substitutions, deletions, or insertions by the MMR system. In eukaryotic cells, there are at least five pathways to repair DNA double-strand breaks: non-homologous end-joining (NHEJ), alternative non-homologous end-joining, single-strand annealing, break-induced replication, and homologous recombination repair (HRR) [1–3].

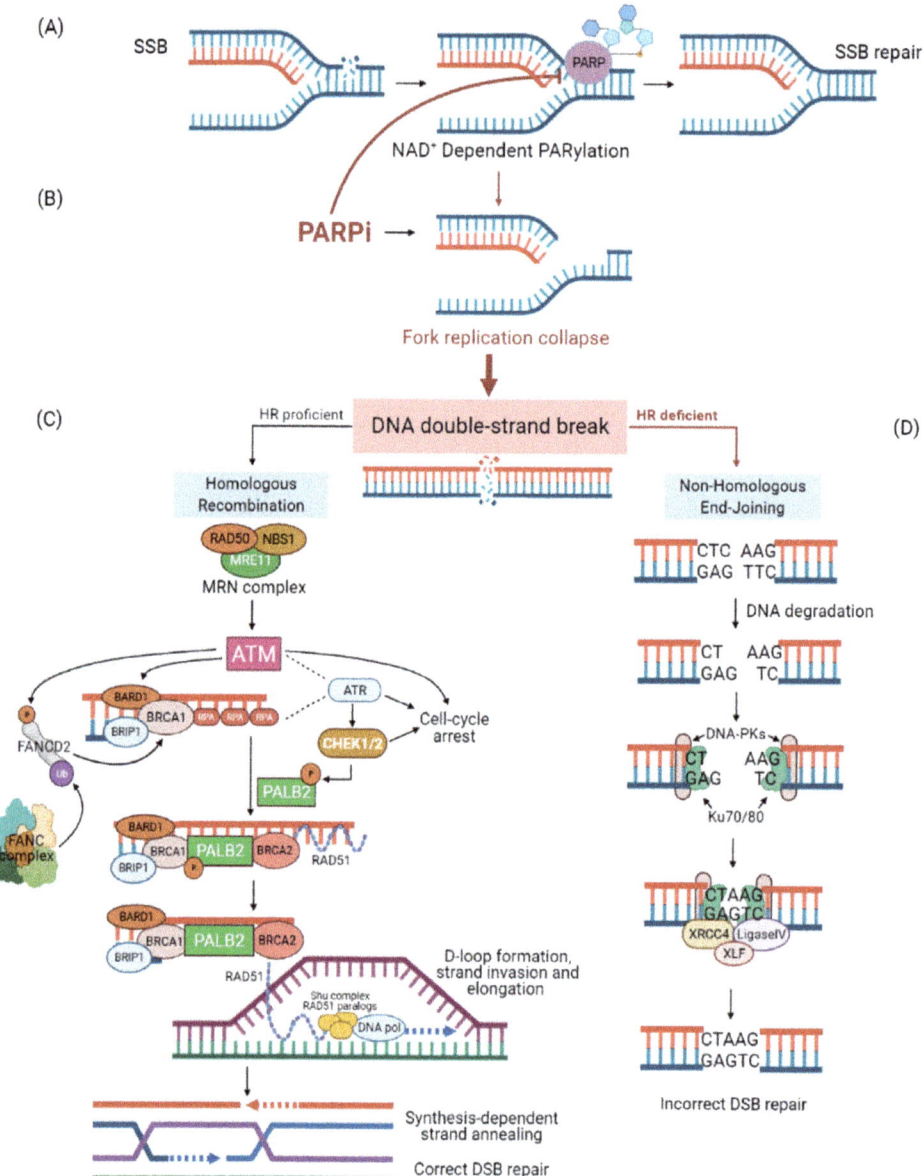

Figure 1. Overview of DNA double-strand break repair mechanisms and PARP inhibitor function. When DNA single-strand break (SSB) occurs, poly (ADP-ribose) polymerase (PARP) recruitment and activation leads to SSB repair through NAD+poly(ADP-ribosyl)ation (PARylation) of histones and chromatin remodeling enzymes and recruitment of PARP-dependent DNA-repair proteins (**A**). In the presence of PARP inhibitor (PARPi), PARP recruited to DNA SSB is no longer able to activate PARP-dependent repair systems and to dissociate from DNA-determining fork replication collapse during DNA replication (**B**). The collapsed replication fork creates a DNA double-strand break (DSB) that, in homologous recombination (HR)-proficient cells, is mainly repaired by the error-free mechanism of HR. MRN complex (Mre11, Rad50, and Nbs1) initiates DNA end resection, leading to the formation of single-strand DNA (ssDNA) at the extremity of the DSB; ssDNA is

protected from degradation by the loading of replication protein A (RPA). The MRN complex recruits and activates ataxia telangiectasia mutated (ATM); ATM and RPA contribute to ataxia telangiectasia and Rad3-related (ATR) activation. Once activated, ATM and ATR phosphorylate several proteins involved in the HR pathway, such as checkpoint kinases 1 and 2 (CHEK1/2). Besides, ATM, ATR, and CHEK1/2 regulate cell cycle arrest after the DSB. Fanconi anemia complementation group D2 (FANCD2) contributes to breast cancer 1 (BRCA1) activation once monoubiquitinated by Fanconi anemia complementation (FANC) and phosphorylated by ATM. The complex BRCA1- BRCA1-associated RING domain 1 (BARD1) facilitates DNA end resection and interacts with the bridging protein partner and localizer of BRCA2 (PALB2) phosphorylated by CHEK2. PALB2 promotes the recruitment of breast cancer 2 (BRCA2). PALB2 and BRCA2 remove RPA and facilitate the assembly of the RAD51 recombinase nucleoprotein filament. RAD51 nucleoprotein filament, Shu complex (which consists of four proteins, Shu1, Shu2, Csm2, and Psy3), and RAD51 paralogs mediate the D-loop formation and strand invasion of ssDNA into the intact sister chromatid, searching a homologous template for DNA synthesis by DNA polymerase (DNA pol). The repaired DNA is resolved by synthesis-dependent strand annealing (**C**). In HR-deficient cells, DSB is mainly repaired by the more error-prone template-independent mechanism of non-homologous end-joining (NHEJ). DNA ends are recognized by the Ku70/80 heterodimer, which recruits DNA-dependent protein kinases (DNA-PKs). The X-ray repair cross complementing 4 (XRCC4)-DNA Ligase IV-XRCC4-like factor (XLF) ligation complex seals the break. However, DNA ends can degrade, leading to incorrect DSB repair (**D**).

The most accurate of all, HRR, uses the intact sister chromatid as a template for error-free DNA double-strand break repair, mainly during the S/G2 phase of the cell cycle. DNA damage response is fundamentally mediated by the kinases belonging to the phosphatidylinositol 3-kinase-like protein kinase family, which include ataxia telangiectasia mutated (ATM), ataxia telangiectasia and Rad3-related (ATR), and DNA-PK (DNA-dependent protein kinase). While DNA-PK activates the more error-prone template-independent mechanism of NHEJ [4], both ATM and ATR orchestrate the initial phase of the HRR pathway and mediate cell cycle arrest [5]. In detail, the MRN complex (Mre11, Rad50, and Nbs1) initiates DNA end resection from 5' to 3' leading to the formation of single-strand DNA (ssDNA) at the extremity of the DNA double-strand break repair. ssDNA is protected from degradation by the loading of replication protein A (RPA) [6]. The MRN complex recruits and activates ATM [7], while the sensor protein RPA finally drives ATR activation [8]. Once activated, ATM and ATR phosphorylate several proteins involved in the HRR pathway such as checkpoint kinase 2 (CHEK2) [5]. On the other hand, the tumor suppressor complex Breast Cancer 1 (BRCA1) and (BRCA1-associated RING domain 1 (BARD1) facilitates DNA end resection and interacts with the bridging protein partner and localizer of BRCA2 (PALB2) which in turn promotes the recruitment of breast cancer 2 (BRCA2) [9]. PALB2 and BRCA2 remove RPA and facilitate the assembly of the RAD51 recombinase nucleoprotein filament. RAD51 nucleoprotein filament mediates the invasion of ssDNA into the intact sister chromatid, searching for a homologous template for DNA synthesis and faithful repair of DNA [10] (Figure 1C,D).

1.2. PARP Inhibitor Treatments

We well know that tumor cells with *BRCA1/2* germline mutations are targeted by PARP inhibitor (PARPi) therapies through synthetic lethality. During DNA replication, PARPi induces the single arm of the fork interruption, producing a collapsed fork (Figure 1B). If PARP enzymes are inhibited in cells lacking functional BRCA1/2 proteins, DNA double-strand breaks can only be repaired by the NHEJ pathway. However, the error-prone nature of this template-independent repair pathway ultimately leads to tumor cell death [11]. Since 2009, when a first-in-human clinical trial of olaparib confirmed the synthetic lethal interaction between inhibition of PARP1, a key sensor of DNA damage, and *BRCA1/2* deficiency [12], PARPi therapies have been approved for the use in several cancers. Based on Study 19 [13], Study 42 [14], and SOLO2 studies [15], olaparib has been approved for the response maintenance treatment of germline/somatic *BRCA1/2*-mutated high-grade serous ovarian cancers (including fallopian tube or primary peritoneal cancers) after first-line platinum-based chemotherapy and for the treatment of germline *BRCA1/2* (g*BRCA1/2*) mutated ovarian cancer progressing to three or more prior lines of chemotherapy. Besides, another two PARP inhibitors, niraparib [16], and rucaparib [17] have been granted approval in the maintenance setting of ovarian cancer, regardless of BRCA1/2 status. Furthermore, both olaparib [18] and talazoparib [19] are approved in human epidermal growth factor receptor 2 (HER2)-negative, gBRCA1/2-mutation-associated metastatic breast cancer [20]. Finally, several trials of olaparib in patients with gBRCA1/2 mutations identified responders beyond ovarian or breast cancer patients, suggesting that other HRR-defective tumors could be suitable for PARPi treatment [14].

1.3. PARPi Targeting HRR Genes other Than BRCA

Regarding breast cancer, in addition to the known high-penetrance pathogenic variants of BRCA1/2, mutations in other high- or intermediate-penetrance genes can increase the risk of cancer [21] and the most common non-BRCA pathogenic or likely pathogenic variants affect PALB2, ATM, and CHEK2 genes [22]. Individuals carrying heterozygous pathogenic variants of ATM have a 33% cumulative lifetime risk of breast cancer by 80 years of age [23]. Nevertheless, ATM heterozygous pathogenic variants have also been reported in some cases of familial ovarian, pancreatic, and prostate cancer [21]. Certain variants in CHEK2 are associated with increased breast cancer risk, with a cumulative lifetime risk ranging from 28% to 37%, depending on family history [24]. Within families carrying pathogenic CHEK2 variants, there is also an increased risk of other malignancies including colon, prostate, kidney, bladder, and thyroid cancers [25].

With the aim of testing the hypothesis that olaparib would also have efficacy in germline mutation in an HRR-related gene other than BRCA1/2, the TBCRC-048 study was designed in metastatic breast cancer patients. In this study, eligible patients had germline mutations in non-BRCA1/2 HRR-related genes (cohort 1) or somatic mutations in these genes or BRCA1/2 (cohort 2). Fifty-four patients received olaparib 300 mg orally twice a day until progression. Exclusion criteria included platinum refractory disease or progression on more than two chemotherapy regimens in the metastatic setting. Examining cohort 1, this phase II trial found that the olaparib provided an impressive objective response rate (82%) in patients with germline PALB2 (gPALB2) mutation compared to germline ATM (gATM) and germline CHEK2 (gCHEK2) mutation carriers [26]. Therefore, olaparib could be used in gPALB2 mutation carriers beyond patients with gBRCA1/2 mutations, significantly expanding the number of patients with metastatic breast cancer who would benefit from PARPi. Moreover, since gPALB2 mutations also predispose to pancreatic and ovarian cancers [27,28], these results may have significant implications for the treatment of other gPALB2-associated cancers. Reasons why gPALB2 mutation carriers are so highly responsive to olaparib compared to gATM and gCHEK2 have not been fully explained. Nonetheless, similar data have been found in a phase II trial that evaluated talazoparib in patients with advanced HER2-negative breast cancer or other solid tumors with a germline or somatic alteration in HRR-related genes other than BRCA1/2. Patients who received at least one prior therapy in the advanced setting and without progression on or within 8 weeks of their last platinum dose were eligible. They were treated with talazoparib 1 mg daily until disease progression. Twenty patients were enrolled: 13 breast cancers (12 luminal and 1 triple negative) and 7 other solid cancers (pancreas, colon, uterine, testicular, and parotid salivary). Of 12 breast cancer patients evaluated, 6 showed a response or stable disease (clinical benefit rate equal to 50%), of which 3 were gPALB2 mutation carriers. No responses were observed in non-breast tumors. This proof-of-concept phase II study with talazoparib as the single agent demonstrated activity in HER2-negative advanced breast cancer patients with an HR pathway mutation beyond BRCA1/2 [29].

The study by Yadav et al. [30] evaluated the clinical characteristics of pancreatic ductal adenocarcinoma in germline mutation carriers of HRR genes and the implications of these mutations on overall survival (OS) by analyzing 37 cancer predisposition genes in 3078 patients. One hundred seventy-five HRR mutation carriers and 2730 noncarriers were compared, finding a younger age and more metastatic disease at diagnosis in HRR mutation carriers. In a multivariable model adjusting for sex, age at diagnosis, and tumor staging, patients with germline HRR mutations had a significantly longer OS compared with noncarriers (HR, 0.83; 95% confidence interval (CI), 0.70–0.97; $p = 0.02$). Further, gene-level analysis demonstrated that germline *ATM* mutation carriers had longer OS compared with patients without germline mutations in any of the 37 genes (HR, 0.72; 95% CI, 0.55–0.94; $p = 0.01$).

The primary aim of our commentary was to discuss whether germline mutations in an HRR-related gene other than *BRCA1/2* have to be considered as prognostic factors or predictive to therapies by discussing the results of the abovementioned TBCRC-048 study by Tung et al. [25] and of the study by Yadav et al. [30].

2. The Different Role of High- and Moderate-Penetrance Genes

The role of *PALB2* as a high/moderate-penetrance gene has been extensively discussed. The risk of breast cancer development in g*PALB2* mutations is lower than in g*BRCA1/2* mutation carriers, reaching 53% at 80 years [31]. However, breast cancer risk appears higher than in g*ATM* or g*CHEK2* mutation carriers, where it is 2/3-fold higher than in the general population [23,24]. The difference between high- and moderate-risk genes is that in the latter case, both endogenous (genomic variations) and exogenous (e.g., environmental exposures and lifestyle) factors contribute to cancer development. It is likely that in cases of cancer in g*ATM* and g*CHEK2* mutation carriers, olaparib needs to be supported by the modification of environmental factors such as diet or lifestyle in order to improve its efficacy. It might be of interest to evaluate the addition of a methionine-choline-deficient diet to PARPi treatment. In a murine model of non-alcoholic fatty liver disease, a methionine- and choline-deficient diet attenuated PARP activation, enhancing the benefits of olaparib [32].

As previously described, *PALB2* represents a key gene in the HRR system, as the signal mediator between BRCA1 and the BRCA2/RAD51 complex. PALB2 purification studies [33,34] revealed that PALB2 uses two DNA-binding domains to interact directly with D-loop and ssDNA structures, and that the recombinase RAD51 interacts with PALB2 through its amino-terminal region, which leads to the enhancement of RAD51 activity. In its carboxyl-terminal region, PALB2 presents a WD40 domain through which PALB2 interacts with both BRCA2 and RAD51 [34,35]. Being an important player in different steps of HRR, PALB2 is strictly regulated by ubiquitylation and histone acetylation [36], as well as at a post-transcriptional level, being phosphorylated initially by cyclin-dependent kinases (CDKs) [37] and later by ATM [38]. As in *BRCA1/2* mutation carriers, the lack of both *PALB2* alleles causes the activation of the NHEJ with a consequent genomic instability and cancer cell death [11].

On the other hand, ATM has multiple functions in cancer development, such as cell cycle checkpoint modulation, DNA double-strand break repair, metabolic regulation, migration, and chromatin remodeling [39]. Following exposure to stress, ATM acts as a cell cycle checkpoint regulating G1/S arrest, S phase, and G2-M arrest after the DNA double-strand break repair through different pathways. CHEK2 is also involved in the cell cycle arrest, being activated by ATM [40]. In case of g*ATM* or g*CHEK2* mutation, their role in cell cycle arrest can be overcome by ATR, which blocks the cell cycle, allowing the HRR before the cell enters into replication and mitosis phases. In detail, while ATM identifies and amplifies the signal generated by DNA double-strand break repair, ATR is activated by ssDNA or interstrand DNA crosslinking (both of which lead to stalled replication forks), or by resected DNA double-strand break repair. The principal substrates of ATM and ATR are the checkpoint kinases CHEK2 and CHEK1, respectively, which block cell cycle progression to allow repair. In particular, CHEK2 triggers the G1-S checkpoint by phosphorylation of the tumor-suppressor protein p53 which in turn inhibits the cyclin-dependent kinase 2 (CDK2)-CCNE1 (cyclin E1) interaction. In contrast, CHEK1 is mainly involved in the intra-S checkpoint and the G2-M checkpoint [41]. It is therefore likely that in both germline mutations, the PARPi needs to be added to ATR or CHEK1 inhibitors to work more effectively than in the case of g*PALB2* mutations. Besides, the ATR–CHEK1 pathway is often upregulated in human neoplasms, especially CHEK1, whose promoter activity is believed to promote tumor growth. Nevertheless, some evidence indicates that ATR and CHEK1 may also behave as haploinsufficient oncosuppressors, at least in a specific genetic background. Interestingly, the inactivation of ATM–CHEK2 and ATR–CHEK1 pathways in preclinical studies has been shown to efficiently sensitize malignant cells to radiotherapy and chemotherapy [41].

On these grounds, we can conclude that gPALB2 mutations represent a predictive factor for treatment. However, can we also consider gPALB2 mutations as having a prognostic role? The prognostic versus predictive nature of HRR defect deserves special attention. Recent results from the study by Yadav et al. [30] showed a significantly longer OS in patients with germline HRR (gHRR) mutations compared to non-carriers in pancreatic ductal adenocarcinoma. This is particularly evident in gATM mutation carriers, although patients with gHRR mutations more often present metastatic disease at the diagnosis. Molecular studies previously showed that gHRR mutations are more frequently associated to the wild-type KRAS gene, which is one of the best prognostic factors in pancreatic ductal adenocarcinoma. Therefore, the pancreatic ductal adenocarcinoma with wild-type KRAS seems to have the most favorable prognosis when accomplished by gHRR mutations, which is probably responsible for the best response to therapy.

3. Results

3.1. How to Improve the Access to Genetic Counseling and Testing

All trials that explore the efficacy of PARPi in high-penetrance risk genes (BRCA1/2, PALB2) have shown activity in those genes, definitely introducing in the metastatic breast cancer therapeutic algorithm a new standard treatment for germline mutation carriers. Unfortunately, patients with breast cancer who may be eligible for PARP inhibitor therapy are often missed, even when using established diagnostic guidelines and techniques. In the USA, only 2.7% of eligible women reported the uptake of genetic counseling and testing [42,43]. Eligibility for and uptake of gHRR testing varies among countries [44,45], and the use of international testing criteria is not feasible for all countries owing to disparities in resources and ethnicities [46].

There are potential barriers to gHRR testing and genetic counseling for eligible women with or without a diagnosis of breast cancer: lack of understanding and knowledge about genetic counseling and testing by physicians and patients; lack of perceived benefits of counseling; lack of perceived risk of having a mutation; cost of testing; and fear of insurance discrimination [47–50]. Patients' attitudes to gHRR testing (the predisposing factor), income (the enabling factor), and risk of carrying a mutation (the need factor) predict uptake of testing [51]. There are multiple ways that the uptake of gHRR testing may be increased: provision of free genetic counseling; greater dissemination of information to at-risk individuals; genetic counseling that covers strategies for individuals to discuss their diagnosis with family members; and awareness and implementation of population-based testing as a preventive measure [52,53].

Future avenues to identify patients with gHRR mutations who may benefit from treatment with PARP inhibitors are under evaluation in clinical trials, and have yet to gain approval from licensing authorities, including the FDA and EMA. Moreover, in order to increase the detection of actionable genetic mutations at earlier stages of disease, a wider access to multiple-gene panel testing and the validation of predictive models to establish probabilities of having gene mutations are needed [54,55]. The evaluation of mutations in various HRR genes could be fundamental to identify patients suitable for PARP inhibitor therapy. Accordingly, a suite of biomarkers correlating with PARP activity have recently been identified in human cancer cell lines, and these could be used as patient selection criteria for expanding the clinical development of PARP inhibitors [56,57].

Interestingly, gHRR mutations also represent a favorable factor in pancreatic ductal adenocarcinoma, being more often associated to the wild-type KRAS gene. Hence, sequencing of gHRR genes other than BRCA1/2 should be routinely offered as part of the biological characterization of pancreatic ductal adenocarcinoma. For all of these reasons, there is an urgent need for new techniques to aid in diagnosis, staging, and clinical-therapeutic decisions. Finally, since gastroenterology providers interface with patients who develop pancreatic ductal adenocarcinoma, they should have an understanding of genetic counseling and should be able to interpret multigene panel test results.

3.2. How to Improve PARPi Response in gHRR Mutation Carriers

Many efforts need to be made in gHRR mutations other than gBRCA1/2, for example by preventing breast cancer development with lifestyle modifications or by treating genetic tumors adding other DNA damage repair gene inhibitors to PARPi. Several recent studies have indicated the potential involvement of PARP activity in promoting metabolic dysfunction [58,59]. Interestingly, various metabolic disorders have been associated with elevated oxidative stress and DNA damage, which can subsequently induce PARP activity, which is also true in some cancers [32]. A methionine- and choline-deficient diet could increase the PARP inhibitor activity in gHRR mutation carriers, avoiding the development of breast cancer. A strong relationship can be observed between genetic and behavioral risk factors, underlining the prognostic role of moderate-penetrance genes.

On the other hand, as already shown, alterations in non-BRCA1/2 HRR genes may confer sensitivity not only to PARP inhibitors but also to the WEE1 checkpoint inhibitor or the ataxia telangiectasia and Rad3-related protein inhibitor. The goal for the use of HRR-targeted agents in cancer treatment should be to maximize DNA damage in G1 and S phase, and to prevent repair in G2 phase, in order to ensure the damage is taken through into mitosis where the effects will manifest. Patients carrying HRR gene mutations, who are unable to repair the DNA double-strand break, obtain the most efficient cure by G1/S checkpoint abrogation and G2/M checkpoint prevention. Achieving similar successes in the clinic should be possible using targeted HRR agents, but most likely in combination with other targeted therapies, and will require the correct identification of cancer-specific genetic deficiencies that will be associated with susceptibility to the specific HRR-targeted agent. In addition, in order to target the right tumors with HRR agents, it will also be important to maximize the therapeutic window by identifying the correct dose and schedule for treating patients, and this in turn will require an understanding of the drug mechanism of action, target engagement, and downstream pharmacodynamic biomarkers that can be used in the clinic.

The combination of PARP inhibitors and WEE1 or ATM inhibitors is under investigation in different studies with the aim of exploiting the replication stress in these mutation carriers. For instance, the Violette trial is an ongoing study with olaparib monotherapy versus olaparib in combination with an inhibitor of ATR (ceralasertib [AZD6738]) and olaparib monotherapy versus olaparib in combination with an inhibitor of WEE1 (adavosertib [AZD1775]), in the second- or third-line setting, in patients with triple-negative breast cancer prospectively stratified by qualifying tumor mutations in genes involved in the HRR pathway [60]. Another interesting phase I study is currently evaluating the addition of adavosertib to olaparib in refractory solid tumors [61].

Additionally, other ongoing trials are evaluating PARP inhibitors in pancreatic ductal adenocarcinoma patients with non-BRCA DNA damage responsive gene deficiencies, as well as PARP inhibitors in combination with other agents (i.e., immune checkpoint inhibitors) to expand the group of patients that might derive benefit from this treatment.

4. Conclusions

To conclude, gHRR mutations represent an interesting predictive factor for treatment with DNA damage repair agents, particularly in tumors where current standard therapies are insufficient, such as in the case of pancreatic ductal adenocarcinoma. Indeed, several DNA damage repair agents are under development in order to improve the therapeutic paraphernalia in rare cancer diseases. We believe that future research should be directed to better clarifying the biological rationale underpinning the mechanism of action of moderate-

and high-penetrance risk genes. A deeper knowledge of these molecular pathways is key to better understanding and exploiting the huge potential of PARP inhibitors as therapeutic agents for a wider but targeted population of cancer patients.

Author Contributions: Writing—original draft preparation, L.C. and C.P.; writing—review and editing, A.T. All authors have read and agreed to the published version of the manuscript.

Funding: This work was supported by Associazione Angela Serra per la Ricerca sul Cancro, Modena (Angela Serra Association for Cancer Research).

Institutional Review Board Statement: Not applicable.

Informed Consent Statement: Not applicable.

Data Availability Statement: No new data were created or analyzed in this study. Data sharing is not applicable to this article.

Acknowledgments: We would like to thank and express our gratitude to Tamara Sassi and Johanna Chester for their editorial assistance.

Conflicts of Interest: L.C.: Honoraria: AstraZeneca, MSD, Pfizer; Consulting or Advisory Role: Pfizer, Novartis, Tesaro, Clovis. A.T.: Consulting or Advisory Role: Lilly, Novartis. No other potential conflicts of interest were reported.

References

1. Ciccia, A.; Elledge, S.J. The DNA damage response: Making it safe to play with knives. *Mol. Cell* **2010**, *40*, 179–204. [CrossRef]
2. Chapman, J.R.; Taylor, M.R.; Boulton, S.J. Playing the end game: DNA double-strand break repair pathway choice. *Mol. Cell* **2012**, *47*, 497–510. [CrossRef] [PubMed]
3. Ceccaldi, R.; Sarangi, P.; D'Andrea, A.D. The Fanconi anaemia pathway: New players and new functions. *Nat. Rev. Mol. Cell Biol.* **2016**, *17*, 337–349. [CrossRef] [PubMed]
4. Falck, J.; Coates, J.; Jackson, S.P. Conserved modes of recruitment of ATM, ATR and DNA-PKcs to sites of DNA damage. *Nature* **2005**, *434*, 605–611. [CrossRef]
5. Matsuoka, S.; Ballif, B.A.; Smogorzewska, A.; McDonald, E.R.; Hurov, K.E.; Luo, J.; Bakalarski, C.E.; Zhao, Z.; Solimini, N.; Lerenthal, Y.; et al. ATM and ATR substrate analysis reveals extensive protein networks responsive to DNA damage. *Science* **2007**, *316*, 1160–1166. [CrossRef] [PubMed]
6. Myler, L.R.; Gallardo, I.F.; Soniat, M.M.; Deshpande, R.A.; Gonzalez, X.B.; Kim, Y.; Paull, T.T.; Finkelstein, I.J. Single-Molecule Imaging Reveals How Mre11-Rad50-Nbs1 Initiates DNA Break Repair. *Mol. Cell* **2017**, *67*, 891–898.e4. [CrossRef]
7. Lee, J.H.; Paull, T.T. Direct activation of the ATM protein kinase by the Mre11/Rad50/Nbs1 complex. *Science* **2004**, *304*, 93–96. [CrossRef]
8. Kumagai, A.; Lee, J.; Yoo, H.Y.; Dunphy, W.G. TopBP1 activates the ATR-ATRIP complex. *Cell* **2006**, *124*, 943–955. [CrossRef] [PubMed]
9. Prakash, R.; Zhang, Y.; Feng, W.; Jasin, M. Homologous recombination and human health: The roles of BRCA1, BRCA2, and associated proteins. *Cold Spring Harb. Perspect. Biol.* **2015**, *7*, a016600. [CrossRef]
10. Ducy, M.; Sesma-Sanz, L.; Guitton-Sert, L.; Lashgari, A.; Gao, Y.; Brahiti, N.; Rodrigue, A.; Margaillan, G.; Caron, M.C.; Côté, J.; et al. The Tumor Suppressor PALB2: Inside Out. *Trends Biochem. Sci.* **2019**, *44*, 226–240. [CrossRef]
11. Sun, Y.; McCorvie, T.J.; Yates, L.A.; Zhang, X. Structural basis of homologous recombination. *Cell Mol. Life Sci.* **2020**, *77*, 3–18. [CrossRef]
12. Fong, P.C.; Boss, D.S.; Yap, T.A.; Tutt, A.; Wu, P.; Mergui-Roelvink, M.; Mortimer, P.; Swaisland, H.; Lau, A.; O'Connor, M.J.; et al. Inhibition of poly(ADP-ribose) polymerase in tumors from BRCA mutation carriers. *N. Engl. J. Med.* **2009**, *361*, 123–134. [CrossRef]
13. Ledermann, J.; Harter, P.; Gourley, C.; Friedlander, M.; Vergote, I.; Rustin, G.; Scott, C.; Meier, W.; Shapira-Frommer, R.; Safra, T.; et al. Olaparib maintenance therapy in platinum-sensitive relapsed ovarian cancer. *N. Engl. J. Med.* **2012**, *366*, 1382–1392. [CrossRef]
14. Kaufman, B.; Shapira-Frommer, R.; Schmutzler, R.K.; Audeh, M.W.; Friedlander, M.; Balmaña, J.; Mitchell, G.; Fried, G.; Stemmer, S.M.; Hubert, A.; et al. Olaparib monotherapy in patients with advanced cancer and a germline BRCA1/2 mutation. *J. Clin. Oncol.* **2015**, *33*, 244–250. [CrossRef]
15. Pujade-Lauraine, E.; Ledermann, J.A.; Selle, F.; Gebski, V.; Penson, R.T.; Oza, A.M.; Korach, J.; Huzarski, T.; Poveda, A.; Pignata, S.; et al. Olaparib tablets as maintenance therapy in patients with platinum-sensitive, relapsed ovarian cancer and a BRCA1/2 mutation (SOLO2/ENGOT-Ov21): A double-blind, randomised, placebo-controlled, phase 3 trial. *Lancet Oncol.* **2017**, *18*, 1274–1284. [CrossRef]

16. Mirza, M.R.; Monk, B.J.; Herrstedt, J.; Oza, A.M.; Mahner, S.; Redondo, A.; Fabbro, M.; Ledermann, J.A.; Lorusso, D.; Vergote, I.; et al. Niraparib Maintenance Therapy in Platinum-Sensitive, Recurrent Ovarian Cancer. *N. Engl. J. Med.* **2016**, *375*, 2154–2164. [CrossRef]
17. Coleman, R.L.; Oza, A.M.; Lorusso, D.; Aghajanian, C.; Oaknin, A.; Dean, A.; Colombo, N.; Weberpals, J.I.; Clamp, A.; Scambia, G.; et al. Rucaparib maintenance treatment for recurrent ovarian carcinoma after response to platinum therapy (ARIEL3): A randomised, double-blind, placebo-controlled, phase 3 trial. *Lancet* **2017**, *390*, 1949–1961. [CrossRef]
18. Robson, M.; Im, S.A.; Senkus, E.; Xu, B.; Domchek, S.M.; Masuda, N.; Delaloge, S.; Li, W.; Tung, N.; Armstrong, A.; et al. Olaparib for Metastatic Breast Cancer in Patients with a Germline BRCA Mutation. *N. Engl. J. Med.* **2017**, *377*, 523–533. [CrossRef] [PubMed]
19. Litton, J.K.; Rugo, H.S.; Ettl, J.; Hurvitz, S.A.; Gonçalves, A.; Lee, K.H.; Fehrenbacher, L.; Yerushalmi, R.; Mina, L.A.; Martin, M.; et al. Talazoparib in Patients with Advanced Breast Cancer and a Germline BRCA Mutation. *N. Engl. J. Med.* **2018**, *379*, 753–763. [CrossRef]
20. Cortesi, L.; Rugo, H.S.; Jackisch, C. An Overview of PARP Inhibitors for the Treatment of Breast Cancer. *Target Oncol.* **2021**. [CrossRef] [PubMed]
21. Desmond, A.; Kurian, A.W.; Gabree, M.; Mills, M.A.; Anderson, M.J.; Kobayashi, Y.; Horick, N.; Yang, S.; Shannon, K.M.; Tung, N.; et al. Clinical actionability of multigene panel testing for hereditary breast and ovarian cancer risk assessment. *JAMA Oncol.* **2015**, *1*, 943–951. [CrossRef] [PubMed]
22. Kapoor, N.S.; Curcio, L.D.; Blakemore, C.A.; Bremner, A.K.; McFarland, R.E.; West, J.G.; Banks, K.C. Multigene panel testing detects equal rates of pathogenic BRCA1/2 mutations and has a higher diagnostic yield compared to limited BRCA1/2 analysis alone in patients at risk for hereditary breast cancer. *Ann. Surg. Oncol.* **2015**, *22*, 3282–3288. [CrossRef] [PubMed]
23. Marabelli, M.; Cheng, S.C.; Parmigiani, G. Penetrance of ATM Gene Mutations in Breast Cancer: A Meta-Analysis of Different Measures of Risk. *Genet. Epidemiol.* **2016**, *40*, 425–431. [CrossRef]
24. Cybulski, C.; Wokołorczyk, D.; Jakubowska, A.; Huzarski, T.; Byrski, T.; Gronwald, J.; Masojć, B.; Deebniak, T.; Górski, B.; Blecharz, P.; et al. Risk of breast cancer in women with a CHEK2 mutation with and without a family history of breast cancer. *J. Clin. Oncol.* **2011**, *29*, 3747–3752. [CrossRef]
25. Cybulski, C.; Górski, B.; Huzarski, T.; Masojć, B.; Mierzejewski, M.; Debniak, T.; Teodorczyk, U.; Byrski, T.; Gronwald, J.; Matyjasik, J.; et al. CHEK2 is a multiorgan cancer susceptibility gene. *Am. J. Hum. Genet.* **2004**, *75*, 1131–1135. [CrossRef]
26. Tung, N.M.; Robson, M.E.; Ventz, S.; Santa-Maria, C.A.; Nanda, R.; Marcom, P.K.; Shah, P.D.; Ballinger, T.J.; Yang, E.S.; Vinayak, S.; et al. TBCRC 048: Phase II Study of Olaparib for Metastatic Breast Cancer and Mutations in Homologous Recombination-Related Genes. *J. Clin. Oncol.* **2020**, *38*, 4274–4282. [CrossRef] [PubMed]
27. Jones, S.; Hruban, R.H.; Kamiyama, M.; Borges, M.; Zhang, X.; Parsons, D.W.; Lin, J.C.; Palmisano, E.; Brune, K.; Jaffee, E.M.; et al. Exomic sequencing identifies PALB2 as a pancreatic cancer susceptibility gene. *Science* **2009**, *324*, 217. [CrossRef]
28. Norquist, B.M.; Harrell, M.I.; Brady, M.F.; Walsh, T.; Lee, M.K.; Gulsuner, S.; Bernards, S.S.; Casadei, S.; Yi, Q.; Burger, R.A.; et al. Inherited Mutations in Women With Ovarian Carcinoma. *JAMA Oncol.* **2016**, *2*, 482–490. [CrossRef]
29. Gruber, J.J.; Afghahi, A.; Hatton, A.; Scott, D.; McMillan, A.; Ford, J.M.; Telli, M.L. Talazoparib beyond BRCA: A phase II trial of talazoparib monotherapy in BRCA1 and BRCA2 wild-type patients with advanced HER2-negative breast cancer or other solid tumors with a mutation in homologous recombination (HR) pathway genes. *J. Clin. Oncol.* **2019**, *37*, 3006. [CrossRef]
30. Yadav, S.; Kasi, P.M.; Bamlet, W.R.; Ho, T.P.; Polley, E.C.; Hu, C.; Hart, S.N.; Rabe, K.G.; Boddicker, N.J.; Gnanaolivu, R.D.; et al. Effect of Germline Mutations in Homologous Recombination Repair Genes on Overall Survival of Patients with Pancreatic Adenocarcinoma. *Clin. Cancer Res.* **2020**, *26*, 6505–6512. [CrossRef] [PubMed]
31. Yang, X.; Leslie, G.; Doroszuk, A.; Schneider, S.; Allen, J.; Decker, B.; Dunning, A.M.; Redman, J.; Scarth, J.; Plaskocinska, I.; et al. Cancer Risks Associated With Germline PALB2 Pathogenic Variants: An International Study of 524 Families. *J. Clin. Oncol.* **2020**, *38*, 674–685. [CrossRef] [PubMed]
32. Gariani, K.; Ryu, D.; Menzies, K.J.; Yi, H.S.; Stein, S.; Zhang, H.; Perino, A.; Lemos, V.; Katsyuba, E.; Jha, P.; et al. Inhibiting poly ADP-ribosylation increases fatty acid oxidation and protects against fatty liver disease. *J. Hepatol.* **2017**, *66*, 132–141. [CrossRef]
33. Buisson, R.; Dion-Côté, A.M.; Coulombe, Y.; Launay, H.; Cai, H.; Stasiak, A.Z.; Stasiak, A.; Xia, B.; Masson, J.Y. Cooperation of breast cancer proteins PALB2 and piccolo BRCA2 in stimulating homologous recombination. *Nat. Struct. Mol. Biol.* **2010**, *17*, 1247–1254. [CrossRef] [PubMed]
34. Dray, E.; Etchin, J.; Wiese, C.; Saro, D.; Williams, G.J.; Yu, X.; Galkin, V.E.; Liu, D.; Tsai, M.; Sy, S.M.H.; et al. Enhancement of the RAD51 Recombinase Activity by the Tumor Suppressor PALB2. *Nat. Struct. Mol. Biol.* **2011**, *17*, 1255–1259. [CrossRef]
35. Oliver, A.W.; Swift, S.; Lord, C.J.; Ashworth, A.; Pearl, L.H. Structural basis for recruitment of BRCA2 by PALB2. *EMBO Rep.* **2009**, *10*, 990–996. [CrossRef]
36. Nepomuceno, T.C.; De Gregoriis, G.; de Oliveira, F.M.B.; Suarez-Kurtz, G.; Monteiro, A.N.; Carvalho, M.A. The Role of PALB2 in the DNA Damage Response and Cancer Predisposition. *Int. J. Mol. Sci.* **2017**, *18*, 1886. [CrossRef]
37. You, Z.; Bailis, J.M. DNA damage and decisions: CtIP coordinates DNA repair and cell cycle checkpoints. *Trends Cell Biol.* **2010**, *20*, 402–409. [CrossRef]
38. Guo, Y.; Feng, W.; Sy, S.M.H.; Huen, M.S.Y. ATM-dependent phosphorylation of the Fanconi anemia protein PALB2 promotes the DNA damage response. *J. Biol. Chem.* **2015**, *290*, 27545–27556. [CrossRef]

39. Stracker, T.H.; Roig, I.; Knobel, P.A.; Marjanović, M. The ATM signaling network in development and disease. *Front. Genet.* **2013**, *4*, 37. [CrossRef]
40. Guleria, A.; Chandna, S. ATM kinase: Much more than a DNA damage responsive protein. *DNA Repair* **2016**, *39*, 1–20. [CrossRef] [PubMed]
41. Manic, G.; Obrist, F.; Sistigu, A.; Vitale, I. Trial Watch: Targeting ATM–CHK2 and ATR–CHK1 pathways for anticancer therapy. *Mol. Cell Oncol.* **2015**, *2*, e1012976. [CrossRef] [PubMed]
42. Rajagopal, P.S.; Nielsen, S.; Olopade, O.I. USPSTF recommendations for BRCA1 and BRCA2 testing in the context of a transformative national cancer control plan. *JAMA Netw. Open* **2019**, *2*, e1910142. [CrossRef]
43. Hull, L.E.; Haas, J.S.; Simon, S.R. Provider discussions of genetic tests with U.S. women at risk for a BRCA mutation. *Am. J. Prev. Med.* **2018**, *54*, 221–228. [CrossRef] [PubMed]
44. National Comprehensive Cancer Network. Genetic/Familial High-Risk Assessment: Breast, Ovarian, and Pancreatic (Version 2–20 November 2020). Available online: https://www.nccn.org/professionals/physician_gls/pdf/genetics_bop.pdf (accessed on 24 February 2021).
45. Paluch-Shimon, S.; Cardoso, F.; Sessa, C.; Balmana, J.; Cardoso, M.J.; Gilbert, F.; Senkus, E.; ESMO Guidelines Committee. Prevention and screening in BRCA mutation carriers and other breast/ovarian hereditary cancer syndromes: ESMO Clinical Practice Guidelines for cancer prevention and screening. *Ann. Oncol.* **2016**, *27*, v103–v110. [CrossRef] [PubMed]
46. Shaw, J.; Bulsara, C.; Cohen, P.A.; Gryta, M.; Nichols, C.B.; Schofield, L.; O'Sullivan, S.; Pachter, N.; Hardcastle, S.J. Investigating barriers to genetic counseling and germline mutation testing in women with suspected hereditary breast and ovarian cancer syndrome and Lynch syndrome. *Patient Educ. Couns.* **2018**, *101*, 938–944. [CrossRef]
47. PDQ Cancer Genetics Editorial Board. Cancer Genetics Risk Assessment and Counseling (PDQ®): Health Professional Version. 4 December 2020. Available online: https://www.ncbi.nlm.nih.gov/books/NBK65817/ (accessed on 24 February 2021).
48. Vogel, R.I.; Niendorf, K.; Lee, H.; Petzel, S.; Lee, H.Y.; Geller, M.A. A qualitative study of barriers to genetic counseling and potential for mobile technology education among women with ovarian cancer. *Hered. Cancer Clin. Pract.* **2018**, *16*, 13. [CrossRef]
49. Hann, K.E.J.; Freeman, M.; Fraser, L.; Waller, J.; Sanderson, S.C.; Rahman, B.; Side, L.; Gessler, S.; Lanceley, A.; PROMISE Study Team. Awareness, knowledge, perceptions, and attitudes towards genetic testing for cancer risk among ethnic minority groups: A systematic review. *BMC Public Health* **2017**, *17*, 503. [CrossRef]
50. Jones, T.; McCarthy, A.M.; Kim, Y.; Armstrong, K. Predictors of BRCA1/2 genetic testing among Black women with breast cancer: A population-based study. *Cancer Med.* **2017**, *6*, 1787–1798. [CrossRef]
51. Godard, B.; Kääriäinen, H.; Kristoffersson, U.; Tranebjaerg, L.; Coviello, D.; Aymé, S. Provision of genetic services in Europe: Current practices and issues. *Eur. J. Hum. Genet.* **2003**, *11*, S13–S48. [CrossRef]
52. Scherr, C.L.; Bomboka, L.; Nelson, A.; Pal, T.; Vadaparampil, S.T. Tracking the dissemination of a culturally targeted brochure to promote awareness of hereditary breast and ovarian cancer among Black women. *Patient Educ. Couns.* **2017**, *100*, 805–811. [CrossRef]
53. Cohen, S.A.; Bradbury, A.; Henderson, V.; Hoskins, K.; Bednar, E.; Arun, B.K. Genetic Counseling and Testing in a Community Setting: Quality, Access, and Efficiency. *Am. Soc. Clin. Oncol. Educ. Book* **2019**, *39*, e34–e44. [CrossRef]
54. Katsanis, S.H.; Katsanis, N. Molecular genetic testing and the future of clinical genomics. *Nat. Rev. Genet.* **2013**, *14*, 415–426. [CrossRef]
55. Di Resta, C.; Galbiati, S.; Carrera, P.; Ferrari, M. Next-generation sequencing approach for the diagnosis of human diseases: Open challenges and new opportunities. *EJIFCC* **2018**, *29*, 4–14.
56. Oplustilova, L.; Wolanin, K.; Mistrik, M.; Korinkova, G.; Simkova, D.; Bouchal, J.; Lenobel, R.; Bartkova, J.; Lau, A.; O'Connor, M.J.; et al. Evaluation of candidate biomarkers to predict cancer cell sensitivity or resistance to PARP-1 inhibitor treatment. *Cell Cycle* **2012**, *11*, 3837–3850. [CrossRef]
57. Michels, J.; Vitale, I.; Saparbaev, M.; Castedo, M.; Kroemer, G. Predictive biomarkers for cancer therapy with PARP inhibitors. *Oncogene* **2014**, *33*, 3894–3907. [CrossRef] [PubMed]
58. Szántó, M.; Bai, P. The role of ADP-ribose metabolism in metabolic regulation, adipose tissue differentiation, and metabolism. *Genes Dev.* **2020**, *34*, 321–340. [CrossRef]
59. Ke, Y.; Wang, C.; Zhang, J.; Zhong, X.; Wang, R.; Zeng, X.; Ba, X. The Role of PARPs in Inflammation-and Metabolic-Related Diseases: Molecular Mechanisms and Beyond. *Cells* **2019**, *8*, 1047. [CrossRef]
60. Tutt, A.; Stephens, C.; Frewer, P.; Pierce, A.; Rhee, J.; So, K.; Ottesen, L.; Dean, E.; Hollingsworth, S.J. VIOLETTE: A randomized phase II study to assess DNA damage response inhibitors in combination with olaparib (Ola) vs Ola monotherapy in patients (pts) with metastatic, triple-negative breast cancer (TNBC) stratified by alterations in homologous recombination repair (HRR)-related genes. *J. Clin. Oncol.* **2018**, *36*. [CrossRef]
61. Hamilton, E.; Falchook, G.S.; Wang, J.S.; Fu, S.; Oza, A.; Karen, S.; Imedio, E.R.; Kumar, S.; Ottesen, L.; Mugundu, G.M.; et al. Abstract CT025: Phase Ib study of adavosertib in combination with olaparib in patients with refractory solid tumors: Dose escalation. *Cancer Res.* **2019**, *79* (Suppl. 13), CT025.

Tumor Infiltrating Neutrophils Are Frequently Found in Adenocarcinomas of the Biliary Tract and Their Precursor Lesions with Possible Impact on Prognosis

Vittorio Branchi [1,†], Benedict Jürgensen [1,†], Laura Esser [2], Maria Gonzalez-Carmona [3], Tobias J. Weismüller [3], Christian P. Strassburg [3], Jonas Henn [1], Alexander Semaan [1], Philipp Lingohr [1], Steffen Manekeller [1], Glen Kristiansen [2], Jörg C. Kalff [1], Marieta I. Toma [2] and Hanno Matthaei [1,*]

1 Department of General, Visceral, Thoracic and Vascular Surgery, University Hospital Bonn, 53127 Bonn, Germany; vittorio.branchi@ukbonn.de (V.B.); benedict.juergensen@ukbonn.de (B.J.); jonas.henn@ukbonn.de (J.H.); alexander.semaan@ukbonn.de (A.S.); philipp.lingohr@ukbonn.de (P.L.); steffen.manekeller@ukbonn.de (S.M.); joerg.kalff@ukbonn.de (J.C.K.)
2 Institute of Pathology, University Hospital Bonn, 53127 Bonn, Germany; laura.esser@ukbonn.de (L.E.); glen.kristiansen@ukbonn.de (G.K.); marieta.toma@ukbonn.de (M.I.T.)
3 Department of Internal Medicine I, University Hospital Bonn, 53127 Bonn, Germany; maria.gonzalez-carmona@ukbonn.de (M.G.-C.); tobias.weismueller@ukbonn.de (T.J.W.); christian.strassburg@ukbonn.de (C.P.S.)
* Correspondence: hanno.matthaei@ukbonn.de
† These authors contributed equally to this work.

Abstract: Biliary tract cancer (BTC) is characterized by an intense stromal reaction and a complex landscape of infiltrating immune cells. Evidence is emerging that tumor-infiltrating neutrophils (TINs) have an impact on carcinogenesis and tumor progression. TINs have also been associated with outcomes in various solid malignant tumors but their possible clinical role in BTC is largely unknown. Tissue samples from patients with sporadic BTC ("spBTC" cohort, $N = 53$) and BTC in association with primary sclerosing cholangitis ("PSC-BTC" cohort, $N = 7$) were collected. Furthermore, tissue samples from 27 patients with PSC who underwent liver transplantation ("PSC-LTX" cohort) were investigated. All specimens were assessed for TIN density in invasive and precancerous lesions (biliary intraepithelial neoplasia, BilIN). Most spBTC showed low TIN density (LD, 61%). High TIN density (HD) was detected in 16% of the tumors, whereas 23% were classified as intermediate density (ID); the majority of both HD and ID groups were in T1–T2 tumors (83% and 100%, $p = 0.012$). TIN density in BilIN lesions did not significantly differ among the three groups. The HD group had a mean overall survival (OS) of 53.5 months, whereas the mean OS in the LD and ID groups was significantly shorter (LD 29.5 months vs. ID 24.6 months, log-rank $p < 0.05$). The results of this study underline the possible prognostic relevance of TINs in BTC and stress the complexity of the immune cell landscape in BTC. The prognostic relevance of TINs suggests a key regulator role in inflammation and immune landscape in BTC.

Keywords: cholangiocarcinoma; biliary tract cancer; prognosis; neutrophils

1. Introduction

Biliary tract cancers (BTC) are a heterogeneous group of malignancies arising from the epithelial cells of the intra- and extrahepatic biliary ductal system and gallbladder. These tumors account for approximately 3% of all gastrointestinal cancers and represent the second most common primary liver tumor [1,2]. Hence, BTC are rare, while in particular the incidence of intrahepatic cholangiocarcinoma is on the rise in Western countries [3]. BTC is one of the most aggressive cancer entities and radical surgery represents the only curative option [4]. However, only about 30% of patients with BTC are resectable at the time of first presentation [5]. Even after radical surgery, the median overall survival barely reaches three years [6].

Several risk factors for the development of BTC have been identified, such as chronic inflammation through primary sclerosing cholangitis (PSC), viral hepatitis, liver cirrhosis, and liver fluke [7]. In fact, BTC is histologically characterized by an intense stromal reaction while the stroma is densely populated by cancer-associated fibroblasts (CAF) and various infiltrating immune cells such as monocytes and tumor-associated macrophages (TAM). These inflammatory cells likely play a predominant role in tumor development and progression [8,9]. Thus, a biomarker function of easily obtainable systemic inflammation markers such as C-reactive protein (CRP), neutrophils to lymphocytes ratio (NLR), and platelets to lymphocytes ratio (PLR) has been intensely investigated in BTC in the recent years with remarkable success [10–14]. Neutrophils are the most abundant white blood cell subtype, thereby representing a crucial component of the innate immune system. While the main function of neutrophils is to fight infections by phagocytosis and elimination of microorganisms, a chronic neutrophilic inflammation has been associated with the early phase of various epithelial cancers. Interestingly, evidence is emerging that tumor-infiltrating neutrophils (TINs) are impacting progression and spread in later phases of the disease. Apparently, malignant tumors have the ability to induce myelopoiesis and to attract neutrophils to the tumor microenvironment. Here, these cells gather a protumorigenic, immunosuppressive phenotype, whereas the exact mechanisms and possible targeted therapies are currently under investigation [15]. Not surprisingly, TINs have been associated with outcome in various solid tumors [16,17]. However, their presence and possible prognostic role in BTC is still largely unknown and focus of the present study.

2. Methods

2.1. Patients and Tissues

For this monocentric retrospective study, data from three different patient cohorts were collected and analyzed.

2.1.1. Patients with Surgically Resected Sporadic Biliary Tract Cancer (spBTC Cohort)

Tissue samples from 53 patients who underwent surgical resection for sporadic BTC (spBTC) between 2013 and 2018 at the Department of Surgery, Bonn University Hospital, were collected. Only patients without previous radiochemotherapy were selected. All patients were operated on in the absence of clinical signs of an acute infection. Patient serum was obtained shortly before surgery and analyzed for carcinoembryonic antigen (CEA), carbohydrate antigen 19.9 (CA19.9), and C reactive protein (CRP). Therapy options for every patient were discussed in our weekly interdisciplinary tumor board and all patients included were offered surgical resection. Demographic and clinical data, including age, gender, postoperative complications, hospital stay, and adjuvant chemotherapy were retrieved from the patients' records. Tumor samples from the resected specimens were fixed in formalin and embedded in paraffin (FFPE) according to a standardized protocol. Survival data were available for all patients. The usage of archived diagnostic left-over tissues for tissue microarray (TMA) manufacturing, the analysis for research purposes, and patient data analysis were approved by the ethics committee, Bonn University Hospital (IRB number: 417/17). The study was carried out in compliance with the Helsinki Declaration.

2.1.2. Patients with Primary Sclerosing Cholangitis and BTC (PSC-BTC Cohort)

Tissue samples from 7 patients with primary sclerosing cholangitis and BTC (PSC-BTC) were retrieved from archived diagnostic left-over FFPE tissue. All patients were operated on between 2010 and 2017 at the Department of Surgery, Bonn University Hospital. All tumor samples were obtained for diagnostic reasons during radical tumor resection or explorative laparotomy and open biopsy. A survival analysis was not performed in this cohort due to the small number of patients.

2.1.3. Patients with PSC Who Underwent Liver Transplantation (PSC-LTX Cohort)

Tissue samples from 27 patients with PSC who underwent liver transplantation between 2003 and 2017 at the Department of Surgery, Bonn University Hospital, were collected from FFPE left-over tissue. A mean of 12 samples per patient, each from different localizations along the biliary ductal system, were analyzed. A survival analysis was not performed in this cohort due to the small number of patients.

2.2. Tissue Microarray Construction and Tumor-Infiltrating Neutrophil (TIN) Density Score Analysis in Sporadic BTC

For spBTC, a tissue microarray (TMA) was constructed according to standardized protocols. Briefly, four to six different 1 mm cores were taken from every tissue sample. For internal controls, normal kidney and normal liver tissue cores were included in each TMA block. A 2 µm section was stained following a standard hematoxylin and eosin staining protocol. Neutrophils were counted in each core by an experienced pathologist, who was blinded to tumor stage and patient characteristics. Apoptotic neutrophils, as well as neutrophils found inside the lumen of blood vessels were excluded. Then, the mean value was calculated for each tumor, as well as the 60 and the 85 percentile which we used as cut-offs. The use of these cut-offs was arbitrary in order to classified samples into "low density" if the TIN density score was lower than the 60th percentile (LD, score 0), "intermediate density", if the TIN density score was between the 60th and 85th percentiles (ID, score 1), or "high density" if the TIN density score was higher than the 85th percentile (HD, score 2).

2.3. Neutrophils Density Analysis in Biliary Intraepithelial Neoplasia (BilIN)

For spBTC and PSC-BTC cohorts, diagnostic slides were reviewed for the presence of high-grade biliary intraepithelial neoplasia (BilIN) in the tumor proximity. For the PSC patients with PSC who underwent liver transplantation (PSC-LTX) cohort, all diagnostic slides were reviewed for the presence of high-grade BilIN in bile ducts. In the presence of multiple BilIN lesions, one representative high-grade BilIN was randomly selected. The total number of neutrophils in six 40× microscopic fields (three intraepithelial/intratumoral fields and three in periepithelial stroma) were assessed. Neutrophils that were identified in blood vessels were not counted. The mean value for each localization was then calculated.

2.4. BTC and BilIN Classification

All tumors were reclassified according to the UICC (Union for International Cancer Control) TNM classification system by the International Union Against Cancer, 8th Edition [18]. BilINs were classified according to established histopathological characteristics such as degree of cellular and structural atypia as recommended [19,20].

2.5. Statistical Analysis

Statistical analysis was performed in the R environment (RStudio Version 1.3, package survminer version 0.4.8) and SPSS Statistics Version 22 (IBM, Armonk, New York, NY, USA) [21,22]. Continuous variables are shown as mean or median with interquartile range (IQR). Univariate analysis was performed, and Kaplan–Meier (KM) plots were generated for overall survival (OS). KM curves were compared using the log-rank test. Multivariate analyses for OS were performed using the Cox regression method. Variables which were significant in the univariate analysis were included in the Cox regression model. Mean OS was indicated if the median OS was not reached. Comparisons between groups were made with Fisher's exact test or Anova test, as appropriate. Pearson's correlation analysis for TIN density in BilIN was performed and displayed as scatter plot. Statistical significance was assumed at a p-value < 0.05.

3. Results

3.1. Patient Characteristics

A total of 53 patients (29 females and 24 males, median age 67, range 38–81) were enrolled in the spBTC cohort. A majority of tumors was diagnosed as intrahepatic cholangiocarcinoma (IHC, N = 19, 36%), followed by distal cholangiocarcinoma (DC, N = 14, 26%), and perihilar cholangiocarcinoma (PHC, N = 13, 24%). A gallbladder carcinoma (GBCA) was diagnosed in seven patients (13%). Median preoperative CA19.9 and CEA levels were 53.6 kU/L (IQR 26.9–359 kU/L) and 2.2 ng/mL (IQR 1.2–3.0 ng/mL), respectively. Median preoperative CRP level was 17.2 mg/L (IQR 7.2–59.5 mg/L). Most primary tumors were classified pT2 (N = 19, 36%) or pT3 (N = 19, 36%), whereas 28% of the patients were staged pT1 (N = 15, 28%). A positive nodal status was found in 57% of the patients (N1, N = 30). Four patients (7%) with apparently resectable disease had to be classified M1 according to the final pathology report due to peritoneal carcinomatosis. Most tumors were moderately differentiated (G2, N = 31, 58%). Postoperative adjuvant chemotherapy was administered in a majority of patients (N = 33, 62%). Characteristics of the spBTC cohort are summarized in Table 1.

Table 1. Patient's characteristics according to the extent of tumor-infiltrating neutrophils (TINs) in resected biliary tract cancer (BTC).

		All Patients N = 53 n, mean, median (%, SD, or IQR)	TIN Density Low N = 31 n, mean, median (%, SD, or IQR)	TIN Density Intermediate N = 12 n, mean, median (%, SD, or IQR)	TIN Density High N = 8 n, mean, median (%, SD, or IQR)	p *
Sex	W	29 (54.7)	18 (58.1)	5 (41.7)	4 (50.0)	0.624
	M	24 (45.3)	13 (41.9)	7 (58.3)	4 (50.0)	
Age	≤67	28 (52.8)	16 (51.6)	7 (58.3)	4 (50.0)	0.925
	>67	25 (47.2)	15 (48.4)	5 (41.7)	4 (50.0)	
CA19-9		53.6 (26.9–359.0)	53.6 (28.3–160.4)	61.8 (20.3–360.4)	36.4 (29.7–1164.6)	0.325
CEA		2.2 (1.2–3.0)	2.4 (1.4–3.3)	2.2 (1.1–4.6)	1.2 (0.9–1.3)	0.080
CRP		17.2 (7.2–59.5)	24.7 (9.50–75.50)	11.0 (4.9–31.2)	19.4 (6.2–26.7)	0.396
Localization	IHC	19 (35.8)	10 (32.3)	5 (41.7)	4 (50.0)	0.312
	PHC	13 (24.5)	6 (19.4)	2 (16.7)	3 (37.5)	
	DC	14 (26.4)	8 (25.8)	5 (41.7)	1 (12.5)	
	GBC	7 (13.2)	7 (22.6)	0 (0.0)	0 (0.0)	
T	T1	15 (28.3)	6 (19.4)	4 (33.3)	4 (50.0)	0.012
	T2	19 (35.8)	8 (25.8)	6 (50.0)	4 (50.0)	
	T3	19 (35.8)	17 (54.8)	2 (16.7)	0 (0.0)	
	T4	0 (0)	0 (0.0)	0 (0.0)	0 (0.0)	
N	N0	23 (43.4)	9 (29.3)	9 (75.0)	4 (50)	0.025
	N1	30 (56.6)	22 (71.0)	3 (25.0)	4 (50)	
M	M0	49 (92.5)	27 (87.1)	12 (100.0)	8 (100.0)	0.462
	M1	4 (7.5)	4 (12.9)	0 (0.0)	0 (0.0)	
L	L0	39 (73.6)	22 (71.0)	9 (75.0)	7 (87.5)	0.743
	L1	14 (26.4)	9 (29.0)	3 (25.0)	1 (12.5)	
V	V0	44 (83.0)	24 (77.4)	11 (91.7)	7 (87.5)	0.671
	V1	9 (17.0)	7 (22.6)	1 (8.3)	1 (12.5)	
Pn	Pn0	24 (45.3)	13 (41.9)	6 (50.0)	3 (37.5)	0.851
	Pn1	29 (54.7)	18 (58.9)	6 (50.0)	5 (62.5)	
G	G1	3 (5.7)	2 (6.5)	1 (8.3)	0 (0.0)	0.517
	G2	31 (58.5)	18 (58.1)	8 (66.7)	3 (37.5)	
	G3	19 (35.8)	11 (35.5)	3 (25.0)	5 (62.5)	
R	R0	42 (79.2)	25 (80.6)	11 (91.7)	5 (62.5)	0.285
	R+	11 (20.8)	6 (19.4)	1 (8.3)	3 (37.5)	
Stage	Stage I	9 (17.0)	1 (3.2)	4 (33.3)	3 (37.5)	0.010
	Stage II	19 (35.8)	12 (38.7)	6 (50.0)	1 (12.5)	
	Stage III	20 (37.7)	14 (45.2)	1 (8.3)	4 (50.0)	
	Stage IV	5 (9.4)	4 (12.9)	1 (8.3)	0 (0.0)	
Postoperative Complications	Yes	28 (52.8)	16 (51.6)	6 (50.0)	5 (62.5)	0.837
	No	25 (47.2)	15 (48.4)	6 (50.0)	3 (37.5)	
Chemotherapy	Yes	33 (62.3)	22 (71.0)	6 (50.0)	4 (50.0)	0.356
	No	20 (37.7)	9 (29.0)	6 (50.0)	4 (50.0)	

3.2. Correlation of TIN Density with Clinicopathologic Parameters

Among the tumor samples, 16% were classified as tumors with a high TIN density ($N = 8$), while 23% were classified as intermediate ($N = 12$), and 61% were classified as low TIN-density tumors ($N = 31$). Two samples had to be excluded from the analysis because of tissue fragmentation during TMA preparation. Representative images of tumor sections with different TIN densities are displayed in Figure 1.

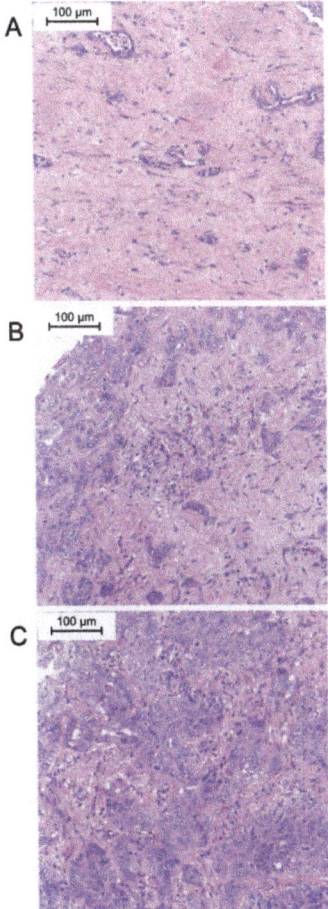

Figure 1. Examples of high-resolution microscopy images of biliary tract cancer with low (**A**), intermediate (**B**), and high (**C**) TIN density (hematoxylin and eosin staining).

The demographics of the three groups were similar regarding age (mean age 67 in the LD group vs. 66 in the ID group vs. 67 in the HD group) and gender (58% females and 42% males in the LD group vs. 42% females and 58% males in the ID group and 50% females vs. 50% males in the HD group). Tumor stage distribution differed significantly in the three groups, since in the LD group the most represented T stage was T3 ($N = 17$, 55%). In the ID group, the majority of the patients had T1–T2 tumors ($N = 10, 83\%$) and 17% ($N = 2$), also in the HD group, all had a comparatively smaller T1–T2 primary tumor ($p = 0.012$). The rate of N+ tumors was also significantly different in the three groups. In the LD group, 71% ($N = 22$) had a positive nodal status as compared with 25% ($N = 3$) in the ID group and 50% ($N = 4$) in the HD group ($p = 0.025$). No difference was observed regarding preoperative CA19.9, CEA, CRP, tumor location, M stage, grading, as well as lymphovascular and perineural invasion. Most of the tumors in the LD were IHC ($N = 10$, 32%) followed by DC ($N = 8$, 26%), GBC ($N = 7$, 23%), and PHC ($N = 6$, 19%). In the ID group, IHC and DC were the most represented tumor localizations ($N = 5$, 42%), followed by PHC ($N = 2$, 17%). In the HD group, IHC were the most frequent tumors ($N = 4$, 50%), followed by PHC ($N = 3$, 37%) and DC ($N = 1$, 12%) The LD group was the only group with samples from GBCA patients. The abovementioned varying TIN densities according to T stage and positive nodal status were mirrored in the respective UICC stages. In fact, in the LD group, most patients had advanced UICC stages III or IV, in the ID group the majority of the patients had earlier UICC stages I or II, and in the HD group 50% had a UICC stage I or II ($p = 0.010$). Clinicopathological characteristics of the three groups are summarized in Table 1.

3.3. Correlation of TIN Density with Outcome

Median follow-up time was 19.4 months (range 0.2–60 months). The HD group had a mean OS of 53.5 months (standard error (SE) 6.0, 95% confidence interval (CI) 41.7–65.4), whereas the mean OS in the LD and ID groups was significantly shorter (LD group, 29.5 months, SE 3.9, 95% CI 21.7–37.3, log-rank $p < 0.05$ and ID group, 24.6 months, SE 6.0, 95% CI 11.8–37.4, log-rank $p < 0.05$). The Kaplan–Meier plot in Figure 2 displays OS probabilities stratified for neutrophil density.

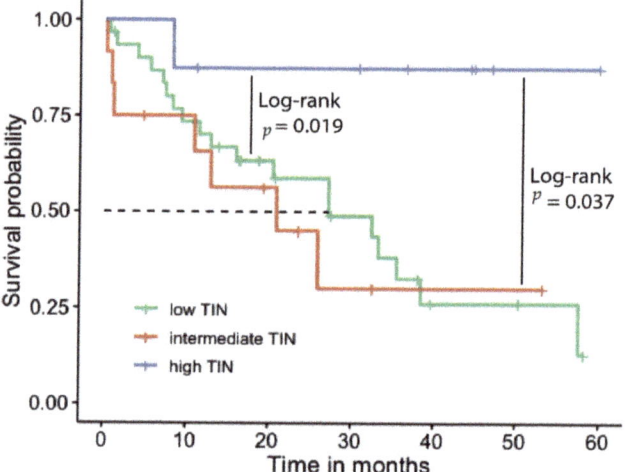

Figure 2. Kaplan–Meier (KM) plot showing survival probability stratified for tumor infiltrating neutrophiles (TIN) density. From the log-rank, only significant p-values are displayed.

In the univariate survival analysis, a correlation with poor prognosis in HD vs. ID (hazard ratio (HR) 10.10, 95% confidence interval (CI) 1.22–83.50, $p = 0.032$) was found. When comparing HD vs. LD, a similar correlation with prognosis was found (HR 7.66, 95% CI 1.02–57.53, $p = 0.048$). In addition, univariate analysis showed that a UICC stage III was significantly associated with poorer prognosis as compared with UICC stage I (HR 4.48, 95% CI 1.01–19.92, $p = 0.049$). The results of the univariate analyses are summarized in Table 2. The results of the multivariate analysis are summarized in Supplementary Table S1.

Table 2. Results of the univariate analysis.

Endpoint	Subgroup	HR	CI 95%	p
	Age > 67 vs. ≤67	1.17	0.55–2.47	0.678
	Female vs. Male	1.02	0.48–2.14	0.963
	CEA high vs. low	1.75	0.73–4.20	0.207
	CA19.9 high vs. low	1.78	0.82–3.84	0.145
	TIN intermediate vs. high	10.10	1.22–83.50	0.032
	TIN low vs. high	7.66	1.02–57.53	0.048
	Complications Yes vs. No	1.30	0.61–2.78	0.498
	G2 vs. G1	1.63	0.22–12.34	0.636
	G3 vs. G1	1.72	0.22–13.66	0.607
	T2 vs. T1	0.83	0.31–2.23	0.706
	T3 vs. T1	1.26	0.51–3.11	0.612
	N1 vs. N0	1.69	0.79–3.62	0.179
	M1 vs. M0	1.07	0.25–4.53	0.927
	Stage 2 vs. Stage 1	3.23	0.71–14.66	0.128
	Stage 3 vs. Stage 1	4.48	1.01–19.92	0.049
	Stage 4 vs. Stage 1	3.15	0.44–22.51	0.254
	R1 vs. R0	1.30	0.52–3.25	0.579
	V1 vs. V0	1.74	0.70–4.34	0.234
	L1 vs. L0	0.82	0.33–2.05	0.676
	Pn1 vs. Pn0	1.39	0.65–2.95	0.394
	Chemotherapy Yes vs. No	0.62	0.29–1.31	0.208

3.4. Neutrophil Infiltration in BTC-Associated BilIN

In the spBTC cohort, 23% of the patients ($N = 12$) had at least one high-grade BilIN lesion in the analyzed slides displaying their primary adenocarcinoma. In the PSC-BTC cohort, 57% of the patients ($N = 4$) had at least one high-grade BilIN lesion near the tumor. In the PSC-LTX cohort, at least one BilIN lesion was found in 25% of the explanted liver samples ($N = 7$). The mean TINs in the BilIN lesions from the cohort of patients with PSC who underwent LTX did not significantly differ from the mean TINs of BilIN lesions adjacent to sporadic BTC and PSC-associated BTC (7.0, standard deviation (SD) 8.1 vs. 4.9, SD 5.7 vs. 4.0, SD 2.5, $p > 0.05$) (Figure 3).

A positive correlation between intraepithelial TIN and stromal TIN was observed (Pearson's $R = 0.51$, $p = 0.025$). The number of TINs in spBTC and PSC-BTC lesions did not correlate with the number of neutrophils infiltrating adjacent BilIN lesions (Pearson's $R = 0.16$, $p = 0.63$). Patient characteristics of the PSC-LTX and PSC-BTC cohorts are summarized in the Supplementary Table S2.

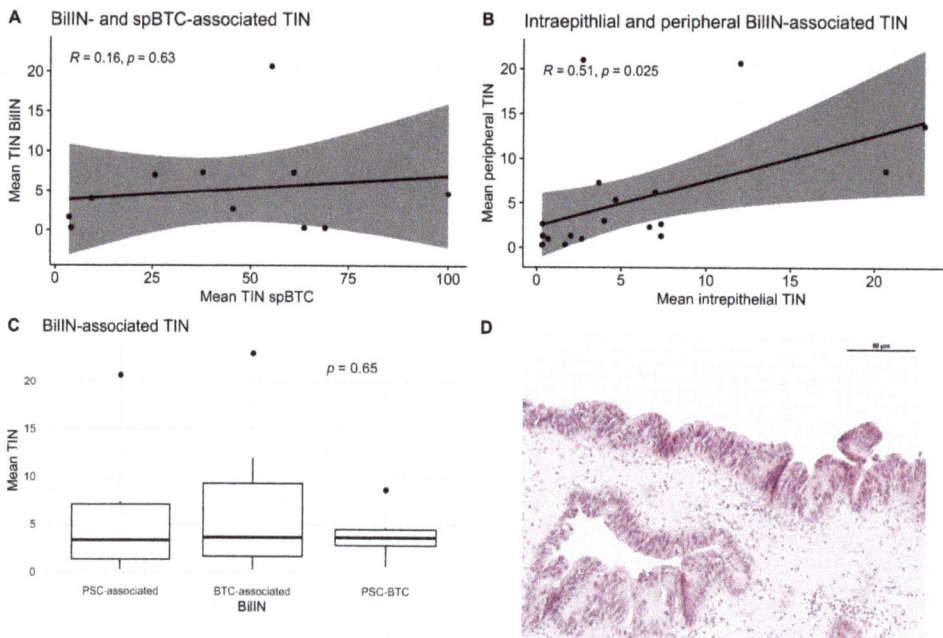

Figure 3. Scatter plot showing the relationship between tumor-infiltrating neutrophils (TINs) in spBTC and BTC-associated biliary intraepithelial neoplasia (BilIN) (**A**) and between intraepithelial and peripheral (stromal) TINs in BilIN lesions (**B**). Best-fitting lines and 95% confidence intervals as well as R coefficients and *p* values are displayed. Boxplots displaying mean infiltrating neutrophils (TINs) in BilIN from patients with primary sclerosing cholangitis (PSC), in sporadic BTC-associated BilIN and in PSC-related, BTC-associated BilIN (PSC-BTC). The lower and upper hinges correspond to the 25th and 75th percentiles. The upper/lower whiskers represent the largest/smallest observation less/greater than or equal to upper/lower hinge +/− 1.5 times the interquartile range (**C**). Exemplary section of a high-grade BilIN lesion from a patient with BTC. (hematoxylin/eosin staining) (**D**).

4. Discussion

Neutrophils are a crucial component of the human innate immunity and the first circulating cellular responders in the case of acute tissue damage and infections. In cancer, neutrophils play a pivotal role in the tumor microenvironment and can acquire an antitumor (N1) or a protumor (N2) phenotype [23].

Several soluble factors produced by tumor cells promote TIN recruitment. Among others, CXCL1, CXCL2, CXCL5, CXCL6, IL17, IL 8, and CCL3 have been found to act as potent TIN chemoattractants [23]. TIN recruitment is followed by a polarization in either N1 or N2 phenotype due to a complex cytokine stimulation promoted directly from tumor cells and other tumor microenvironment cells [24]. Transforming growth factor-β (TGF-β) and interferon-β (IFN-β) have been found to be one of the most important promoters of neutrophil polarization in mice [25,26]. Therefore, some studies have addressed the possible use of TGF-β inhibition as a therapeutic approach in cancer [26]. However, the N1/2 polarization as well as the role of TINs in human cancers are still controversial [27].

Inflammation and inflammatory mediators are the hallmark of several risk factors associated with BTC [7]. In PSC, chronic inflammation of the bile ducts has been linked to the increased risk of BTC in this population [28]. Choledocholithiasis and cholecystolithiasis are characterized by cholestasis and chronic inflammation and are also considered risk factors for BTC [29]. Liver fluke infections, viral infections, and cirrhosis are similarly linked to cholangiocarcinogenesis [28].

Neutrophil infiltration has been evidenced and comprehensively investigated in various solid tumors revealing heterogeneous results. As such, high neutrophil infiltration proved to be related to chemosensitivity and longer recurrence-free survival in high-grade ovarian cancer [30]. Furthermore, high levels of intratumoral granulocytes negatively correlates with cancer-specific survival in patients with clear cell renal cell carcinoma [31]. In hepatocellular carcinoma, neutrophil infiltration has been shown to be a negative prognosticator after curative resection, correlating with angiogenesis progression and tumor recurrence in this entity [32–34]. Ino et al. described similar results in patients with resected adenocarcinomas of the pancreas [35]. The role of TINs has also been investigated in BTC. Gu et al. found that presence of TINs was significantly associated with adverse OS in a cohort of intrahepatic cholangiocarcinomas [36]. Another study found that a high density of CD15 (a carbohydrate epitope expressed on neutrophils) positive neutrophils correlated with shorter OS in cholangiocarcinoma [37]. In our cohort, we observed that patients with tumors with higher neutrophil infiltration had a better prognosis as compared with those with tumors of low or intermediate neutrophil infiltration. Our results regarding OS in resected BTC revealed intriguing aspects. On the one hand, tumors with the highest infiltration showed a longer OS as compared with the group with intermediate infiltration. On the other hand, the group with intermediate TIN infiltration had a tendency of worse OS as compared with the group with low TIN infiltration. However, in the group with high TIN infiltration, there were only T1 and T2 tumors. Moreover, the group with low TINs had a significantly higher N+ tumors as compared with the other groups. This could represent an important confounding factor, and therefore the results of the survival analysis should be interpreted with caution. A multivariate survival analysis of a larger cohort with matched groups could address this topic, provide more robust results, and reduce the bias. The different prognosis among the groups could also be explained based on the complexity of the tumor immune microenvironment in BTC, which includes tumor-associated fibroblasts, tumor-associated macrophages (TAM), dendritic cells, natural killer cells, and myeloid-derived suppressor cells. All these cells contribute to both tumor immunosurveillance and immunosuppressive functions. The tumors with high TINs in our cohort may represent a subgroup with a high immunological antitumoral activity. In fact, previous studies have reported that tumor-associated neutrophils could have a dual role. On the one hand, in early tumors, neutrophils could play a role in stimulating T-cell response [38]. On the other hand, neutrophils have an immunosuppressive activity in advanced tumors [39]. In our cohort, the tumors with high TINs were T1 and T2 tumors, whereas in the group with intermediate TIN, T1 to T3 stage tumors were represented. However, this could confirm previous observations about the dual role of TINs in cancer. Interestingly, the number of infiltrating neutrophils in BilINs did not significantly differ from those adjacent to sporadic BTC and those found in patients with PSC with or without BTC. Therefore, it is reasonable to think that neutrophils play a role in the development of a subset of BTC from BilIN towards invasive carcinoma, thus, underlying their tumor-promoting activity in early stage, possibly independent of predisposition.

Our study has some limitations. Firstly, our monocentric cohort was too small to build a proper validation of our preliminary findings which we anticipate in the future. In particular, due to the small BTC cohort and the small number of samples per group, a definitive conclusion about the prognostic role of TINs cannot be reached. A multicentric research effort could potentially address this limitation. Moreover, a multivariate survival analysis of matched groups could help by reducing the bias deriving from unbalanced groups. The retrospective design of this study carries intrinsic limitations, which should be taken into account when interpreting the results. In addition, our study did not focus on further TIN characterization. It is already known that infiltrating neutrophils have different phenotypes and capabilities, which lead to heterogeneous inflammatory responses [40]. This topic has not yet been deeply investigated in BTC and represents an intriguing research field with promising translational implications. Nonetheless, the phenotypical characterization of TINs was not the aim of the present study which mainly focused on prognostic implication. Furthermore, we enrolled patients with BTC irrespective of anatomical localization. This may be relevant when assessing prognostic factors for this tumor. However, some authors have described similar outcome for patients with BTC from different localizations but with comparable pathological characteristics [41]. BTCs are believed to be a stem cell-based disease and there are probably several different BTC stem cell populations involved in carcinogenesis [42,43]. In addition, there is growing evidence of a heterogeneous genetic landscape in BTC [44]. Due to the rareness and similar clinical behavior, we should find a prognostic factor that could be useful to the entire population of BTC patients, despite the proven heterogeneity of BTC.

5. Conclusions

In summary, the results of this study underline the frequency and possible prognostic relevance of TINs in BTC. Our clinically apparent, though somewhat ambivalent, results stress the complexity of the immune cell landscape in this fatal cancer entity that deserves further scientific dedication. The role of TINs as a prognostic factor in BTC remains unclear. The prognostic relevance of TINs should be further investigated in order to determine if neutrophils may act as a key regulator of inflammation and immune status in BTC. Further studies addressing the role of TINs would hopefully provide new insights to elucidate the associated tumor microenvironment for clinical implications in BTC.

Supplementary Materials: The following are available online at https://www.mdpi.com/2075-4426/11/3/233/s1, Table S1: Patient characteristics of the PSC-LTX and PSC-BTC cohort, Table S2: Multivariate analysis.

Author Contributions: Conceptualization, V.B., B.J., M.I.T., and H.M.; Data curation, V.B., B.J., J.H., S.M., M.I.T., and H.M.; Formal analysis, V.B., B.J., L.E., and M.I.T.; Methodology, M.I.T. and H.M.; Project administration, H.M.; Supervision, J.C.K., M.I.T., and H.M.; Writing—original draft, V.B., B.J., L.E., and H.M.; Writing—review and editing, M.G.-C., T.J.W., C.P.S., J.H., A.S., P.L., S.M., G.K., and J.C.K. All authors have read and agreed to the published version of the manuscript.

Funding: V.B. received a post-doctoral fellowship grant from the Else-Kröner Fresenius Stiftung (grant number 2014_Kolleg.05).

Institutional Review Board Statement: All the procedures in this study involving human participants were performed in accordance with the ethical standards of the institutional and national research committee and with the 1964 Helsinki Declaration and its later amendments or comparable ethical standards. The usage of archived diagnostic left-over tissues for TMA manufacturing, the analysis for research purposes, and patient data analysis were approved by the ethics committee, Bonn University Hospital (IRB number 417/17).

Informed Consent Statement: Patient consent was waived due to the retrospective character of the study and the usage of archived diagnostic left-over tissues.

Data Availability Statement: The data presented in this study are available upon reasonable request from the corresponding author.

Acknowledgments: The authors would like to express their gratitude to Kerstin Fuchs and Seher Aktekin for their outstanding technical support.

Conflicts of Interest: The authors declare no conflict of interest.

References

1. Fitzmaurice, C.; Dicker, D.; Pain, A.; Hamavid, H.; Moradi-Lakeh, M.; MacIntyre, M.F.; Allen, C.; Hansen, G.; Woodbrook, R.; Wolfe, C.; et al. The global burden of cancer 2013. *JAMA Oncol.* **2015**, *1*, 505. [CrossRef] [PubMed]
2. Siegel, R.L.; Miller, K.D.; Jemal, A. Cancer statistics, 2020. *CA Cancer J. Clin.* **2020**, *70*, 7–30. [CrossRef] [PubMed]
3. Saha, S.K.; Zhu, A.X.; Fuchs, C.S.; Brook, S.G.A. Forty-year trends in cholangiocarcinoma incidence in the U.S.: Intrahepatic disease on the rise. *Oncologist* **2016**, *21*. [CrossRef] [PubMed]
4. Valle, J.W.; Borbath, I.; Khan, S.A.; Huguet, F.; Gruenberger, T.; Arnold, D. ESMO guidelines committee biliary cancer: ESMO clinical practice guidelines for diagnosis, treatment and follow-up. *Ann. Oncol. Off. J. Eur. Soc. Med. Oncol.* **2016**, *27*, v28–v37. [CrossRef]

5. Bridgewater, J.; Galle, P.R.; Khan, S.A.; Llovet, J.M.; Park, J.W.; Patel, T.; Pawlik, T.M.; Gores, G.J. Guidelines for the diagnosis and management of intrahepatic cholangiocarcinoma. *J. Hepatol.* **2014**, *60*, 1268–1289. [CrossRef]
6. Endo, I.; Gonen, M.; Yopp, A.C.; Dalal, K.M.; Zhou, Q.; Klimstra, D.; D'Angelica, M.; DeMatteo, R.P.; Fong, Y.; Schwartz, L.; et al. Intrahepatic cholangiocarcinoma: Rising frequency, improved survival, and determinants of outcome after resection. *Ann. Surg.* **2008**, *248*, 84–96. [CrossRef]
7. Boonstra, K.; Weersma, R.K.; van Erpecum, K.J.; Rauws, E.A.; Spanier, B.W.M.; Poen, A.C.; van Nieuwkerk, K.M.; Drenth, J.P.; Witteman, B.J.; Tuynman, H.A.; et al. Population-based epidemiology, malignancy risk, and outcome of primary sclerosing cholangitis. *Hepatology* **2013**, *58*, 2045–2055. [CrossRef]
8. Hasita, H.; Komohara, Y.; Okabe, H.; Masuda, T.; Ohnishi, K.; Lei, X.F.; Beppu, T.; Baba, H.; Takeya, M. Significance of alternatively activated macrophages in patients with intrahepatic cholangiocarcinoma. *Cancer Sci.* **2010**, *101*, 1913–1919. [CrossRef]
9. Cadamuro, M.; Morton, S.D.; Strazzabosco, M.; Fabris, L. Unveiling the role of tumor reactive stroma in cholangiocarcinoma: An opportunity for new therapeutic strategies. *Transl. Gastroenterol. Cancer* **2013**, *2*, 130–144. [CrossRef]
10. McNamara, M.G.; Templeton, A.J.; Maganti, M.; Walter, T.; Horgan, A.M.; McKeever, L.; Min, T.; Amir, E.; Knox, J.J. Neutrophil/lymphocyte ratio as a prognostic factor in biliary tract cancer. *Eur. J. Cancer Oxf. Engl. 1990* **2014**, *50*, 1581–1589. [CrossRef]
11. Chen, Q.; Yang, L.-X.; Li, X.-D.; Yin, D.; Shi, S.-M.; Chen, E.-B.; Yu, L.; Zhou, Z.-J.; Zhou, S.-L.; Shi, Y.-H.; et al. The elevated preoperative neutrophil-to-lymphocyte ratio predicts poor prognosis in intrahepatic cholangiocarcinoma patients undergoing hepatectomy. *Tumour Biol. J. Int. Soc. Oncodev. Biol. Med.* **2015**, *36*, 5283–5289. [CrossRef]
12. Zhang, Y.; Jiang, C.; Li, J.; Sun, J.; Qu, X. Prognostic significance of preoperative neutrophil/lymphocyte ratio and platelet/lymphocyte ratio in patients with gallbladder carcinoma. *Clin. Transl. Oncol. Off. Publ. Fed. Span. Oncol. Soc. Natl. Cancer Inst. Mex.* **2015**, *17*, 810–818. [CrossRef]
13. Lin, G.; Liu, Y.; Li, S.; Mao, Y.; Wang, J.; Shuang, Z.; Chen, J.; Li, S. Elevated neutrophil-to-lymphocyte ratio is an independent poor prognostic factor in patients with intrahepatic cholangiocarcinoma. *Oncotarget* **2016**, *7*, 50963–50971. [CrossRef]
14. Yeh, Y.-C.; Lei, H.-J.; Chen, M.-H.; Ho, H.-L.; Chiu, L.-Y.; Li, C.-P.; Wang, Y.-C. C-Reactive Protein (CRP) is a promising diagnostic immunohistochemical marker for intrahepatic cholangiocarcinoma and is associated with better prognosis. *Am. J. Surg. Pathol.* **2017**, *41*, 1630–1641. [CrossRef]
15. Rapoport, B.L.; Steel, H.C.; Theron, A.J.; Smit, T.; Anderson, R. Role of the neutrophil in the pathogenesis of advanced cancer and impaired responsiveness to therapy. *Molecules* **2020**, *25*, 1618. [CrossRef]
16. Zhang, H.; Liu, H.; Shen, Z.; Lin, C.; Wang, X.; Qin, J.; Qin, X.; Xu, J.; Sun, Y. Tumor-infiltrating neutrophils is prognostic and predictive for postoperative adjuvant chemotherapy benefit in patients with gastric cancer. *Ann. Surg.* **2018**, *267*, 311–318. [CrossRef]
17. Zeindler, J.; Angehrn, F.; Droeser, R.; Däster, S.; Piscuoglio, S.; Ng, C.K.Y.; Kilic, E.; Mechera, R.; Meili, S.; Isaak, A.; et al. Infiltration by myeloperoxidase-positive neutrophils is an independent prognostic factor in breast cancer. *Breast Cancer Res. Treat.* **2019**, *177*, 581–589. [CrossRef]
18. Brierley, J.D.; Gospodarowicz, M.K.; Wittekind, C. *TNM Classification of Malignant Tumours*, 8th ed.; John Wiley & Sons: Hoboken, NJ, USA, 2017; ISBN 978-1-119-26354-8.
19. Zen, Y.; Adsay, N.V.; Bardadin, K.; Colombari, R.; Ferrell, L.; Haga, H.; Hong, S.-M.; Hytiroglou, P.; Klöppel, G.; Lauwers, G.Y.; et al. Biliary intraepithelial neoplasia: An international interobserver agreement study and proposal for diagnostic criteria. *Mod. Pathol.* **2007**, *20*, 701–709. [CrossRef]
20. Basturk, O.; Aishima, S.; Esposito, I. Biliary intraepithelial neoplasia. In *WHO Classification of Tumours: Digestive System Tumours*; WHO Classification of Tumours Editorial Board, International Agency for Research on Cancer: Lyon, France, 2019; Volume 1, ISBN 978-92-832-4499-8.
21. R Core Team. *R: A Language and Environment for Statistical Computing*; R Core Team: Vienna, Austria, 2020.
22. Kassambara, A.; Kosinski, M.; Biecek, P. *Survminer: Drawing Survival Curves Using "Ggplot2"*, 2020.
23. Masucci, M.T.; Minopoli, M.; Carriero, M.V. Tumor associated neutrophils. Their role in tumorigenesis, metastasis, prognosis and therapy. *Front. Oncol.* **2019**, *9*, 1146. [CrossRef]
24. Powell, D.R.; Huttenlocher, A. Neutrophils in the tumor microenvironment. *Trends Immunol.* **2016**, *37*, 41–52. [CrossRef]
25. Fridlender, Z.G.; Sun, J.; Kim, S.; Kapoor, V.; Cheng, G.; Ling, L.; Worthen, G.S.; Albelda, S.M. Polarization of tumor-associated neutrophil phenotype by TGF-β: "N1" versus "N2" TAN. *Cancer Cell* **2009**, *16*, 183–194. [CrossRef]
26. Flavell, R.A.; Sanjabi, S.; Wrzesinski, S.H.; Licona-Limón, P. The polarization of immune cells in the tumour environment by TGFβ. *Nat. Rev. Immunol.* **2010**, *10*, 554–567. [CrossRef]
27. Eruslanov, E.B.; Singhal, S.; Albelda, S.M. Mouse versus human neutrophils in cancer: A major knowledge gap. *Trends Cancer* **2017**, *3*, 149–160. [CrossRef]
28. Roy, S.; Glaser, S.; Chakraborty, S. Inflammation and progression of cholangiocarcinoma: Role of angiogenic and lymphangiogenic mechanisms. *Front. Med.* **2019**, *6*, 293. [CrossRef]
29. Schottenfeld, D.; Beebe-Dimmer, J. Chronic inflammation: A common and important factor in the pathogenesis of Neoplasia. *CA Cancer J. Clin.* **2006**, *56*, 69–83. [CrossRef]

30. Posabella, A.; Köhn, P.; Lalos, A.; Wilhelm, A.; Mechera, R.; Soysal, S.; Muenst, S.; Güth, U.; Stadlmann, S.; Terracciano, L.; et al. High density of CD66B in primary high-grade ovarian cancer independently predicts response to chemotherapy. *J. Cancer Res. Clin. Oncol.* **2020**, *146*, 127–136. [CrossRef]
31. Stenzel, P.J.; Schindeldecker, M.; Tagscherer, K.E.; Foersch, S.; Herpel, E.; Hohenfellner, M.; Hatiboglu, G.; Alt, J.; Thomas, C.; Haferkamp, A.; et al. Prognostic and predictive value of tumor-infiltrating leukocytes and of immune checkpoint molecules PD1 and PDL1 in clear cell renal cell carcinoma. *Transl. Oncol.* **2020**, *13*, 336–345. [CrossRef]
32. Li, Y.-W.; Qiu, S.-J.; Fan, J.; Zhou, J.; Gao, Q.; Xiao, Y.-S.; Xu, Y.-F. Intratumoral neutrophils: A Poor prognostic factor for hepatocellular carcinoma following resection. *J. Hepatol.* **2011**, *54*, 497–505. [CrossRef] [PubMed]
33. Kuang, D.-M.; Zhao, Q.; Wu, Y.; Peng, C.; Wang, J.; Xu, Z.; Yin, X.-Y.; Zheng, L. Peritumoral neutrophils link inflammatory response to disease progression by fostering angiogenesis in hepatocellular carcinoma. *J. Hepatol.* **2011**, *54*, 948–955. [CrossRef] [PubMed]
34. Zhou, S.-L.; Dai, Z.; Zhou, Z.-J.; Wang, X.-Y.; Yang, G.-H.; Wang, Z.; Huang, X.-W.; Fan, J.; Zhou, J. Overexpression of CXCL5 mediates neutrophil infiltration and indicates poor prognosis for hepatocellular carcinoma. *Hepatology* **2012**, *56*, 2242–2254. [CrossRef] [PubMed]
35. Ino, Y.; Yamazaki-Itoh, R.; Shimada, K.; Iwasaki, M.; Kosuge, T.; Kanai, Y.; Hiraoka, N. Immune cell infiltration as an indicator of the immune microenvironment of pancreatic cancer. *Br. J. Cancer* **2013**, *108*, 914–923. [CrossRef]
36. Gu, F.-M.; Gao, Q.; Shi, G.-M.; Zhang, X.; Wang, J.; Jiang, J.-H.; Wang, X.-Y.; Shi, Y.-H.; Ding, Z.-B.; Fan, J.; et al. Intratumoral IL-17+ cells and neutrophils show strong prognostic significance in intrahepatic cholangiocarcinoma. *Ann. Surg. Oncol.* **2012**, *19*, 2506–2514. [CrossRef]
37. Mao, Z.-Y.; Zhu, G.-Q.; Xiong, M.; Ren, L.; Bai, L. Prognostic value of neutrophil distribution in cholangiocarcinoma. *World J. Gastroenterol.* **2015**, *21*, 4961–4968. [CrossRef]
38. Eruslanov, E.B.; Bhojnagarwala, P.S.; Quatromoni, J.G.; Stephen, T.L.; Ranganathan, A.; Deshpande, C.; Akimova, T.; Vachani, A.; Litzky, L.; Hancock, W.W.; et al. Tumor-associated neutrophils stimulate t cell responses in early-stage human lung cancer. *J. Clin. Invest.* **2014**, *124*, 5466–5480. [CrossRef]
39. Wu, P.; Wu, D.; Ni, C.; Ye, J.; Chen, W.; Hu, G.; Wang, Z.; Wang, C.; Zhang, Z.; Xia, W.; et al. ΓδT17 cells promote the accumulation and expansion of myeloid-derived suppressor cells in human colorectal cancer. *Immunity* **2014**, *40*, 785–800. [CrossRef]
40. Singhal, S.; Bhojnagarwala, P.S.; O'Brien, S.; Moon, E.K.; Garfall, A.L.; Rao, A.S.; Quatromoni, J.G.; Stephen, T.L.; Litzky, L.; Deshpande, C.; et al. Origin and role of a subset of tumor-associated neutrophils with antigen-presenting cell features in early-stage human lung cancer. *Cancer Cell* **2016**, *30*, 120–135. [CrossRef]
41. Ercolani, G.; Dazzi, A.; Giovinazzo, F.; Ruzzenente, A.; Bassi, C.; Guglielmi, A.; Scarpa, A.; D'Errico, A.; Pinna, A.D. Intrahepatic, peri-hilar and distal cholangiocarcinoma: Three different locations of the same tumor or three different tumors? *Eur. J. Surg. Oncol.* **2015**, *41*, 1162–1169. [CrossRef]
42. Cardinale, V.; Renzi, A.; Carpino, G.; Torrice, A.; Bragazzi, M.C.; Giuliante, F.; DeRose, A.M.; Fraveto, A.; Onori, P.; Napoletano, C.; et al. Tumorigenesis and neoplastic progression profiles of cancer stem cell subpopulations in cholangiocarcinomas. *Am. J. Pathol.* **2015**, *185*. [CrossRef]
43. Mayr, C.; Ocker, M.; Ritter, M.; Pichler, M.; Neureiter, D.; Kiesslich, T. Biliary tract cancer stem cells-Translational options and challenges. *World J. Gastroenterol.* **2017**, *23*, 2470–2482. [CrossRef]
44. Andersen, J.B.; Spee, B.; Blechacz, B.R.; Avital, I.; Komuta, M.; Barbour, A.; Conner, E.A.; Gillen, M.C.; Roskams, T.; Roberts, L.R.; et al. Genomic and Genetic characterization of cholangiocarcinoma identifies therapeutic targets for tyrosine kinase inhibitors. *Gastroenterology* **2012**, *142*, 1021–1031.e15. [CrossRef]

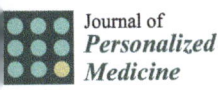

Article

Gender Differences in Patients with Metastatic Pancreatic Cancer Who Received FOLFIRINOX

Jinkook Kim [1], Eunjeong Ji [2], Kwangrok Jung [1], In Ho Jung [1], Jaewoo Park [1], Jong-Chan Lee [1], Jin Won Kim [1], Jin-Hyeok Hwang [1] and Jaihwan Kim [1,*]

1 Department of Internal Medicine, Seoul National University Bundang Hospital, Seoul National University College of Medicine, Seongnam 13620, Korea; newscboy@naver.com (J.K.); herojkr@hanmail.net (K.J.); andpassion@naver.com (I.H.J.); jaewoo0604@naver.com (J.P.); ljc0316@naver.com (J.-C.L.); jwkim@snubh.org (J.W.K.); jhhwang@snubh.org (J.-H.H.)
2 Medical Research Collaborating Center, Seoul National University Bundang Hospital, Seoul National University College of Medicine, Seongnam 13620, Korea; 99145@snubh.org
* Correspondence: drjaihwan@snu.ac.kr; Tel.: +82-31-787-7075 or +82-10-8937-5645; Fax: +82-31-787-4051

Abstract: Background: The combination of 5-fluorouracil, leucovorin, irinotecan, and oxaliplatin (FOLFIRINOX) is a very effective chemotherapeutic regimen for unresectable pancreatic cancer. Previous studies have reported that female gender may be a predictor of a better response to FOLFIRINOX. This study was aimed at investigating the clinical outcomes and dose modification patterns of FOLFIRINOX by gender. Methods: Patients with metastatic pancreatic cancer (MPC) who began FOLFIRINOX as the first-line therapy at Seoul National University Bundang Hospital between 2013 and 2018 were enrolled. The patients received at least four chemotherapy cycles. Local regression and a linear mixed model were used to analyze dose modification patterns by gender. Results: Ninety-seven patients with MPC (54 men; 43 women) were enrolled. In the first FOLFIRINOX cycle, there were significant differences in age and body surface area between the genders (58.8 (men) and 64.9 years (women), $p = 0.005$; 1.7 (men) and 1.6 m^2 (women), $p < 0.001$, respectively). The median progression-free survival (PFS) and overall survival (OS) were 10.8 and 18.0 months, respectively. There was a trend of longer PFS (10.3 (men) and 11.9 months (women), $p = 0.153$) and a significantly longer OS (17.9 (men) and 25.9 months (women), $p = 0.019$) in female patients. During the first year of FOLFIRINOX treatment, there was a significant difference of the age-corrected dose reduction pattern by gender (a mean of 95.6% dose at the initial cycle and −0.35% of dose reduction per week in men versus a mean of 90.7% dose at the initial cycle and −0.53% of dose reduction per week in women, p-value of the slope: <0.001). There was no difference in the adverse event rates between the genders. Conclusions: Female patients showed longer OS despite a more rapid dose reduction during each cycle. Gender differences should be considered during FOLFIRINOX treatment.

Keywords: pancreatic cancer; FOLFIRINOX; chemotherapy; gender

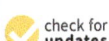

Citation: Kim, J.; Ji, E.; Jung, K.; Jung, I.H.; Park, J.; Lee, J.-C.; Kim, J.W.; Hwang, J.-H.; Kim, J. Gender Differences in Patients with Metastatic Pancreatic Cancer Who Received FOLFIRINOX. *J. Pers. Med.* **2021**, *11*, 83. https://doi.org/10.3390/jpm11020083

Academic Editor: Ari VanderWalde
Received: 7 January 2021
Accepted: 28 January 2021
Published: 30 January 2021

Publisher's Note: MDPI stays neutral with regard to jurisdictional claims in published maps and institutional affiliations.

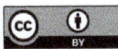

Copyright: © 2021 by the authors. Licensee MDPI, Basel, Switzerland. This article is an open access article distributed under the terms and conditions of the Creative Commons Attribution (CC BY) license (https://creativecommons.org/licenses/by/4.0/).

1. Introduction

Pancreatic cancer is a lethal malignancy and the fourth leading cause of cancer-related death in the United States, with a current 5-year survival rate of only approximately 9% [1]. In up to 85% of patients, pancreatic cancer is diagnosed at an advanced stage because of infiltration of the surrounding vessels or distant metastasis [2]. In patients with metastatic pancreatic cancer (MPC), the combination of 5-fluorouracil (5-FU), leucovorin, irinotecan, and oxaliplatin (FOLFIRINOX) or gemcitabine and nab-paclitaxel resulted in significantly longer overall survival (OS) than that associated with gemcitabine monotherapy [3,4]. Furthermore, FOLFIRINOX has shown excellent efficacy in not only palliative but also adjuvant settings [5], and this regimen has been used as the neoadjuvant chemotherapy in several phase III clinical trials [6]. The mechanism of FOLFIRINOX is regarded as synergistic activity of irinotecan when it is administered before fluorouracil and leucovorin and synergistic activity of irinotecan and oxaliplatin [3]. However, the regimen has been associated with a high incidence of adverse events, including grade 3 or 4 neutropenia and fatigue.

The effects of gender in cancer treatment are not generally considered in preclinical experiments, clinical trials, or real clinical settings. However, there are differences in the efficacies and toxicities of chemotherapeutic agents between male and female patients [7]. For example, 5-FU, which is the backbone of the FOLFIRINOX regimen, degraded more slowly and was associated with higher toxicity in female patients [8,9]. In addition, a previous study reported that female gender may be a predictor of a better response to FOLFIRINOX. In this study, female gender was associated with a significantly higher disease control rate and showed a tendency towards a longer median progression-free survival (PFS) [10]. However, a secondary analysis within the PRODIGE 4/ACCORD 11 trial did not conclusively show a possible effect of gender on the prognosis of patients receiving FOLFIRINOX, because median OS and PFS results in female were superior to those in males, without statistical significance [11]. Therefore, the association remains controversial and elucidation is necessary for further evaluation of the effects of gender. The current study was aimed at investigating gender differences in clinical outcomes and dose modification patterns during FOLFIRINOX chemotherapy in patients with MPC.

2. Materials and Methods

2.1. Patients

Patients with MPC who received the first-line FOLFIRINOX treatment between January 2013 and December 2018 at the Seoul National University Bundang Hospital were retrospectively included. Metastatic pancreatic cancer is defined as cancer that started in the pancreas and spread to areas outside the pancreas, such as the liver, peritoneum, lungs, or distant lymph nodes. The exclusion criteria were as follows: (1) less than four cycles of FOLFIRINOX due to treatment intolerability, adverse events, or a loss to follow up; (2) resectable, borderline resectable, or locally advanced pancreatic cancer at the time of diagnosis; (3) use of FOLFIRINOX as the second-line or later chemotherapy; (4) a history of radiation therapy prior to FOLFIRINOX use; and (5) an Eastern Cooperative Oncology Group Performance Score (ECOG PS) of 2 or higher. The clinical and pathological records of the patients were obtained from a retrospective review of electronic medical records and pathologic reports. Treatment response was evaluated according to response evaluation criteria in solid tumors (RECIST) and the carbohydrate antigen 19 (CA 19-9) was used as a supplementary tool. This study was approved by the institutional review board of Seoul National University Bundang Hospital (IRB# B-1907/550-112).

2.2. Calculation of the Modified Dose of FOLFIRINOX

The FOLFIRINOX regimen was administered in 14 day cycles according to the PRODIGE 4/ACCORD 11 trial [3], with dose reduction or increases of the intervals between cycles decided by a physician. The response to chemotherapy was evaluated every 8 to 12 weeks by using contrast-enhanced computerized tomography and by determining the carbohydrate antigen 19 (CA 19-9) levels. Magnetic resonance imaging or positron emission tomography was also used for evaluation if necessary. FOLFIRINOX administration was continued until the patients showed disease progression or treatment intolerability. The relative dose intensity (RDI) of FOLFIRINOX was defined according to its definition in a previous study performed by our group (Figure 1) [12], in which a modified Hryniuk calculation method was used [13]. Single-agent RDI is the simple proportion of the actual dose delivered compared to the standard dose of each agent (85, 180, 400, and 2400 mg/m^2 for oxaliplatin, irinotecan, 5-FU as a bolus, and 5-FU via continuous intravenous injection, respectively), and the multi-drug RDI was the mathematical average of single-agent RDIs.

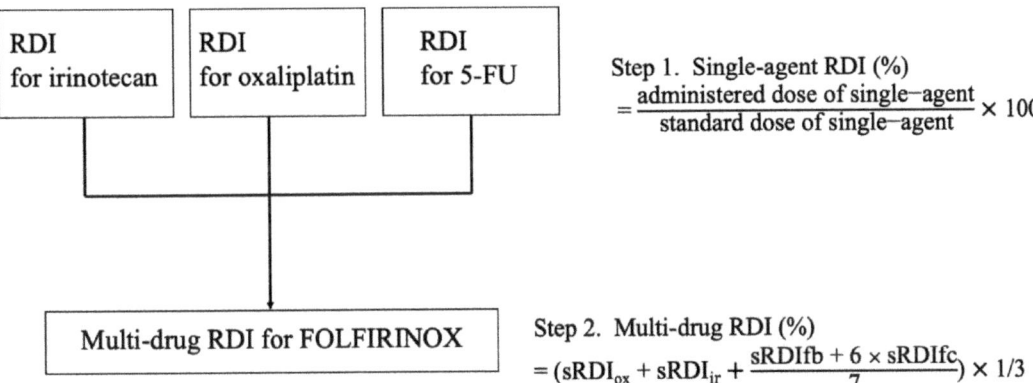

Figure 1. The modified Hryniuk model. 5-FU could be divided into sRDIfb and sRDIfc. The effect of the administration was not considered, which means that only the dose (mg) was used for calculations. RDI, relative dose intensity; ox, oxaliplatin; ir, irinotecan; fb, 5-FU bolus; fc, 5-FU continuous intravenous (Figure modified from reference 12).

2.3. Study Objectives

The primary outcomes were OS and progression-free survival (PFS). The secondary outcomes were the dose modification pattern of FOLFIRINOX according to time and adverse events. Data on adverse events were collected according to the National Cancer Institute Common Terminology Criteria for Adverse Events version 5.0.

2.4. Statistical analysis

All statistical analyses were performed using R version 3.6.2. Chi-square or Fisher's exact test was used for a comparative analysis of categorical data. According to the time, the dose modification pattern of FOLFIRINOX was evaluated with a local regression method (locally estimated scatterplot smoothing—LOESS), namely a linear mixed model. A LOESS plot is a non-parametric regression method that combines multiple regression models. To identify the marginal effect of time, the linear mixed model was adjusted by the average effect of age. Univariable analyses for OS and PFS were performed using the Kaplan–Meier method with log-rank tests. Statistical significance was defined as $p < 0.05$.

3. Results

3.1. Baseline Patient and Tumor Characteristics

A total of 97 patients with MPC (54 men and 43 women) were enrolled in this study. The baseline characteristics of the patients are summarized in Table 1. The median age at diagnosis was 61.1 years (range, 41.0–85.5 years). The male patients were significantly younger than the female patients (58.8 and 64.9 years, respectively; $p = 0.005$). Furthermore, the male patients had a significantly larger body surface area than did the female patients (1.7 and 1.6 m^2, respectively; $p < 0.001$). However, there were no differences in other characteristics such as the location of the primary tumor, metastatic sites, body mass index, initial CA 19-9 level, or ECOG PS between the genders. Granulocyte colony-stimulating factor was used more than once in 84 patients (86.6%). During chemotherapy, five patients received surgery as following: two patients received pylorus-preserving pancreaticoduodenectomy, two received distal pancreatectomy, and one received explorative laparotomy. After progression was noted, despite FOLFIRINOX, 50 patients (51.5%) received the second-line chemotherapy: 40 patients (41.2%) received gemcitabine-based combination chemotherapy and 10 (10.3%) received TS-1.

Table 1. Baseline characteristics of the patients.

	Men (N = 54)	Women (N = 43)	Total (N = 97)	p
Age, years				0.005
Median	58.8	64.9	61.1	
Range	55.0–64.2	58.7–69.9	55.9–68.7	
Tumor location, no. (%)				0.211
Head	19 (35.8)	21 (48.8)	40 (41.7)	
Body	7 (13.2)	6 (14)	13 (13.5)	
Tail	26 (49.1)	13 (30.2)	39 (40.6)	
Multiple	1 (1.9)	3 (7)	4 (4.2)	
Metastatic site, no. (%)				0.704
Liver	30 (37.0)	23 (36.5)	53 (36.8)	
Peritoneum	19 (23.5)	10 (15.9)	29 (20.1)	
Lung	7 (8.6)	9 (14.3)	16 (11.1)	
Lymph node	22 (27.2)	19 (30.2)	41 (28.5)	
Bone	3 (3.7)	2 (3.2)	5 (3.5)	
BMI (kg/m^2)				0.248
Median	22.7	24.1	23.1	
Range	20.5–24.9	20.8–26	20.7–25.7	
BSA (m^2)				<0.001
Median	1.7	1.6	1.6	
Range	1.6–1.8	1.5–1.6	1.5–1.8	
CA 19-9 (U/mL)				0.413
Median	900.0	620.0	760.0	
Range	192.6–3800.0	64.0–2100.0	118.0–2100.0	
ECOG PS score (%)				0.326
0	21 (38.9)	21 (48.8)	42 (43.3)	
1	33 (61.1)	22 (51.2)	55 (56.7)	
Use of G-CSF				0.647
Yes	46 (85.2)	38 (88.4)	84 (86.6)	
No	8 (14.8)	5 (11.6)	13 (13.4)	
Surgery (%)				0.793
Yes	2 (3.7)	3 (7.0)	5 (5.2)	
No	52 (96.3)	40 (93.0)	92 (94.8)	
Second-line chemotherapy, no. (%)				0.733 *
Gemcitabine	4 (7.4)	3 (7.0)	7 (7.2)	
Gemcitabine plus erlotinib	8 (14.8)	4 (9.3)	12 (12.4)	
Gemcitabine plus cisplatin	4 (7.4)	2 (4.7)	6 (6.2)	
Gemcitabine plus nab-paclitaxel	8 (14.8)	7 (16.3)	15 (15.5)	
TS-1	3 (5.6)	7 (16.3)	10 (10.3)	
None	27 (50.0)	20 (46.5)	47 (48.5)	

Table 1. BMI, body mass index; BSA, body surface area; CA 19-9, carbohydrate antigen 19-9; ECOG PS, Eastern Cooperative Oncology Group performance score; G-CSF, granulocyte colony-stimulating factor; *, second-line chemotherapy vs. no additional chemotherapy.

3.2. PFS and OS

The median PFS and OS in this study were 10.8 and 18.0 months, respectively. The median PFS values for the male and female patients were 10.3 and 11.9 months, respectively; the intergroup difference was not significant (p = 0.153, Figure 2A). The median OS values for the male and female patients were 17.9 and 25.9 months, respectively; the intergroup difference was not significant (p = 0.019, Figure 2B). The 1- and 2-year survival rates in male patients were 61.3% and 23.6%, respectively; the corresponding percentages in female patients were 72.9% and 56.8%. Four patients (one male and three female patients) survived for more than 3 years. Of these, three patients showed local invasion of other organs (e.g., the stomach or spleen) and peritoneal seeding at the time of diagnosis and one patient showed a few tiny hepatic metastases.

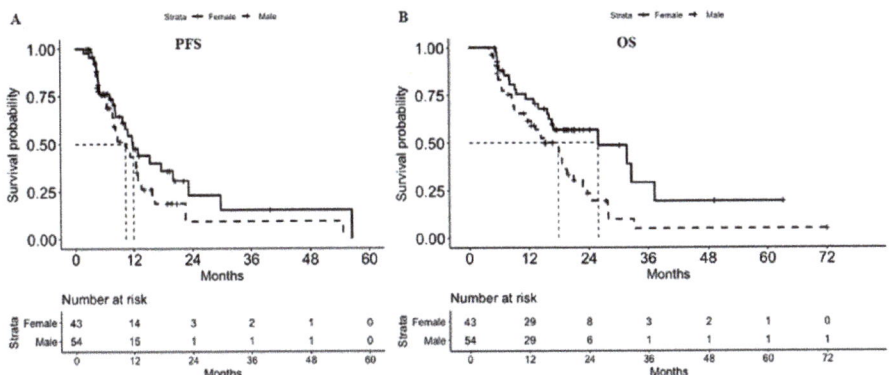

Figure 2. Median progression-free survival (**A**) and overall survival (**B**). (**A**) The median PFS values for male and female patients were 10.3 and 11.9 months, respectively ($p = 0.153$). (**B**) The median OS values for male and female patients were 17.9 and 25.9 months, respectively ($p = 0.019$). PFS, progression-free survival; OS, overall survival.

3.3. FOLFIRINOX Dose Modification Pattern

During a year of FOLFIRINOX chemotherapy, the dose modification pattern was determined with regression analyses. According to the LOESS regression, there was a difference in the dose reduction patterns of chemotherapy in a year between male and female patients (Figure 3A). For statistical comparison of the dose reduction patterns between male and female patients, the linear mixed model was used. Before correction for age, male patients received a mean FOLFIRINOX dose of 95.8% as the initial cycle and the slope of dose reduction was −0.33% per week (p-value of the slope: <0.001; Figure 3B). However, female patients received a mean dose of 89.8% and the slope was −0.52% per week. After correction for mean age (61.2 years old), the slopes for male and female patients were −0.35% and −0.53% per week, respectively (p-value of the slope: <0.001); and the doses for the male and female patients in the initial cycle were 95.6% and 90.7%, respectively (p-value of the slope: <0.001; Figure 3C).

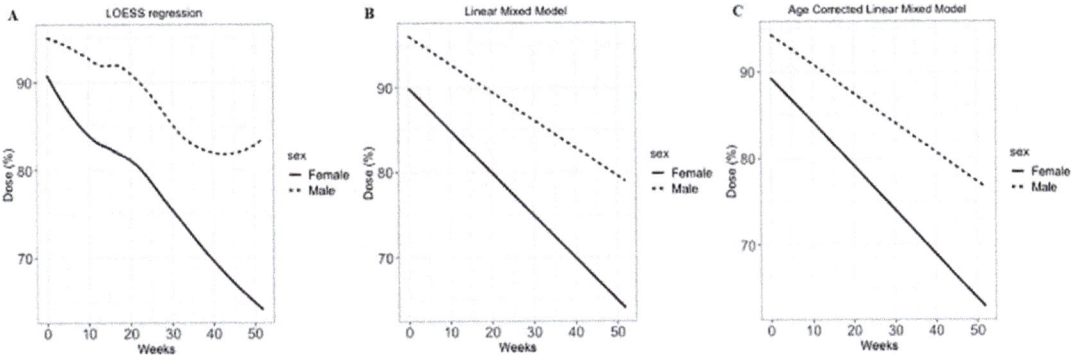

Figure 3. FOLFIRINOX dose modification model. There was a significant difference in the slopes between plots B and C ($p < 0.001$). (**A**) Local regression (LOESS) plot. (**B**) Linear mixed model without age correction. (**C**) Linear mixed model with marginal effect of time (corrected by mean age).

3.4. Treatment-Related Adverse Events and the Number of Visits to the Emergency Department

During a year of chemotherapy, the most common grade 3 or 4 chemotherapy-related adverse event was neutropenia (Table 2). Nausea, febrile neutropenia, and sensory neuropathy also occurred in more than 10% of the patients. There was no difference in grade 3 or 4 treatment-related adverse events between male and female patients. Due to the chemotherapy-related adverse events, 36 patients had to visit the emergency department and five patients visited the emergency department more than three times (Table 3). However, there was no difference in the number of visits to the emergency department between male and female patients.

Table 2. Treatment-related grade 3 or 4 adverse events.

	Men (N = 54)	Women (N = 43)	Total (N = 97)	p
Hematologic				
Neutropenia	17 (31.5)	20 (46.5)	37 (38.1)	0.192
Febrile neutropenia	6 (11.1)	9 (20.9)	15 (15.5)	0.296
Anemia	0 (0.0)	1 (2.3)	1 (1.0)	0.909
Thrombocytopenia	1 (1.9)	4 (9.3)	5 (5.2)	0.235
Non-hematologic				
Anorexia	1 (1.9)	1 (2.3)	2 (2.1)	>0.99
Nausea	12 (22.2)	8 (18.6)	20 (20.6)	0.853
Vomiting	6 (11.1)	3 (7.0)	9 (9.3)	0.730
Diarrhea	4 (7.4)	2 (4.7)	6 (6.2)	0.892
Fatigue	0 (0.0)	2 (4.7)	2 (2.1)	0.378
Sensory neuropathy	7 (13.0)	3 (7.0)	10 (10.3)	0.531

Table 3. Number of visits to the emergency department due to chemotherapy-related adverse events.

	Men (N = 54)	Women (N = 43)	Total (N = 97)	p
				0.239
0	36 (66.7)	25 (58.1)	61 (62.9)	
1~2	17 (31.5)	14 (32.6)	31 (32.0)	
More than 3	1 (1.9)	4 (9.3)	5 (5.2)	

4. Discussion

FOLFIRINOX is a 5-FU–based combination chemotherapeutic regimen and is very effective for patients with unresectable pancreatic cancer [3]. However, the regimen is associated with considerable grade 3 or 4 toxicities, and dose modification during the treatment is very common. The current study aimed to assess differences in FOLFIRINOX outcomes by gender with regard to not only efficacy but also the amount of chemotherapeutic agents delivered.

Factors such as tumor biology, the immune system, body composition, and drug disposition differ between genders. These differences are associated with sex chromosomes, the levels of sex hormones, and environmental factors such as nutrition and microbiota [14]. The incidences of several cancers differ by gender, including esophageal and colorectal cancers. Besides differences in incidence and tumor location, drug pharmacology also differs. Fat-free body mass is approximately 80% and 65% in male and female patients, respectively; body composition also differs between the genders [15]. However, the current doses of chemotherapy are based on body surface area or body mass index, and gender is not considered in the calculation of chemotherapy doses [14].

5-FU is a drug with substantial inter-individual variability in clearance; the impact of gender on 5-FU clearance is significant, with the exposure in female patients being 26% higher than that in male patients [16]. A previous study showed that women were at a higher risk of grade 3 or 4 hematologic toxicities of 5-FU, and the higher clearance of 5-FU in men likely explains the higher toxicity of 5-FU in women with colorectal cancer [9]. It was also reported that the clearance of irinotecan in female patients is 30 to 38% less than that in male patients [17–19]. Consequently, adverse events were more frequently observed in women for most regimens [20].

A recent study about the FOLFIRINOX regimen by gender within the PRODIGE 4/ACCORD 11 trial reported longer median OS (13.1 vs. 10.3 months) and PFS (7.2 vs. 5.9 months) in women, although the differences between the genders were not significant (p = 0.101 and 0.169, respectively) [11]. Similar outcomes were also reported in another study, which showed a longer tendency of PFS (5.0 vs. 3.0 months, p = 0.099) and a higher disease control rate (91.7 vs. 48.0%, p = 0.001) in women [10]. Although these studies failed to conclusively show a definite effect of gender on the FOLFIRINOX regimen, they suggested the possibility of an effect. Compared to these studies, in this study, the median OS in the female patients was significantly longer than that in the male patients (25.9 months vs. 17.9 months, p = 0.019), despite the gender-related differences in PFS being non-significant (11.9 in female patients vs. 10.3 months in male patients, p = 0.153). Therefore, our results also suggested the possibility of better outcomes in female patients who received the FOLFIRINOX regimen. Additional research is necessary to determine whether these different outcomes of the FOLFIRINOX regimen are attributable to gender.

In addition to the chemotherapy response, this study focused on dose modification. Compared to previous studies, which only presented the average or median dose of FOLFIRINOX [12], in this study we calculated the modified dose for each cycle and compared the pattern of dose modification by gender according to time. As a result, female patients on average received 90% of the original dose in the first cycle and 65% of the original dose at 1 year. The doses seemed vastly different from those administered to male patients, who on average received 95% of the original dose in the first cycle and 83% of the original dose at 1 year. For statistical comparison of the dose modification pattern, a linear mixed model was adopted and the negative slopes were significantly different by gender. Considering that there were no differences in the rates of grade 3 or 4 adverse event or number of visits to the emergency department due to chemotherapy-related adverse events, our study suggested that better outcomes could be expected in female patients, even with smaller doses of FOLFIRINOX.

There were several limitations of this study. First, it was a retrospective single-center study. Therefore, further studies are necessary for the generalization of our results. Second, the median OS and PFS in this study seemed longer than those in previous studies because the current study excluded patients who underwent fewer than four cycles of FOLFIRINOX for the comparison of the dose modification pattern. Therefore, there was a possibility of selection bias for a good response in both genders. Third, no pharmacodynamic or pharmacokinetic data were available for the regimen. Lastly, half of the patients received second-line chemotherapy, which was mainly a gemcitabine-based regimen. Therefore, there is a possibility that second-line therapy might contribute to a difference in OS, although the regimens were heterogeneous. In conclusion, female patients showed better survival outcomes in spite of greater reductions in the doses of FOLFIRINOX in this study, and more attention should be focused on the effect of gender on FOLFIRINOX treatment in patients with MPC.

Author Contributions: Data curation, J.K. (Jinkook Kim), K.J., I.H.J., J.P., J.-C.L., J.W.K. and J.K. (Jaihwan Kim); Formal analysis, J.K. (Jinkook Kim), J.-C.L., J.-H.H. and J.K. (Jaihwan Kim); Methodology, E.J., J.-H.H. and J.K. (Jaihwan Kim); Supervision, J.-H.H.; Validation, J.K. (Jaihwan Kim); Writing–original draft, J.K. (Jinkook Kim). All authors have read and agreed to the published version of the manuscript.

Funding: This research received no external funding

Institutional Review Board Statement: The study was conducted according to the guidelines of the Declaration of Helsinki, and approved by the Institutional Review Board of Seoul National University Bundang Hospital (protocol code IRB# B-1907/550-112 approved at July/3/2019).

Informed Consent Statement: Patient consent was waived due to retrospective design of the study.

Conflicts of Interest: The authors declare no conflict of interest.

References

1. Siegel, R.L.; Miller, K.D.; Jemal, A. Cancer statistics, 2019. *CA Cancer J. Clin.* **2019**, *69*, 7–34. [CrossRef] [PubMed]
2. Ryan, D.P.; Hong, T.S.; Bardeesy, N. Pancreatic adenocarcinoma. *N. Engl. J. Med.* **2014**, *371*, 2140–2141. [CrossRef] [PubMed]
3. Conroy, T.; Desseigne, F.; Ychou, M.; Bouche, O.; Guimbaud, R.; Becouarn, Y.; Adenis, A.; Raoul, J.L.; Gourgou-Bourgade, S.; de la Fouchardiere, C.; et al. FOLFIRINOX versus gemcitabine for metastatic pancreatic cancer. *N. Engl. J. Med.* **2011**, *364*, 1817–1825. [CrossRef] [PubMed]
4. Von Hoff, D.D.; Ervin, T.; Arena, F.P.; Chiorean, E.G.; Infante, J.; Moore, M.; Seay, T.; Tjulandin, S.A.; Ma, W.W.; Saleh, M.N.; et al. Increased survival in pancreatic cancer with nab-paclitaxel plus gemcitabine. *N. Engl. J. Med.* **2013**, *369*, 1691–1703. [CrossRef] [PubMed]
5. Conroy, T.; Hammel, P.; Hebbar, M.; Ben Abdelghani, M.; Wei, A.C.; Raoul, J.L.; Chone, L.; Francois, E.; Artru, P.; Biagi, J.J.; et al. FOLFIRINOX or Gemcitabine as Adjuvant Therapy for Pancreatic Cancer. *N. Engl. J. Med.* **2018**, *379*, 2395–2406. [CrossRef] [PubMed]
6. Lambert, A.; Schwarz, L.; Borbath, I.; Henry, A.; Van Laethem, J.L.; Malka, D.; Ducreux, M.; Conroy, T. An update on treatment options for pancreatic adenocarcinoma. *Ther. Adv. Med. Oncol.* **2019**, *11*, 1758835919875568. [CrossRef] [PubMed]
7. Kim, H.I.; Lim, H.; Moon, A. Sex Differences in Cancer: Epidemiology, Genetics and Therapy. *Biomol. Ther. (Seoul)* **2018**, *26*, 335–342. [CrossRef] [PubMed]
8. Milano, G.; Etienne, M.C.; Cassuto-Viguier, E.; Thyss, A.; Santini, J.; Frenay, M.; Renee, N.; Schneider, M.; Demard, F. Influence of sex and age on fluorouracil clearance. *J. Clin. Oncol.* **1992**, *10*, 1171–1175. [CrossRef] [PubMed]
9. Sloan, J.A.; Goldberg, R.M.; Sargent, D.J.; Vargas-Chanes, D.; Nair, S.; Cha, S.S.; Novotny, P.J.; Poon, M.A.; O'Connell, M.J.; Loprinzi, C.L. Women experience greater toxicity with fluorouracil-based chemotherapy for colorectal cancer. *J. Clin. Oncol.* **2002**, *20*, 1491–1498. [CrossRef] [PubMed]
10. Hohla, F.; Hopfinger, G.; Romeder, F.; Rinnerthaler, G.; Bezan, A.; Stattner, S.; Hauser-Kronberger, C.; Ulmer, H.; Greil, R. Female gender may predict response to FOLFIRINOX in patients with unresectable pancreatic cancer: A single institution retrospective review. *Int. J. Oncol.* **2014**, *44*, 319–326. [CrossRef] [PubMed]
11. Lambert, A.; Jarlier, M.; Gourgou Bourgade, S.; Conroy, T. Response to FOLFIRINOX by gender in patients with metastatic pancreatic cancer: Results from the PRODIGE 4/ ACCORD 11 randomized trial. *PLoS ONE* **2017**, *12*, e0183288. [CrossRef] [PubMed]
12. Lee, J.C.; Kim, J.W.; Ahn, S.; Kim, H.W.; Lee, J.; Kim, Y.H.; Paik, K.H.; Kim, J.; Hwang, J.H. Optimal dose reduction of FOLFIRINOX for preserving tumour response in advanced pancreatic cancer: Using cumulative relative dose intensity. *Eur. J. Cancer* **2017**, *76*, 125–133. [CrossRef] [PubMed]
13. Hryniuk, W.; Bush, H. The importance of dose intensity in chemotherapy of metastatic breast cancer. *J. Clin. Oncol.* **1984**, *2*, 1281–1288. [CrossRef] [PubMed]
14. Wagner, A.D.; Oertelt-Prigione, S.; Adjei, A.; Buclin, T.; Cristina, V.; Csajka, C.; Coukos, G.; Dafni, U.; Dotto, G.P.; Ducreux, M.; et al. Gender medicine and oncology: Report and consensus of an ESMO workshop. *Ann. Oncol.* **2019**, *30*, 1914–1924. [CrossRef]
15. Janmahasatian, S.; Duffull, S.B.; Ash, S.; Ward, L.C.; Byrne, N.M.; Green, B. Quantification of lean bodyweight. *Clin. Pharmacokinet.* **2005**, *44*, 1051–1065. [CrossRef] [PubMed]
16. Mueller, F.; Buchel, B.; Koberle, D.; Schurch, S.; Pfister, B.; Krahenbuhl, S.; Froehlich, T.K.; Largiader, C.R.; Joerger, M. Gender-specific elimination of continuous-infusional 5-fluorouracil in patients with gastrointestinal malignancies: Results from a prospective population pharmacokinetic study. *Cancer Chemother. Pharmacol.* **2013**, *71*, 361–370. [CrossRef] [PubMed]
17. Berg, A.K.; Buckner, J.C.; Galanis, E.; Jaeckle, K.A.; Ames, M.M.; Reid, J.M. Quantification of the impact of enzyme-inducing antiepileptic drugs on irinotecan pharmacokinetics and SN-38 exposure. *J. Clin. Pharmacol.* **2015**, *55*, 1303–1312. [CrossRef] [PubMed]
18. Klein, C.E.; Gupta, E.; Reid, J.M.; Atherton, P.J.; Sloan, J.A.; Pitot, H.C.; Ratain, M.J.; Kastrissios, H. Population pharmacokinetic model for irinotecan and two of its metabolites, SN-38 and SN-38 glucuronide. *Clin. Pharmacol. Ther.* **2002**, *72*, 638–647. [CrossRef] [PubMed]
19. Wu, H.; Infante, J.R.; Keedy, V.L.; Jones, S.F.; Chan, E.; Bendell, J.C.; Lee, W.; Zamboni, B.A.; Ikeda, S.; Kodaira, H.; et al. Population pharmacokinetics of PEGylated liposomal CPT-11 (IHL-305) in patients with advanced solid tumors. *Eur. J. Clin. Pharmacol.* **2013**, *69*, 2073–2081. [CrossRef] [PubMed]
20. Cristina, V.; Mahachie, J.; Mauer, M.; Buclin, T.; Van Cutsem, E.; Roth, A.; Wagner, A.D. Association of Patient Sex With Chemotherapy-Related Toxic Effects: A Retrospective Analysis of the PETACC-3 Trial Conducted by the EORTC Gastrointestinal Group. *JAMA Oncol.* **2018**, *4*, 1003–1006. [CrossRef] [PubMed]

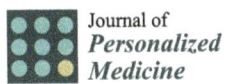

Article

Establishment of a Molecular Tumor Board (MTB) and Uptake of Recommendations in a Community Setting

Ari VanderWalde *, Axel Grothey, Daniel Vaena, Gregory Vidal, Adam ElNaggar, Gabriella Bufalino and Lee Schwartzberg

West Cancer Center and Research Institute, Memphis, TN 38138, USA; agrothey@WESTCLINIC.com (A.G.); DVaena@WESTCLINIC.com (D.V.); gvidal@WESTCLINIC.com (G.V.); AElNaggar@WESTCLINIC.com (A.E.); GBufalino@WESTCLINIC.com (G.B.); lschwartzberg@WESTCLINIC.com (L.S.)
* Correspondence: avanderw@westclinic.com; Tel.: +1-901-683-0055 (ext. 63015)

Received: 13 October 2020; Accepted: 23 November 2020; Published: 27 November 2020

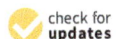

Abstract: In the precision medicine era, molecular testing in advanced cancer is foundational to patient management. Molecular tumor boards (MTBs) can be effective in processing comprehensive genomic profiling (CGP) results and providing expert recommendations. We assessed an MTB and its role in a community setting. This retrospective analysis included patients with MTB recommendations at a community-based oncology practice January 2015 to December 2018; exclusions were death within 60 days of the MTB and/or no metastatic disease. Potentially actionable genomic alterations from CGP (immunohistochemistry, in-situ hybridization, next-generation sequencing) were reviewed bi-weekly by MTB practice experts, pathologists, genetic counselors, and other support staff, and clinical care recommendations were provided. Subsequent chart reviews determined implementation rates of recommendations. In 613 patients, the most common cancers were lung (23%), breast (19%), and colorectal (17%); others included ovarian, endometrial, bladder, and melanoma. Patients received 837 actionable recommendations: standard therapy (37%), clinical trial (31%), germline testing and genetic counseling (17%), off-label therapy (10%), subspecialty multidisciplinary tumor board review (2%), and advice for classifying tumor of unknown origin (2%). Of these recommendations, 36% to 78% were followed by the treating physician. For clinical trial recommendations ($n = 262$), 13% of patients enrolled in a clinical trial. The median time between CPG result availability and MTB presentation was 12 days. A community oncology-based comprehensive and high-throughput MTB provided useful clinical guidance in various treatment domains within an acceptable timeframe for patients with cancer in a large community setting.

Keywords: MTB; precision medicine; cancer; oncology practice; community setting; CGP

1. Introduction

Tumor biology is commonly driven by genomic alterations of oncogenic pathways that regulate processes such as cell differentiation, proliferation, apoptosis, and tumor metabolism [1]. Over the last 20 years, the development of targeted treatments against 'actionable' genomic changes has led to a paradigm shift towards precision medicine across several tumor types [1,2]. Molecular testing therefore allows for tailoring of treatment decisions based on the genomic makeup of a patient's tumor.

Expert consensus clinical practice guidelines have defined requirements for routine molecular testing in many malignancies, including advanced non-small cell lung cancer (NSCLC) [3,4], breast [5], ovarian [6,7], and colorectal cancers [8]. Given the number of different pathogenic mutations, comprehensive genomic profiling (CGP) can identify genomic drivers that are predictive of therapeutic response, and facilitate the timely implementation of treatment guidelines [9,10]. Furthermore, in some cancers, such as NSCLC, guidelines recommend use of CGP over multiple single-gene tests, and the

FDA has approved the use of next-generation sequencing (NGS) testing panels [4,11]. However, cancer centers still have a number of clinical and operational considerations including choice of assay, laboratory, and analysis. Furthermore, the extensive tumor-specific molecular data produced from CGP can lead to uncertain clinical interpretation and utility.

The sheer volume of diverse and continuously evolving data generated by CGP mean effective interpretation and application can be challenging for single-disease focused academic physicians or community oncologists (who are often generalists) [12]. However, molecular tumor boards (MTBs) with multidisciplinary input can provide an effective workflow and expert review process in order to generate precision medicine recommendations for oncology patients. However, implementation of an MTB within the community setting raises additional challenges: limited availability of genetics and genomics expertise, a lack of institutional imperative for an MTB, logistical barriers such as limited staff or meeting timings to ensure all specialties are attending, lack of dedicated expert physicians to screen cases and manage the MTB, and the need for timely submission of cases [13].

This report reviews the clinical utility of CGP and the role of an MTB in a large community oncology clinic on patient treatment decisions and outcomes. We also report the structure, organization, and management of the MTB, including best practices and lessons learned, analysis of patient management decisions based on CGP, and adherence to the MTB decisions.

2. Methods

2.1. Patients and Setting

A systematic program of CGP was initiated in December 2014 at the West Cancer Center, Memphis, TN, USA, a large community-based oncology practice. West Cancer Center physicians were encouraged to offer genomic testing to all patients with newly diagnosed metastatic melanoma, lung, colorectal, breast, and pancreatic cancer to a preferred third-party national testing laboratory. Other types of metastatic or recurrent malignancies were tested at the discretion of the treating provider.

2.2. CGP

Genomic profiling was largely conducted using the Caris MI® Profile test (Caris Life Sciences, Phoenix, AZ, USA), which included multi-platform testing with chromogenic in-situ hybridization (CISH), NGS, and immunohistochemistry (IHC), provided commercially by Caris Life Sciences as part of standard of care testing. The NGS panel included 42 genes through 2015, after which a 592-gene panel was adopted for all samples (Supplementary Table S1). Additional relevant IHC testing was conducted on a tumor-lineage specific basis and could include PD-L1, estrogen receptor, progesterone receptor, androgen receptor, HER2, and others. Fusions were routinely detected using RNA-sequencing for ALK and ROS1, and CISH was used in breast and gastric cancer samples to measure HER2 overexpression.

Mutations were designated as pathogenic, presumed pathogenic, presumed benign, benign, or variant of unknown significance based on the interpretation of available genomic databases. Only pathogenic and presumed pathogenic mutations were reported unless otherwise noted. The criteria used for clinically actionable mutations are described in the Supplementary Material.

2.3. MTB

A bi-weekly, one-hour MTB meeting to review patient cases was set up (Figure 1). The MTB was designed to be comprehensive and high-throughput, with review of at least 50 cases bi-weekly prior to the meeting, and then full MTB review of 10 to 20 cases. All CGP reports were pre-screened for relevant genomic alterations by a MTB member through a testing laboratory-supported, online portal. While the policy was to obtain testing only for patients with newly diagnosed metastatic disease, reports were screened regardless of the timing of testing. Likewise, data from other genomic laboratories testing tissue or liquid biopsy samples were also screened if made available to the screening provider. Cases with genomic alterations that were potentially 'actionable', complicated, or associated with novel treatment decisions not fully incorporated into clinical practice were brought to the MTB for review. Cases could also be referred to the MTB if the treating physician specifically requested clarification of the case or if it was relevant to highlight new data regarding approvals and/or recommendations to the treating physician. Any other cases were omitted from the MTB.

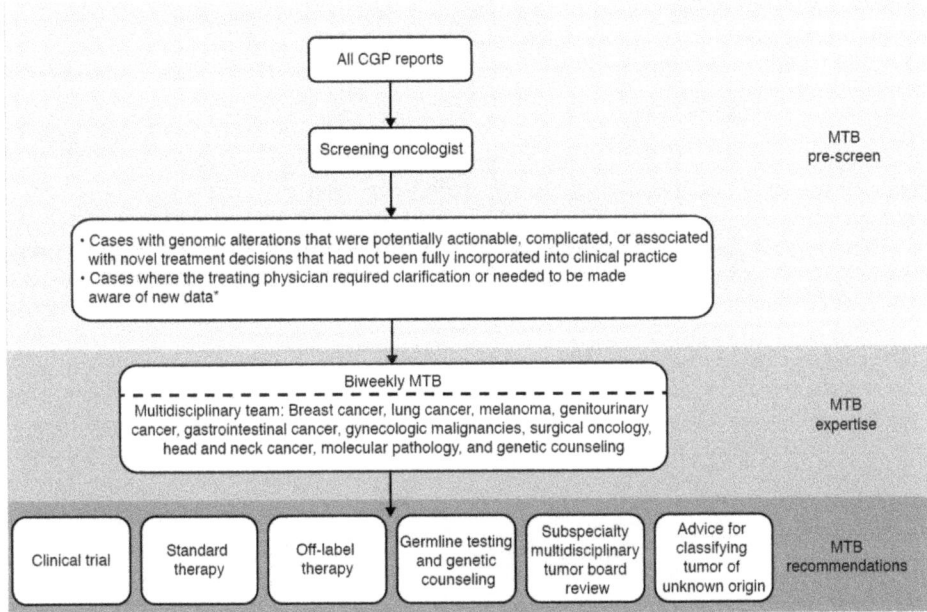

Figure 1. Molecular tumor boards (MTB) workflow and review process. * Data relevant to approvals and/or recommendations for the targeted therapy to be administered. CGP, comprehensive genomic profiling; MTB, molecular tumor board.

MTB meetings were multi-specialty, multi-disciplinary, and open to any interested member of the center. Routine attendance consisted of medical and surgical oncologists with expertise in melanoma, breast, lung, head and neck, gastrointestinal, and genitourinary cancers, gynecologic malignancies, and surgical oncology. Other important members included anatomic and molecular pathologists and genetic counselors. Both the molecular data report and the clinical record from the electronic medical record (EMR) were reviewed and correlated at this live meeting, and the MTB provided recommendations for clinical care within the following six categories: (1) clinical trial; (2) standard therapy; (3) off-label therapy; (4) germline testing and genetic counseling; (5) subspecialty multidisciplinary tumor board review; and (6) advice for classifying tumor of unknown origin.

Recommendations were generally by consensus; any substantial disagreement among the MTB members was reflected in the recommendation summary. Minutes from the MTB were transcribed, input into the patient's EMR, and an email with a summary and recommendations sent to the treating physician.

2.4. Analysis

MTB recommendations by category (Figure 1) and number of recommendations followed by the treating physician were collated and analyzed for all cases presented at the MTB from January 2015 through December 2018. Patients were excluded from the analysis if molecular testing did not meet clinical criteria or if the patient died within 60 days of the MTB, did not have metastatic disease, or was not given recommendations by the MTB.

3. Results

3.1. Patients and MTBs

Over the observation period, the MTB convened 92 times, of which 22, 21, 25, and 24 MTBs occurred in 2015, 2016, 2017, and 2018, respectively. As data were unavailable for four MTBs in 2015 and one MTB in 2018, the data reported include recommendations and follow-up from 87 MTBs. Of an estimated 4438 reported molecular test results, reports and clinical information from 837 patients were selected as potentially benefiting from additional clinical review at the MTB. Of these, 131 patients did not have a follow-up appointment and/or died within 60 days of the MTB, 54 patients did not have metastatic disease, 35 patients did not receive formal recommendations at the MTB, and 4 patients could not be found in the EMR database. As such, 613/4438 patients with recommendations were evaluated (14% of test reports) and received a total of 837 actionable recommendations.

Of the 613 patients analyzed, 58% (n = 355) were female, African Americans comprised 30% (n = 181), with 68% (n = 417) Caucasian, and 2% (n = 15) other ethnicities. The most common cancers were lung (23%), breast (19%), and colorectal (17%). Other malignancies representing more than 20 cases each included ovarian, endometrial, and bladder cancers, and melanoma.

The median time between CGP results becoming available and presentation at the MTB was 12 days (interquartile range, 6 to 18 days). Median time from MTB presentation to last follow-up or date of death was 13.3 months. Among the 508 patients for whom extensive retrospective records were available, the median time from test ordering to result reporting (including time from order to biopsy, biopsy to pathology, pathology shipped to central test, processing, and resulting of the test) was 20 days.

3.2. MTB Recommendations and Adherence to Recommendations

The majority of recommendations from the MTB were for standard therapy (51% of patients), and clinical trials (43% of patients; Table 1). Overall, recommendations followed by the treating physician ranged from 36% to 78%, depending on the category, with the highest compliance for following standard therapy (Figure 2).

Table 1. Recommendations by category from the MTB for all patients analyzed (n = 613).

Recommendation Category	Number of Recommendations	Proportion of Patients Receiving Recommendations [1] (%)
Clinical trial	262	43
Standard therapy	311	51
Off-label therapy	84	14
Germline testing and genetic counseling	143	23
Subspecialty multidisciplinary tumor board review	18	3
Advice for classifying tumor of unknown origin	13	2

[1] Patients could have more than one recommendation. Abbreviations: MTB, molecular tumor board.

MTB recommendations for clinical trial enrollment (n = 262) were followed by the treating physician for 150 (57%) patients, with 35 (13%) patients ultimately enrolling in a clinical trial. Of these clinical trial recommendations, the MTB recommended 167 (64%) patients to enroll immediately, of which 93 (56%) recommendations were followed by the treating physician and 20 (12%) patients enrolled in a trial (Supplementary Figure S1). The remaining MTB recommendations for clinical trial enrollment (n = 95; 36%) were for patients to enroll in future clinical trials upon progression, after standard of care therapy. Of these, 57 (60%) recommendations were followed and 15 (16%) patients enrolled in a clinical trial (Supplementary Figure S1). Among the 115 patients who did not follow the recommendation, the most common reasons for not enrolling included failed screening or ineligibility (34%), declined participation (18%), and lack of follow-up after a preliminary discussion (20%).

MTB recommendations for standard therapy and off-label therapy were followed by the treating physician in 78% ($n = 244$) and 37% ($n = 31$) of cases, respectively. Germline testing and genetic counseling recommendations were followed in 36% ($n = 52$) of cases; of these, 9 (17%) patients declined testing, did not follow-up, or were still deciding, 28 (54%) patients were negative, and 15 (29%) patients were positive for a germline mutation (ATM, $n = 1$; BRCA1, $n = 2$; BRCA2, $n = 6$; CHEK2, $n = 2$; Lynch syndrome, $n = 2$; homozygous MUTYH, $n = 2$).

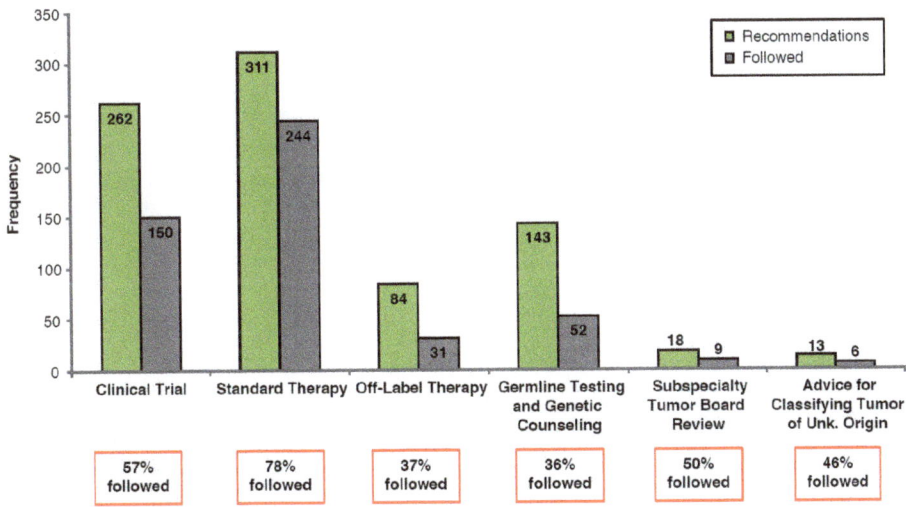

Figure 2. Proportion of MTB recommendations followed by the treating physician for all patients. MTB, molecular tumor board.

The type of recommendation given did not vary by race, with 31% of African American patients and 32% of Caucasian patients receiving the clinical trial recommendation; 40% and 36% were recommended standard therapy, 12% and 10% were recommended off-label therapy, and 15% and 18% were recommended germline testing, respectively. However, there appeared to be minor differences in the following of the recommendations, particularly in germline testing. Recommended germline testing was performed in 27% of African American patients compared with 38% of Caucasian patients. Similar numbers of African American and Caucasian patients followed recommendations for standard therapy (75% vs. 80%), off-label recommendations (32% vs. 39%) and clinical trials (52% vs. 60%); however, these did indicate slightly higher utilization of recommendations by Caucasian patients.

3.3. The Value of MTBs beyond Standard Reporting

The following two cases illustrate how the MTB added value to therapeutic decisions, using combined knowledge of the tumor biology and clinical aspects of cases to guide treatment decisions; treatment suggestions based on molecular alterations would not be adequate in these cases.

In the first case, a 67-year-old woman with a BRCA2 germline mutation (exon 10 I605fs) had surgery for serous carcinoma of the fallopian tube and received adjuvant chemotherapy. She developed liver metastases and subsequently progressed on multiple therapies including endocrine therapy, poly ADP-ribose polymerase (PARP) inhibitors, immunotherapy, and chemotherapy. Following this, molecular analysis revealed new mutations. While circulating free DNA (cfDNA) testing revealed the known germline BRCA2 mutation, it also revealed BRCA2 G602fs (0.2%), BRCA2 c.794-16_797del (0.5%), and BRCA2 c.794-10_794-1del (0.8%). The latter two were described as splice-site indels and felt to represent 'reversal' mutations. Tumor molecular testing revealed the known exon 10 germline mutation but also an additional exon 10 mutation at p.G602E (16% variant frequency), which was described as a variant of uncertain significance and had not been previously present two years prior. Based on the combined data, the patient was referred to a clinical trial with a novel cell cycle regulating agent, to which she began responding.

In the second case, a 49-year-old woman never-smoker was diagnosed with epidermal growth factor receptor (EGFR)-mutated (exon 19 p.E746_A750del) metastatic lung cancer four years prior to MTB presentation. After two years of treatment with EGFR-tyrosine kinase inhibitor (TKI), her tumor developed an EGFR T790M (exon 20) mutation, and she initiated osimertinib treatment. She responded for two years, but ultimately progressed. Repeat tissue molecular profiling showed the presence of a tertiary EGFR mutation (C797S, exon 20) which was notably not seen on liquid biopsy at the time and is associated with acquired resistance to osimertinib. MTB review indicated that similar combinations of mutations also conferred resistance to putative exon 20 inhibitors, but that combining osimertinib with a first-generation EGFR-TKI could possibly be an effective treatment option. However, the patient's health declined as a result of disease progression, and she was unable to receive the recommended combination therapy.

4. Discussion

West Cancer Center was an early adopter of recommending routine CGP for advanced cancers and integrating an MTB to review the results in a timely fashion in a large clinical practice. Here we present four years of data in a pre-planned MTB in a large community setting, reflecting both a large sample size and a broad time-frame (>4400 reviewed reports and >800 patients reviewed in full MTBs). These results show that routine CGP with universal pre-screen review, selection of cases, and presentation at our high-throughput, bi-weekly MTB is feasible as a means of providing clinical guidance to a substantial proportion of cancer patients.

Between 2015 and 2018, MTB recommendations followed by the treating physician ranged from 36% to 78% depending on the recommendation category, with the lowest rate of adherence to recommendations for genetic counseling and germline testing, and highest for standard therapy, similar to acceptance rates reported by other MTBs (27% to 70%) [14,15]. The low rate of germline testing is consistent with that seen in other centers and was likely multifactorial in etiology (patient refusal, provider non-prioritization, poor communication, etc.), although reasons for non-acceptance were not measured in our cohort [16].

The MTB was implemented to provide recommendations on clinical care, increase clinical trial participation, and improve awareness of standard or potential targeted therapies. We found MTB recommendations to be particularly useful in identifying clinical trial eligibility (recommended in 262 cases; 35 patients (13%) ultimately enrolled). This was slightly higher than the 7% rate reported in a community setting in Michigan [17], and similar to that reported by the Institut Curie Molecular Tumor Board, an academic medical center in a more centralized health care system where, among the 442 patients who underwent CGP, 10% were ultimately enrolled in a clinical trial [18]. Clinical trial enrollment in the present study was restricted by failed clinical trial screening, lack of follow-up after initial discussion regarding clinical trial enrollment, and patients declining participation.

Our experience showed that turnaround times for molecular analysis and the delivery of recommendations were favorable in this community-based MTB compared with that reported in academic models. The median time from molecular diagnostic results being received and MTB patient presentation was 12 days. Moreover, overall turnaround time from time of request of molecular tests through to the provision of MTB recommendations was comparable with previous studies (median, 33 days) [19,20].

Rather than performing a 'gate-keeper' role [20], West Cancer Center MTB reviewed each case for appropriateness and the availability of tumor tissue prior to testing to avoid unnecessary testing and associated costs. In our institution, a clinic-wide policy dictated which cases should be sent for tissue-based CGP, namely common malignancies at first diagnosis of metastatic disease. Due to the timing of this approach, recommendations could be made for virtually all lines of therapy with the highest chance of identifying clinical trial opportunities while minimizing disruption to patients, as biopsies are performed at this time point for other clinical purposes. However, this approach can be problematic as molecular results may need to be recalled by the treating physician if the patient qualifies for a clinical trial as they progress through therapy. An additional challenge is that 'upfront' testing underestimates the future development of heterogeneous disease or acquired resistance mutations.

West Cancer Center MTB was innovative by adding a pre-screening step following the CGP report, allowing the MTB to focus only on those cases for which recommendations were of ultimate benefit to the patient. This is in contrast to other MTBs where physicians choose when and whether to present the case. Our methodology, therefore, created a high-throughput model where cases were not missed and maximum utility was maintained. Additionally, it led to cases being presented early in the clinical course, so that recommendations could take into account standard therapies for each disease and targeted actions after standard therapies failed.

There are several noteworthy limitations to our study. The number of 'actionable' molecular alterations reported may be conservative due to changes in actionability and the development of new targeted therapies over the period of the study (2015 to 2018), in addition to the evolution in genomic sequencing. Pre-screening of cases prior to presentation in the MTB was completed by a single physician and relied on their assessment of current clinic practices and baseline knowledge of individual physician practices, therefore the choice of which cases were 'actionable' was somewhat subjective and changed over time with the integration of new molecular-guided therapies into practice. This could have led to changes in what the screening physician decided could be considered of benefit to the treating physicians. We also acknowledge the financial implications involved in broad testing of patients; however, our study was designed to assess the role and feasibility of implementing an MTB in a community setting, and cost was not a key focus.

As personalized/precision medicine becomes integrated into standard clinical practice, MTBs are playing an increasingly important role in supporting decision making by the treating physician. Robust, reproducible, and comprehensive bioinformatics analyses and close interactions between physicians and bioinformaticians are critical to the success of targeted therapy [21,22]. Our MTB was designed to be multi-omic, multi-specialty, and multi-disciplinary; we found that implementation of this comprehensive, collaborative approach led to increased clinical trial participation and more focused use of off-label targeted therapy within our institution. Moreover, the MTB meetings provided an educational opportunity and facilitated increased awareness among physicians of targeted therapies to match genomic alterations.

In conclusion, our comprehensive and high-throughput bi-weekly MTB was feasible as a means to providing clinical guidance within an acceptable timeframe for patients with cancer in a large community setting. It may therefore be useful to adopt similar models in other cancer centers.

Supplementary Materials: The following are available online at http://www.mdpi.com/2075-4426/10/4/252/s1, Figure S1: MTB recommendations for clinical trial enrollment and resulting patient management, Table S1: Caris MI® gene panel.

Author Contributions: Concept and design, A.V., L.S., D.V., and A.G.; data acquisition and analysis, A.V. and G.B.; data interpretation, A.V., L.S., G.V., D.V., A.G., A.E., and G.B.; manuscript preparation, all. All authors have read and agreed to the published version of the manuscript.

Funding: This research received no external funding.

Acknowledgments: The authors would like to acknowledge Natasha Cary, BSc, of iMed Comms, Macclesfield, UK, an Ashfield Company, part of UDG Healthcare plc for medical writing support, under the direction of the authors that was funded by AstraZeneca in accordance with Good Publications Practice (GPP3) guidelines (http://www.ismpp.org/gpp3). No research funding was provided.

Conflicts of Interest: A.V. has received honoraria from Caris Life Sciences and Elsevier; served as a consultant or participated on advisory boards for Bristol-Myers Squibb, AstraZeneca, Medimmune, Compugen, and ConcertoHealthAl. He has also received research funding from Amgen, Genentec, Merck, Bristol-Myers Squibb, AstraZeneca, EliLilly, and Replimune. A.G. has received honoraria from Aptitude Health, Elsevier, and IMEDEX; served as a consultant or participated on advisory boards for Amgen, Array BioPharma, Bayer, Boston Biomedical, Bristol-Myers Squibb, Daiichi Sankyo, Genentech/Roche, and Lilly. He has received research funding from Array BioPharma, Bayer, Boston Biomedical, Daiichi, Sankyo, Eisai, Genentech/Roche, Lilly, and Pfizer; travel and accommodations expenses from Amgen, Array BioPharma, Bayer, Boston Biomedical, Bristol-Myers Squibb, and Genentech/Roche. D.V. has received research funding from Aeglea Biotherapeutics, Amgen, AstraZeneca, BioClin Therapeutics, Bristol-Myers Squibb, Calithera Biosciences, Compugen, Merck, Nektar, Novartis, OBI Pharma, Peloton Therapeutics, T.G. Therapeutics, and Tizona Therapeutics, Inc. He has also served as a consultant or participated on advisory boards for Bayer, Bristol-Myers Squibb, Genomic Health, and received travel and accommodations expenses from Caris Centers of Excellence and Genomic Health. D.V. reports ownership interest with Oncodisc, he has served as a consultant or participated on advisory boards for Eli Lilly, Novartis, Genetech, Puma, Immunomedics, Pfizer, and AstraZeneca; speakers' bureau for Eli Lilly, Pfizer, Puma, and Novartis. He has also received research funding from Merck, Genetech, Roche, BMS, Celcuity, Puma, Eli Lilly, Pfizer, Immunomedics, and Novartis; travel and accommodations expenses from Eli Lilly. A.E. has received reimbursement/research support from Caris Life Sciences. He has served as a consultant or participated on advisory boards for AstraZeneca, Clovis Oncology, Leap Therapeutics, GSK/Tesaro, and AbbVie Pharmaceuticals. He has served as an investigator for studies sponsored by AstraZeneca, Merck, GSK/Tesaro, and Leap Therapeutics. G.B. has no conflict of interest to declare. LS has served as a consultant or participated on advisory boards for Amgen, Pfizer, Helsinn, Genentech, Genomich Health, BMS, Myriad, AstraZeneca, Bayer, Spectrum, and Napo.

References

1. Garraway, L.A. Genomics-driven oncology: Framework for an emerging paradigm. *J. Clin. Oncol.* **2013**, *31*, 1806–1814. [CrossRef] [PubMed]
2. Sholl, L.M.; Do, K.; Shivdasani, P.; Cerami, E.; Dubuc, A.M.; Kuo, F.C.; Garcia, E.P.; Jia, Y.; Davineni, P.; Abo, R.P.; et al. Institutional implementation of clinical tumor profiling on an unselected cancer population. *JCI Insight.* **2016**, *1*, e87062. [CrossRef] [PubMed]
3. Planchard, D.; Popat, S.; Kerr, K.; Novello, S.; Smit, E.F.; Faivre-Finn, C.; Mok, T.S.; Reck, M.; Van Schil, P.E.; Hellmann, M.D.; et al. Metastatic non-small cell lung cancer: ESMO Clinical Practice Guidelines for diagnosis, treatment and follow-up. *Ann. Oncol.* **2019**, *30*, 863–870. [CrossRef] [PubMed]
4. Lindeman, N.I.; Cagle, P.T.; Aisner, D.L.; Arcila, M.E.; Beasley, M.B.; Bernicker, E.; Colasacco, C.; Dacic, S.; Hirsch, F.R.; Kerr, K.; et al. Updated molecular testing guideline for the selection of lung cancer patients for treatment with targeted tyrosine kinase inhibitors: Guideline from the College of American Pathologists, the International Association for the Study of Lung Cancer, and the Association for Molecular Pathology. *Arch. Pathol. Lab. Med.* **2018**, *142*, 321–346. [CrossRef] [PubMed]
5. Manahan, E.R.; Kuerer, H.M.; Sebastian, M.; Hughes, K.S.; Boughey, J.C.; Euhus, D.M.; Boolbol, S.K.; Taylor, W.A. Consensus guidelines on genetic testing for hereditary breast cancer from the American Society of Breast Surgeons. *Ann. Surg Oncol.* **2019**, *26*, 3025–3031. [CrossRef] [PubMed]
6. Food and Drug Administration (FDA). ZEJULA®(niraparib) Prescribing Information. 2017. Available online: https://www.mdpi.com/journal/jpm/special_issues/personalized_oncology (accessed on 22 November 2020).
7. Moore, K.N.; Secord, A.A.; Geller, M.A.; Miller, D.S.; Cloven, N.; Fleming, G.F.; Hendrickson, A.E.W.; Azodi, M.; DiSilvestro, P.; Oza, A.M.; et al. Niraparib monotherapy for late-line treatment of ovarian cancer (QUADRA): A multicentre, open-label, single-arm, phase 2 trial. *Lancet Oncol.* **2019**, *20*, 636–648. [CrossRef]
8. Sepulveda, A.R.; Hamilton, S.R.; Allegra, C.J.; Grody, W.; Cushman-Vokoun, A.M.; Funkhouser, W.K.; Kopetz, S.E.; Lieu, C.; Lindor, N.M.; Minsky, B.D.; et al. Molecular biomarkers for the evaluation of colorectal cancer: Guideline from the American Society for Clinical Pathology, College of American Pathologists, Association for Molecular Pathology, and American Society of Clinical Oncology. *J. Mol. Diagn.* **2017**, *19*, 187–225. [CrossRef] [PubMed]
9. Suh, J.H.; Johnson, A.; Albacker, L.; Wang, K.; Chmielecki, J.; Frampton, G.; Gay, L.; Elvin, J.A.; Vergilio, J.A.; Ali, S.; et al. Comprehensive genomic profiling facilitates implementation of the National Comprehensive Cancer Network Guidelines for lung cancer biomarker testing and identifies patients who may benefit from enrollment in mechanism-driven clinical trials. *Oncologist* **2016**, *21*, 684–691. [CrossRef] [PubMed]
10. Vakiani, E. Molecular testing of colorectal cancer in the modern era: What are we doing and why? *Surg. Pathol. Clin.* **2017**, *10*, 1009–1020. [CrossRef] [PubMed]

11. Food and Drug Administration (FDA). FDA Fact Sheet: CDRH'S Approach to Tumor Profiling Next Generation Sequencing Tests, 2017. Available online: https://www.fda.gov/media/109050/download (accessed on 22 November 2020).
12. Gray, S.W.; Hicks-Courant, K.; Cronin, A.; Rollins, B.J.; Weeks, J.C. Physicians' attitudes about multiplex tumor genomic testing. *J. Clin. Oncol.* **2014**, *32*, 1317–1323. [CrossRef] [PubMed]
13. van der Velden, D.L.; van Herpen, C.M.L.; van Laarhoven, H.W.M.; Smit, E.F.; Groen, H.J.M.; Willems, S.M.; Nederlof, P.M.; Langenberg, M.H.G.; Cuppen, E.; Sleijfer, S.; et al. Molecular tumor boards: Current practice and future needs. *Ann. Oncol.* **2017**, *28*, 3070–3075. [CrossRef] [PubMed]
14. Tafe, L.J.; Gorlov, I.P.; de Abreu, F.B.; Lefferts, J.A.; Liu, X.; Pettus, J.R.; Marotti, J.D.; Bloch, K.J.; Memoli, V.A.; Suriawinata, A.A.; et al. Implementation of a molecular tumor board: The impact on treatment decisions for 35 patients evaluated at Dartmouth-Hitchcock Medical Center. *Oncologist* **2015**, *20*, 1011–1018. [CrossRef] [PubMed]
15. Farhangfar, C.J.; Morgan, O.; Concepcion, C.; Hwang, J.J.; Mileham, K.F.; Carrizosa, D.R.; Dellinger, B.; Farhangfar, F.; Kim, E.S. Utilization of consultative molecular tumor board in community setting. *J. Clin. Oncol.* **2017**, *35*, 6508. [CrossRef]
16. Clark, D.F.; Maxwell, K.N.; Powers, J.; Lieberman, D.B.; Ebrahimzadeh, J.; Long, J.M.; McKenna, D.; Shah, P.; Bradbury, A.; Morrissette, J.J.D.; et al. Identification and confirmation of potentially actionable germline mutations in tumor-only genomic sequencing. *JCO Prec. Oncol.* **2019**, *3*, 1–11. [CrossRef] [PubMed]
17. Reitsma, M.; Fox, J.; Borre, P.V.; Cavanaugh, M.; Chudnovsky, Y.; Erlich, R.L.; Gribbin, T.E.; Anhorn, R. Effect of a collaboration between a health plan, oncology practice, and comprehensive genomic profiling company from the payer perspective. *J. Manag. Care Spec. Pharm.* **2019**, *25*, 601–611. [CrossRef] [PubMed]
18. Basse, C.; Morel, C.; Alt, M.; Sablin, M.P.; Franck, C.; Pierron, G.; Callens, C.; Melaabi, S.; Masliah-Planchon, J.; Bataillon, G.; et al. Relevance of a molecular tumour board (MTB) for patients' enrolment in clinical trials: Experience of the Institut Curie. *ESMO Open* **2018**, *3*, e000339. [CrossRef] [PubMed]
19. Schwaederle, M.; Parker, B.A.; Schwab, R.B.; Fanta, P.T.; Boles, S.G.; Daniels, G.A.; Bazhenova, L.A.; Subramanian, R.; Coutinho, A.C.; Ojeda-Fournier, H.; et al. Molecular tumor board: The University of California-San Diego Moores Cancer Center experience. *Oncologist* **2014**, *19*, 631–636. [CrossRef] [PubMed]
20. Harada, S.; Arend, R.; Dai, Q.; Levesque, J.A.; Winokur, T.S.; Guo, R.; Heslin, M.J.; Nabell, L.; Nabors, L.B.; Limdi, N.A.; et al. Implementation and utilization of the molecular tumor board to guide precision medicine. *Oncotarget* **2017**, *8*, 57845. [CrossRef] [PubMed]
21. Bryce, A.H.; Egan, J.B.; Borad, M.J.; Stewart, A.K.; Nowakowski, G.S.; Chanan-Khan, A.; Patnaik, M.M.; Ansell, S.M.; Banck, M.S.; Robinson, S.I.; et al. Experience with precision genomics and tumor board, indicates frequent target identification, but barriers to delivery. *Oncotarget* **2017**, *8*, 27145. [CrossRef] [PubMed]
22. Singer, J.; Irmisch, A.; Ruscheweyh, H.J.; Singer, F.; Toussaint, N.C.; Levesque, M.P.; Stekhoven, D.J.; Beerenwinkel, N. Bioinformatics for precision oncology. *Briefings Bioinforma.* **2019**, *20*, 778–788. [CrossRef] [PubMed]

Publisher's Note: MDPI stays neutral with regard to jurisdictional claims in published maps and institutional affiliations.

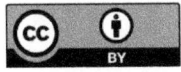

© 2020 by the authors. Licensee MDPI, Basel, Switzerland. This article is an open access article distributed under the terms and conditions of the Creative Commons Attribution (CC BY) license (http://creativecommons.org/licenses/by/4.0/).

Integrin-Linked Kinase Is a Novel Therapeutic Target in Ovarian Cancer

Michael A. Ulm [1], Tiffany M. Redfern [1], Ben R. Wilson [1], Suriyan Ponnusamy [2], Sarah Asemota [2], Patrick W. Blackburn [1], Yinan Wang [3], Adam C. ElNaggar [1] and Ramesh Narayanan [2,*]

[1] Division of Gynecologic Oncology, West Cancer Center and Research Institute, Memphis, TN 38138, USA; mulm@westclinic.com (M.A.U.); tredfern@westclinic.com (T.M.R.); bwilson@westclinic.com (B.R.W.); pblackburn@westclinic.com (P.W.B.); aelnaggar@westclinic.com (A.C.E.)
[2] Department of Medicine, University of Tennessee Health Science Center, Memphis, TN 38163, USA; tponnusa@uthsc.edu (S.P.); vqp741@uthsc.edu (S.A.)
[3] Department of Pathology, University of Tennessee Health Science Center, Memphis, TN 38163, USA; ywang127@uthsc.edu
* Correspondence: rnaraya4@uthsc.edu; Tel.: +1-901-448-2403; Fax: +1-901-448-3910

Received: 5 September 2020; Accepted: 23 November 2020; Published: 26 November 2020

Abstract: Objective: The objective of this study is to identify and validate novel therapeutic target(s) in ovarian cancer. Background: Development of targeted therapeutics in ovarian cancer has been limited by molecular heterogeneity. Although gene expression datasets are available, most of them lack appropriate pair-matched controls to define the alterations that result in the transformation of normal ovarian cells to cancerous cells. Methods: We used microarray to compare the gene expression of treatment-naïve ovarian cancer tissue samples to pair-matched normal adjacent ovarian tissue from 24 patients. Ingenuity Pathway Analysis (IPA) was used to identify target pathways for further analysis. Integrin-linked kinase (ILK) expression in SKOV3 and OV90 cells was determined using Western blot. ILK was knocked down using CRISPR/Cas9 constructs. Subcutaneous xenograft study to determine the effect of ILK knockdown on tumor growth was performed in NOD SCID gamma mice. Results: Significant upregulation of the ILK pathway was identified in 22 of the 24 cancer specimens, identifying it as a potential player that could contribute to the transformation of normal ovarian cells to cancerous cells. Knockdown of ILK in SKOV3 cells resulted in decreased cell proliferation and tumor growth, and inhibition of downstream kinase, AKT (protein kinase B). These results were further validated using an ILK-1 chemical inhibitor, compound 22. Conclusion: Our initial findings validate ILK as a potential therapeutic target for molecular inhibition in ovarian cancer, which warrants further investigation.

Keywords: integrin-linked kinase (ILK); ovarian cancer; sgRNA; gene expression; microarray; xenograft

---

Highlights:

- Integrin-linked kinase (ILK) is upregulated in ovarian cancer specimens relative to normal adjacent tissue specimens.
- ILK siRNA and small-molecule ILK-selective inhibitor (compound 22) inhibited the proliferation of ovarian cancer cells.
- ILK sgRNA lentiviral knockdown in SKOV3 cells resulted in slower tumor growth in NSG mice.
- ILK warrants further investigation as a potential therapeutic target for the treatment of ovarian cancer.

1. Introduction

A hallmark of ovarian cancer is the aggressive and silent nature of metastasis, predominantly through direct extension, into the peritoneal cavity [1]. Metastases are most commonly found within the omentum, the peritoneum, the diaphragm, and bowel surfaces [1,2]. This intraperitoneal dissemination requires detachment, or exfoliation, from the primary tumor on the ovary or fallopian tube [1]. This disruption of integrin–extracellular matrix interactions in normal epithelial cells induces apoptosis [3]. Thus, reduced sensitivity appears to be a hallmark of oncogenic transformation.

It is important to understand epithelial ovarian cancer at the molecular level to determine the underlying causes for its aggressiveness and heterogeneity. Several genome-wide expression studies have been conducted in epithelial ovarian cancer to determine the mechanism for the aggressive phenotype and to identify therapeutic targets [4–6].

Integrin-linked kinase (ILK), a serine-threonine kinase, has multiple functions in cells, such as cell–extracellular matrix interactions, cell cycle, apoptosis, cell proliferation, and cell motility [7–9]. Upregulation of ILK is frequently observed in cancer tissues compared to corresponding normal tissues [10]. Inhibition of ILK has been demonstrated to suppress activation of protein kinase Akt, inducing cell cycle arrest and apoptosis in prostate cancer [11] and colon cancer [12]. ILK is coexpressed with and activates the pro-metastatic enzyme membrane type 1 matrix metalloproteinase (MT1-MMP) in epithelial ovarian cancer cell lines. Downregulation of ILK using siRNA knockdown results in reduced adhesion to and invasion of collagen gels and organotypic meso-mimetic cultures, suggesting that ILK is integral to the development of metastatic disease in ovarian cancer [13].

In this study, we compared differential gene expression of high-grade, treatment-naïve ovarian cancer tissue samples to pair-matched adjacent benign ovarian tissue specimens to identify pathway(s) that are enriched in ovarian cancer tissues compared to adjoining normal ovarian cells. The ILK pathway was identified as the primary pathway that was enriched in cancer tissues compared to adjacent normal tissues. Downregulation of ILK using sgRNA resulted in reduced cell proliferation and tumor growth, confirming ILK as a valid therapeutic target.

2. Materials and Methods

Reagents. TaqMan PCR primers and fluorescent probes, master mixes, and Cells-to-Ct reagents were obtained from Life Technologies (Carlsbad, CA, USA). Cell culture medium and fetal bovine serum were purchased from Fisher Scientific (Waltham, MA, USA). Glyceraldehyde 3-phosphate dehydrogenase (GAPDH) antibody was purchased from Sigma (St. Louis, MO, USA). All other reagents used were of analytical grade. siRNA (Dharmacon Accell on-target plus pool) was ordered from Fisher Scientific. ILK sgRNA CRISPR/Cas9 all-in-one lentiviral vector set (cat. No. K2822105) was procured from Applied Biological Materials Inc. (Richmond, BC, Canada). ILK and pAKT antibodies were procured from Cell Signaling (Danvers, MA, USA). Compound 22 was procured from Millipore (Burlington, MA, USA).

Patient specimen collection. Patient specimens were collected under a University of Tennessee Health Science Center (UTHSC) Institutional Review Board (IRB) approved protocol (14-03113-XP). The Cooperative Human Tissue Network (CHTN) database was searched for ovarian cancer specimens that satisfied the following criteria.

a Histological grade 2 or 3.
b Tumors with adjoining normal ovarian tissue available.
c Treatment naïve.
d Snap frozen to facilitate isolation of high-quality RNA appropriate for microarray.

Out of the more than 10,000 ovarian tumors available in the CHTN database only 24 matched all of these criteria. Three out of the 24 tumors had histological grade less than 3, while the rest are of grade 3. In addition, five specimens were of non-serous epithelial carcinoma type. Histological analysis determined that the tumors contain between 70 and 100% cancer cells.

Microarray. RNA from tumors and benign ovarian specimens was extracted using the Qiagen RNA isolation kit (Qiagen, Hilden, Germany). Quantity was verified using nanodrop and the quality of RNA was verified using the Agilent bioanalyzer. Total RNA (200 ng/sample) from each sample was amplified and labeled using WT Plus Kit from Affymetrix and processed according to Affymetrix protocol. The arrays (Human ST2.0, Affymetrix, Santa Clara, CA, USA) were washed and stained on Affymetrix Fluidics station 450 and scanned on an Affymetrix GCS 3000 scanner. Data from microarrays were normalized using Affymetrix Expression Console. Mean, standard deviation, and variance were calculated across the groups. Fold change from vehicle-treated samples was calculated, and a fold change of 1.5 was used as the cutoff. Pair-wise Student's t-tests were used to determine significance using the cutoff of a p value < 0.05. The false discovery rate (FDR) was calculated using the Benjamini and Hochberg method, and a cutoff for FDR of <0.05 was used to create a significant differential expression list. The gene candidate list was loaded to Ingenuity Pathway Analysis and gene set enrichment analysis (GSEA) was performed for further discovery. Microarray experiments were performed at the UTHSC Molecular Resources Center (MRC), and data analysis was performed by the UTHSC Molecular Bioinformatics core facility. Pathway analysis was also performed using pathway analysis software (Advaita bioinformatics, Ann Arbor, MI). Km plotter was used to obtain Kaplan–Meier plot for ovarian cancer from the Cancer Genome Atlas (TCGA) database [14,15].

Real-time polymerase chain reaction (PCR). Real-time PCR was performed as described previously [16,17]. For RNA isolation and real-time PCR in cells, cells were plated in 96 well plates. RNA was isolated using cells to ct kit and real-time PCR was performed using TaqMan primers and probes on an ABI 7900 real-time PCR machine. RNA from tissues were isolated using RNA isolation kit from Qiagen as described above under the microarray analysis. Total RNA was reverse transcribed into cDNA using reverse transcription kit and real-time PCR was performed for the specified genes using TaqMan real-time PCR primers and probes.

Cell culture. COS7, OV90 and SKOV3 cells were obtained from American Type Culture Collection (ATCC, Manassas, VA, USA). The cells were cultured in accordance with the ATCC recommendations. Respective medium was supplemented with 10% FBS and 1% penicillin-streptomycin. Cells were passaged every third day.

Growth assay. Cells were harvested by trypsinization, counted using a hemocytometer, and plated at 1000 cells per well on 96 well tissue culture plates in quadruplicates. Photomicrographs were taken every four hours using an INCUCYTE live cell imager (Essen Biosciences, AnnArbor, MI, USA) and confluence of the cultures was measured using INCUCYTE software (Essen Biosciences, Ann Arbor, MI, USA) over 72 and 144 h in culture. Simultaneously, cells were plated in 96 well plates. After the indicated period, sulforhodamine blue (SRB) assay was performed to measure the viable cells.

Protein extraction and Western blot. Cells for protein extraction were plated in 60 mm dishes in growth medium. Protein was extracted from tumors and cells as indicated before [16,17]. Protein samples were fractionated on a SDS-PAGE and Western blot was performed with the respective antibodies.

siRNA transfection. A titration starting from 50 nM of accell on-target plus pool siRNA was transfected into the cells using Dharmafect transfection reagent (Dharmacon, Lafayette, CO, USA). Twenty-four hours after transfection, medium was replaced, and the cells were allowed to recover. Efficiency of knockdown was evaluated three and six days after knockdown. GAPDH and scrambled siRNA were used as transfection controls.

CRISPR/Cas9 Lentiviral ILK sgRNA knockdown. Lentivirus carrying ILK sgRNAs (three different CRISPR/Cas9 clones) was produced by packaging in 293FT cells as published previously [18]. SKOV3 cells were plated in 6 well plates at 60% confluence 24 h before viral infection. Twenty-four hours after plating, wells were infected with 1 mL of virus suspension diluted in complete medium with Polybrene to a final concentration of 5–8 µg/mL. Cells were incubated for 48 h and then fed with fresh complete medium without Polybrene. Stable pools of ILK–KO cells were selected with 5 µg/mL puromycin treatment every 3–4 days until drug-resistant colonies were available.

Tumor xenograft experiments. All animal protocols were approved by the UTHSC Institutional Animal Care and Use (IACUC) research committee. Cells (5 million) were implanted subcutaneously in NOD SCID Gamma (NSG) mice. Tumor volume (length * width * width * 0.532) was measured three times weekly. Tumors were collected at sacrifice and stored for further processing. Microarray with Clariom D arrays was performed in the tumor specimens as indicated above. Tumor specimens collected in 10% neutral buffered formalin were sectioned and the sections were stained for hematoxylin and eosin (H&E) and the proliferation marker ki67.

Statistics. Statistical analysis was performed using GraphPad prism software (La Jolla, CA, USA). Experiments containing two groups were analyzed by simple t-test, while those containing more than two groups were analyzed by one-way analysis of variance (ANOVA) followed by Tukey's post-hoc test. All in vitro experiments were performed at least in triplicate. Data are represented as the mean ± S.E. Significance is expressed as * $p < 0.05$, ** $p < 0.01$, and *** $p < 0.001$.

3. Results

ILK is overexpressed in ovarian cancer relative to normal ovarian tissue: To identify reliable therapeutic targets for advanced ovarian cancer, high-grade treatment-naïve ovarian cancer specimens, and pair-matched adjacent normal ovarian tissues were obtained from the CHTN (Figure 1). The patient characteristics are provided in Table 1. Pair-matched normal ovarian specimens were allowed for the determination of alterations that took place in the ovarian cells that led to their transformation into cancerous cells. Out of almost 10,000 ovarian cancer specimens available in the CHTN, only 24 specimens met the criteria described above. Human Transcriptome Array (HT2.0) array was used to determine the genes, small non-coding RNAs, and pathways that were altered in cancer specimens compared to respective normal ovarian tissues. Using 1.5-fold up- or downregulation as a cutoff and an FDR of 0.05, we found that 994 genes and non-coding RNAs were differentially expressed in ovarian cancer specimens compared to pair-matched controls. The most upregulated genes included osteopontin (SPP1), ceruloplasmin (CP), desmoplasmin (DSP), epithelial splicing regulatory proteins (ESRP1), and cadherin (CDH1). The heatmap and unsupervised hierarchical clustering of statistically significant genes shows clustering of normal specimens (except for one normal specimen) to one side and the tumors to the other side (Figure 2).

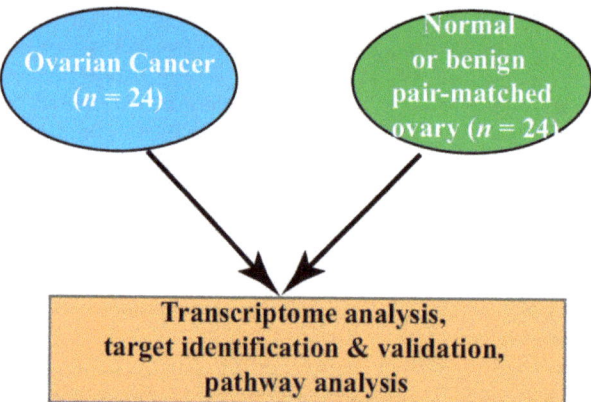

Figure 1. Experiment design. Ovarian cancer specimens (mostly histological grade 3) and adjacent normal tissue specimens ($n = 24$) were used in gene expression microarray experiments and pathway analyses.

Table 1. Patient characteristics.

S. No.	Age	Histology	Hist. Grade	O.S. (Months after Diagnosis)
1	34	Endometrioid adenocarcinoma	1	8
2	41	Endometrioid adenocarcinoma	3	>72
3	57	Serous	3	0.3
4	65	Serous	3	>72
5	74	Serous	3	>72
6	75	Endometrioid adenocarcinoma	3	2
7	77	Serous	3	>72
8	51	Serous	3	48
9	64	Serous	3	24
10	49	Serous	3	7
11	80	Serous	3	8

S. No.—sample number; O.S.—overall survival.

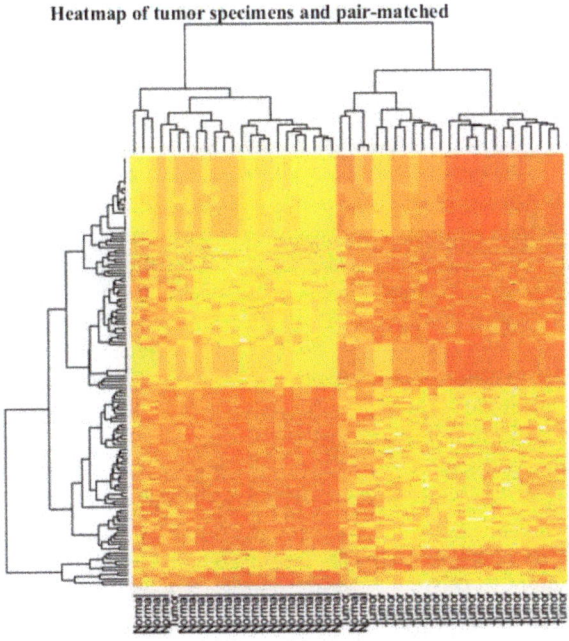

Figure 2. Pathway analysis. Heatmap of differentially regulated genes between tumor specimens and their respective pair-matched control specimens.

The top 100 statistically significant genes were loaded into the Ingenuity Pathway Analysis (IPA) software for the identification of pathways and regulators that were enriched in this dataset (Table 2). The most enriched pathways identified by IPA are the integrin-linked pathway, tryptophan degradation X, putrescine degradation, insulin-like growth factor-1 signaling, and 14-3-3 sigma signaling. A significant enrichment of the ILK pathway was identified in 22 of the 24 cancer specimens, identifying this pathway as a potential player in the transformation of normal ovarian cells to cancerous cells (Table 2). The genes that represent the ILK pathway in the microarray included FOS, DSP, myosin 11 (MYH11), CDH1, mucin 1 (MUC1), and keratin (KRT18). While FOS and MYH11 were lower in the tumor specimens compared to their normal controls, the other genes were more prevalent in the tumor specimens. Interestingly, although c-FOS is a proto-oncogene, counterintuitively its expression was reduced in the cancer specimens. Evidences for c-FOS overexpression as promoting apoptosis and delaying ovarian cancer progression in preclinical models may be supported by the findings in these clinical specimens [19]. MYH11 expression has been shown to be downregulated in cancers, and its downregulation corresponds to poor prognosis and survival [20].

Table 2. Ingenuity Pathway Analysis.

Top Canonical Pathways		Top Upstream Regulators	
Ingenuity Canonical Pathways	$-\log(p\text{-Value})$	Ingenuity Canonical Pathways	$-\log(p\text{-Value})$
Integrin-linked kinase signaling	2.38×10^{-4}	WISP2	1.32×10^{-8}
Tryptophan degradation X	2.63×10^{-3}	PDGF BB	5.45×10^{-8}
Putrescine degradation III	2.63×10^{-3}	LIMA 1	1.30×10^{-7}
Dopamine degradation	4.11×10^{-3}	Estrogen Receptor	2.01×10^{-7}
Noradrenaline & adrenaline degradation	1.03×10^{-2}	NTRK-1	3.77×10^{-7}

The top enriched upstream regulator pathway identified by IPA was the Wnt-1 inducible-signaling pathway (WISP1). The genes that encode the WISP1 pathway identified in the microarray dataset include cluster of differentiation (CD24), CDH1, DSP, KRT18, keratin 8 (KRT8), and MUC1. All of these genes were upregulated in cancer specimens compared to their respective normal controls. The WISP1 pathway is involved in cancer cell proliferation, invasion, and metastasis, and has been shown to be responsible for shorter patient survival [21]. Collectively, the genes enriched in the top canonical pathways and the upstream regulators indicate that the pathways responsible for tumor cell proliferation, metastasis, and invasion are altered to favor cancer growth and metastasis.

Genes and pathways responsible for shorter survival: One of the interesting observations made in the specimens was that some patients survived longer, as much as six years since their first diagnosis, while several others had shorter survival from diagnosis (Table 1). To determine whether the genome-wide expression data provided any indication of the pathways that were contributing to shorter survival, we analyzed the genes based on survival. Unsupervised hierarchical clustering resulted in three subsets with regard to survival. They are patients who survived less than 30 months, those who survived greater than 30 months, and those who were alive at the time of the last data collection. Interestingly, 581 genes were statistically significant in patients who died less than 30 months after diagnosis. The biological pathways that were enriched in the early-death patients were cell adhesion, response to wound healing, and metabolic processes (Figure 3B). The most upregulated gene in the cell adhesion pathway was SPP1, a gene that encodes for osteopontin. Osteopontin that activates interleukin 17 (IL-17) has been shown to be upregulated in ovarian cancer and important for its metastasis [22].

The canonical pathway that was enriched in the patients who were alive at the time of sample collection (greater than six years) was the apelin pathway. Most of the genes in this pathway were downregulated. Considering that the apelin and its ligand apela are oncogenic [23], it is consistent that this pathway was downregulated in patients who survived the longest.

ILK is associated with shorter progression-free survival (PFS): The microarray findings were validated by real-time PCR. All genes that were validated showed reproducible results (Figure 4A). ILK pathway genes DSP and MUC1 were included in the validation. We then determined the effect of ILK-1 high expression on stage III and IV ovarian cancer patients' PFS in the TCGA database using Km plotter (Figure 4B). The probe range was between 32 and 3950 and a cutoff of 1335 was used to define high- vs. low-expression specimens. Ovarian cancer patients with high ILK expression had shorter PFS compared to patients with cancer that expressed lower ILK. The hazard ratio (HR) was 1.36 and the log-rank p was 0.000043. This validated the findings made in our study.

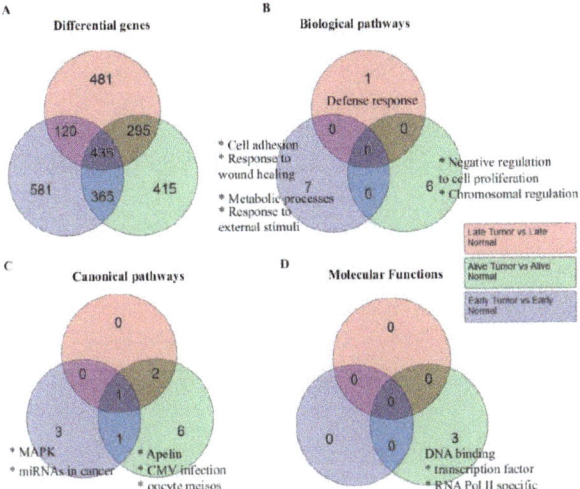

Figure 3. Pathway analysis of the differentially expressed genes with samples segregated based on survival. The numbers in the figures represent the number of genes (**A**) and the enriched pathways (**B**–**D**). The different pathways are represented in each Venn circle. Survival was defined as those patients who survived less than 30 months post-diagnosis (early), more than 30 months (late), and were alive at the time of data collection (alive).

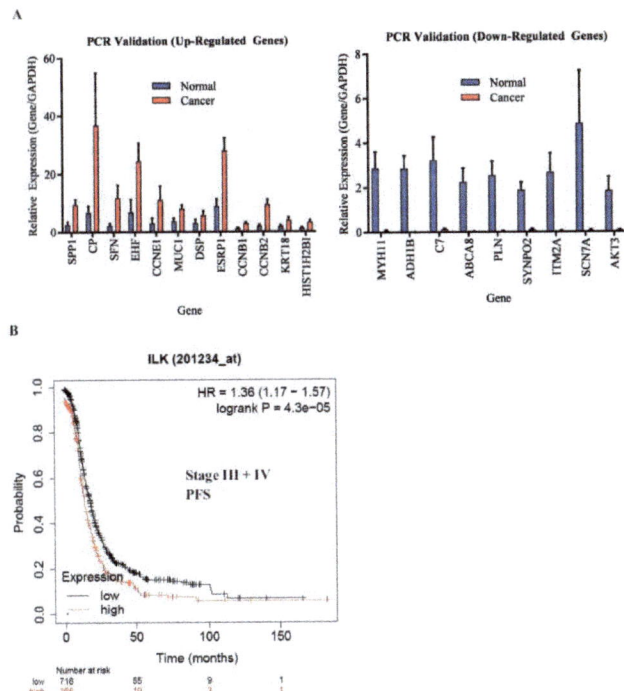

Figure 4. Validation of microarray data by real-time PCR. (**A**) Real-time PCR validation of a subset of genes identified by microarray ($n = 5$/gene). (**B**) Kaplan–Meier plot of the integrin-linked pathway (ILK-1) in the cancer genome atlas (TCGA).

ILK is expressed in ovarian cancer cell lines: To determine whether ILK is expressed in ovarian cancer cell lines, Western blots in SKOV3 and OV90 ovarian cancer cell lines were performed and compared to non-cancerous COS7 cells. SKOV3 cells were chosen as they represented an established, well published serous or epithelial ovarian cancer cell line. OV90 cells were chosen as they are high-grade serous ovarian carcinoma and have an established track record in translational research. Figure 5A shows high expression of ILK in both ovarian cancer cell lines, while COS7 failed to express ILK-1 at detectable levels.

Compound 22 reduces the proliferation of SKOV3 and OV90 cell proliferation: Compound 22 (CP22), is a selective ILK inhibitor that was shown to be antiproliferative in prostate cancer [24]. To characterize the efficacy of CP22, we conducted proliferation studies in SKOV3 and OV90 cell lines in INCUCYTE. A prior dose response study was conducted to narrow down the doses of CP22 to 3 and 10 µM to be used in these experiments. Cells were incubated with DMSO or CP22 at 3 µM or 10 µM and imaged using INCUCYTE. CP22 effectively reduced the proliferation in a dose-dependent manner relative to vehicle control (Figure 5B).

Compound 22 facilitates dephosphorylation of Akt: In order to determine the efficacy of CP22 in ovarian cancer cell lines, Western blot for phosphorylated AKT was performed in SKOV3 and OV90 cells. AKT is a downstream target of ILK [11]. SKOV3 cells were incubated with DMSO or CP22 at 10 µM for 4 h and Western blot for AKT phosphorylation was performed. CP22 effectively inhibited the phosphorylation of AKT (Figure 5C).

siRNA knockdown of ILK reduced SKOV3 cell proliferation: To determine whether knockdown of ILK expression affects ovarian cancer cell proliferation, we transfected SKOV3 cells with ILK siRNA and measured the number of viable cells by SRB assay. Following transfection with siRNA directed against ILK, SKOV3 cells were incubated for 6 days. RT-PCR following siRNA directed knockdown of ILK showed a reduction in ILK expression in transfected cells compared to cells transfected with GAPDH (Figure 5D). A cell proliferation assay was performed following siRNA tranfection that showed a reduced cellular proliferation of SKOV3 cells following ILK siRNA transfection (Figure 5D). The results were comparable when scrambled, instead of GAPDH, siRNA was used as a control.

ILK knockdown in SKOV3 cells results in tumor growth inhibition: To validate the findings obtained using a transient knockdown of ILK-1 using siRNAs, ILK was knocked down stably in SKOV3 cells using CRISPR/Cas9 sgRNA lentiviral constructs. Three sgRNAs to different regions of ILK were used to knockdown ILK. Lentivirus particles containing the CRISPR/Cas9 vectors were prepared and the cells were infected. Western blot showed that all three sgRNAs comparably knocked down ILK (Figure 6A). Control and ILK knockdown SKOV3 cells (clone 1 or virus 1) were implanted subcutaneously in NSG mice and tumor growth was monitored. Since the cells were not labeled with luciferase, subcutaneous, but not orthotopic, model was used to conduct the xenograft studies. ILK knockdown resulted in slower tumor uptake and growth (Figure 6B), confirming the observation made in vitro. Western blot with proteins extracted from tumor tissues confirmed the ILK knockdown and the inhibition of the downstream AKT phosphorylation (Figure 6C).

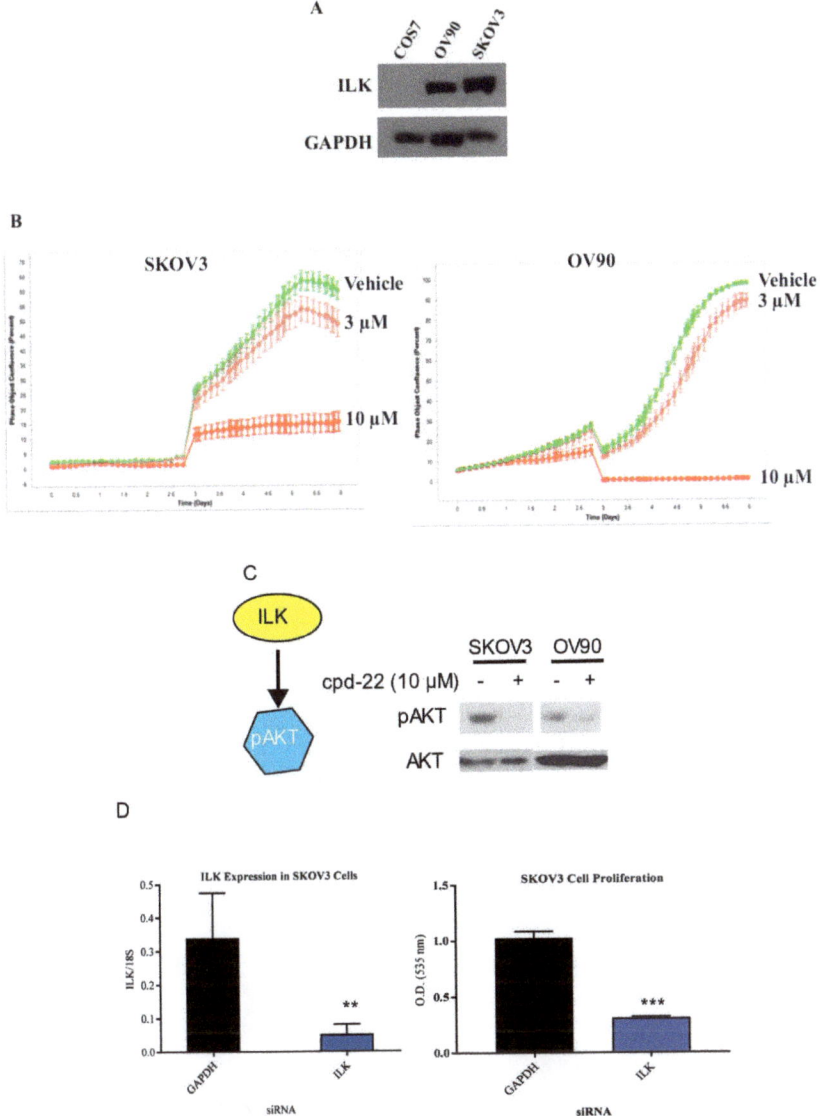

Figure 5. In vitro validation of the ILK pathway. (**A**) Protein expression of ILK-1 in two ovarian cancer cell lines, SKOV3 and OV90 and non-cancerous COS7 cells. Protein was extracted from the cells, fractionated on an SDS-PAGE, and Western blot for ILK-1 and GAPDH was performed. (**B**) INCUCYTE proliferation assay of SKOV3 and OV90 cell lines in the presence of vehicle (DMSO) or 3 or 10 µM ILK inhibitor compound 22. Images were obtained periodically for the indicated time-points. (**C**) Phosphorylation of AKT was inhibited by ILK-1 inhibitor compound 22. SKOV3 and OV90 cells were treated with compound 22 for 4 h. Cells were harvested, protein extracted, and Western blot with phospho-AKT and total AKT antibodies was performed. (**D**) ILK-1 siRNA inhibits SKOV3 cell proliferation. SKOV3 cells were transfected with ILK-1 or GAPDH siRNA. Six days after transfection (re-transfected after day 3) mRNA expression of ILK-1 and 18S (left) and cell proliferation (right) by sulforhodamine B (SRB) assay were measured ($n = 3$). ** $p < 0.01$; *** $p < 0.001$.

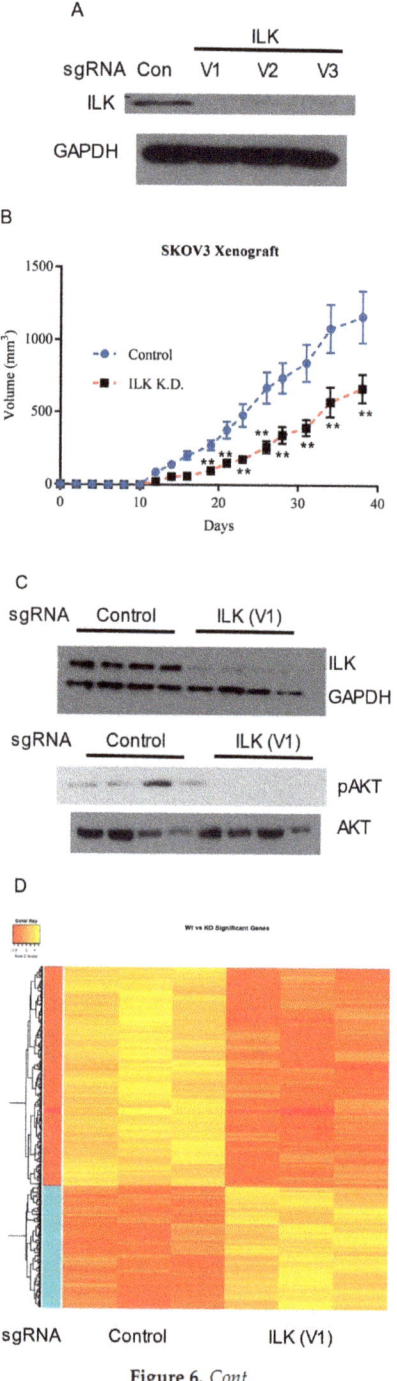

Figure 6. *Cont.*

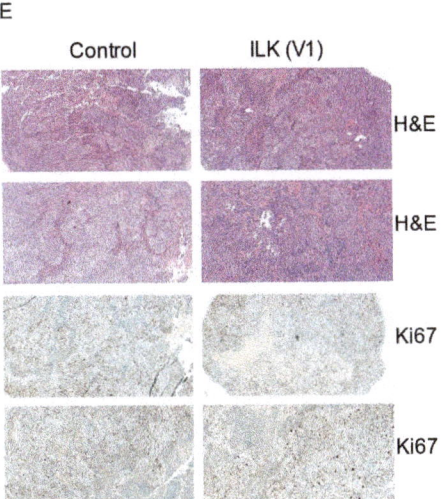

Figure 6. ILK-1 is important for SKOV3 tumor growth. (**A**) ILK-1 was knocked out using three CRISPR/Cas9 sgRNA. Western blot shows the knockout in SKOV3 cells. Control sgRNA was used in the vector-infected group. (**B**) Control and ILK-1 sgRNA knockdown cells (virus 1) were implanted in NSG mice (n = 15/group). Tumor uptake and growth were measured over the course of this study. Animals were sacrificed at the end of this study, tumors were isolated, and stored for further analysis. (**C**) Western blot in the tumors from animals described in panel B is provided. V1 corresponds to virus 1 (clone 1) of the three clones that were screened. (**D**) RNA was isolated from the tumors and the expression of genes in the vector or ILK-1 knockdown tumors (n = 3/group) was measured by microarray. (**E**) Representative H&E and ki67 staining of tumor sections. Statistically different genes between the two groups are represented as heatmap. ** $p < 0.01$.

RNA was isolated from control and ILK knockdown tumors and microarray was performed to determine the effect of ILK knockdown on global gene expression. Knockdown of ILK resulted in alteration of 1301 genes with the hierarchical clustering demonstrating that ILK knockdown tissues clustered together (Figure 6D). The most significant pathway that was altered in ILK knockdown specimens was the ribosomal family of proteins (RPS) genes. Most of the RPS genes were downregulated in ILK knockdown specimens compared to control sgRNA specimens. In addition to the RPS pathway, metabolic pathways were also significantly downregulated in the ILK knockdown tumors.

The FFPE tumors were stained for H&E and ki67. As shown in Figure 6E, the tumor cell proliferation was lower in ILK sgRNA infected cells, matching the results observed with the tumor volume measurement. Representative images are included.

4. Discussion

Epithelial ovarian cancer is a heterologous disease in which the molecular and clinical phenotype can vary significantly between patients [25]. While platinum/taxane chemotherapy remains the standard basis for treatment of this difficult disease, the development of poly-ADP ribose inhibitors (PARPi) has ushered in a new era of molecular therapeutics for the treatment of ovarian cancer, taking advantage of deficiencies in the homologous recombination pathway. PARPi increased survival outcomes for patients with both somatic and germline mutations in BRCA and genes encoding the proteins involved in DNA repair by homologous recombination. For patients without somatic or germline homologous recombination mutations and for those whose cancer have become resistant to PARPi therapy, advances in targeted therapeutics are needed to improve survival of patients with advanced ovarian cancer [26]. Ongoing clinical trials in ovarian cancer are evaluating inhibitors of multiple molecular pathways such as PI3K/AKT, the mTOR pathway, angiogenesis, the MAPK pathway, and the HER/EGFR pathway [27,28]. Our preliminary results showing ILK inhibition in epithelial ovarian cancer highlight a novel pathway for the development of small-molecule inhibitors of this pathway for ovarian cancer treatment.

We discovered a significant upregulation of the ILK pathway through Ingenuity Pathway Analysis, identifying a novel target for molecular inhibition and validating work performed by Ahmed et al. in 2003 [29]. Similarly, upregulation of the ILK pathway is found in colorectal, breast, gastric and pancreatic carcinoma. The association between worse survival in patients with ovarian cancer who exhibit ILK upregulation is also true for these different cancers types as well [9]. In SKOV3 cells, inhibition of ILK using ILK-sgRNA results in upregulation of pro-apoptotic bax gene expression and downregulation of antiapoptotic genes in addition to reduced cell viability, similar to our results [8]. The downstream pathways that are significantly altered when ILK was knocked down include ribosome and metabolic pathways. Previous publications have demonstrated the importance of ribosomal proteins in ovarian cancer. Knockdown of RPS6 resulted in an inhibition of ovarian cancer cell proliferation and invasion [30]. Similarly, the metabolic pathways have been shown to be pivotal for the development of ovarian and other cancers [31]. Several of the ILK pathway genes such as DSP1, FOS, BMP2, and AKT3 that were altered between ovarian cancer and adjacent normal specimens in Figure 2 were altered in the knockdown dataset in Figure 6. These results collectively suggest that ILK is an important mediator of proliferation in ovarian cancer and attempts to deregulate this pathway will provide a bona fide therapeutic approach.

Furthermore, antisense oligonucleotide silencing of ILK expression has been shown to suppress tumor growth in nude mice xenografts [8]. ILK silencing has also been shown to reduce the expression of wnt ligands (wnt3a, wnt4, and wnt5a) and β-catenin in epithelial ovarian cancer cells [32]. Prior studies evaluating Compound 54 (CP54), a non-selective ILK inhibitor, failed to demonstrate activity in vivo due to its lack of specificity [33,34]. CP22 was developed as a highly selective inhibitor of ILK and was shown to have antiproliferative effects in both in vitro and in vivo experiments in prostate cancer [24]. Reyes-Gonzalez et al. showed that both ILK-siRNA and CP22 reduced cell growth, invasion ability and increased apoptosis in both cisplatin-sensitive and cisplatin-resistant ovarian cancer cell lines [35]. They also showed that high ILK expression in tumors from patients with ovarian cancer was associated with worse survival compared to patients with low ILK expression. Li et al. also showed that after transfection with ILK-antisense oligonucleotides, HO-8910 cells spent more time in in the G0/G1 phase, delayed tumor formation and decreased tumor growth compared to controls in xenograft models [36]. The HO-9810 cell line was originally thought to be derived from a 51 year old patient with serous ovarian cancer but was later found to be a derivation of the HeLa cell line, and is not an ovarian cancer model for validation of potential molecular targets for the treatment of ovarian cancer [37]. Our findings expanded on the findings of Reyes-Gonzalez et al. by validating that ILK silencing results in reduced in vivo tumor growth in a validate ovarian cancer cell line. The efficacy of CP22 in epithelial ovarian cancer cell lines and in vivo patient-derived xenografts validates the ability of small-molecule inhibitors to successfully target the ILK pathway in ovarian cancer and warrants further study. At the time of tissue collection, our goal was to obtain tissue from high-grade serous ovarian cancer specimens. The hypothesis regarding fallopian tube origin of high-grade serous ovarian carcinoma had not widely been accepted and thus fallopian tube was not considered normal matched paired tissue [38]. Although two specimens were ultimately found to be clear cell and transitional carcinoma in the analysis and recognize that these likely have different molecular signatures, they represented 2 out of the 24 specimens and we do not feel that their inclusion compromised our analysis. The normal adjacent tissue specimens contained epithelial, stroma and ovarian stem cells as well, not just epithelial tissue. ILK inhibition in ovarian cancer, however, has been shown to affect apoptotic, proliferative, and metastatic pathways.

The introduction of poly ADP-ribose (PARP) inhibition represented a paradigm shift in the traditional approach to ovarian cancer management by ushering in a new era where patient survival can be improved by delivering individualized therapeutics based upon germline and/or somatic testing [39]. Developing a similar understanding of response to ILK inhibition requires better understanding of the genetic alterations that predispose an individual's tumor to respond. Murine models of patient-derived ovarian cancer tissue that have undergone next-generation sequencing are currently under development and will provide insight into the molecular profiles of tumors that respond to ILK inhibition. As more targeted therapeutics become available for patients with homologous recombination deficiency and mismatch repair deficiency, there is an increasing need for a large subset of patients who are not candidates for these targeted, life-saving therapies. ILK represents a potential pathway that may provide a promising alternative to PARPi or immunotherapy in patients who are homologous repair proficient and mismatch repair proficient.

Author Contributions: M.A.U., T.M.R., B.R.W., S.P., S.A., P.W.B. and Y.W. performed the experiments. A.C.E. and R.N. designed the experiments and oversaw the project. M.A.U. and R.N. drafted the manuscript. M.A.U., T.M.R., B.R.W. and A.C.E. edited the manuscript. All authors have read and agreed to the published version of the manuscript.

Funding: This research received no external funding.

Conflicts of Interest: No authors have any relevant conflict of interest to disclose.

References

1. Lengyel, E. Ovarian Cancer Development and Metastasis. *Am. J. Pathol.* **2010**, *177*, 1053–1064. [CrossRef] [PubMed]
2. Raspagliesi, F.; Ditto, A.; Martinelli, F.; Haeusler, E.A.; Lorusso, D. Advanced ovarian cancer: Omental bursa, lesser omentum, celiac, portal and triad nodes spread as cause of inaccurate evaluation of residual tumor. *Gynecol. Oncol.* **2013**, *129*, 92–96. [CrossRef]
3. Aharoni, D.; Meiri, I.; Atzmon, R.; Vlodavsky, I.; Amsterdam, A. Differential effect of components of the extracellular matrix on differentiation and apoptosis. *Curr. Biol.* **1997**, *7*, 43–51. [CrossRef]
4. Sallinen, H.; Janhonen, S.; Pölönen, P.; Niskanen, H.; Liu, O.H.; Kivelä, A.; Hartikainen, J.M.; Anttila, M.; Heinäniemi, M.; Yla-Herttuala, S.; et al. Comparative transcriptome analysis of matched primary and distant metastatic ovarian carcinoma. *BMC Cancer* **2019**, *19*, 1121. [CrossRef] [PubMed]
5. Ye, X. Confluence analysis of multiple omics on platinum resistance of ovarian cancer. *Eur. J. Gynaecol. Oncol.* **2015**, *36*, 514–519.
6. Cohen, S.; Mosig, R.; Moshier, E.; Pereira, E.; Rahaman, J.; Prasad-Hayes, M.; Halpert, R.; Billaud, J.-N.; Dottino, P.; Martignetti, J.A. Interferon regulatory factor 1 is an independent predictor of platinum resistance and survival in high-grade serous ovarian carcinoma. *Gynecol. Oncol.* **2014**, *134*, 591–598. [CrossRef]
7. Dedhar, S.; Williams, B.; Hannigan, G. Integrin-linked kinase (ILK): A regulator of integrin and growth-factor signalling. *Trends Cell Biol.* **1999**, *9*, 319–323. [CrossRef]
8. Liu, Q.; Xiao, L.; Yuan, D.; Shi, X.; Li, P. Silencing of the integrin-linked kinase gene induces the apoptosis in ovarian carcinoma. *J. Recept. Signal Transduct.* **2012**, *32*, 120–127. [CrossRef]
9. Zheng, C.-C.; Hu, H.-F.; Hong, P.; Zhang, Q.-H.; Xu, W.W.; He, Q.-Y.; Li, B. Significance of integrin-linked kinase (ILK) in tumorigenesis and its potential implication as a biomarker and therapeutic target for human cancer. *Am. J. Cancer Res.* **2019**, *9*, 186–197.
10. Attwell, S.; Roskelley, C.; Dedhar, S. The integrin-linked kinase (ILK) suppresses anoikis. *Oncogene* **2000**, *19*, 3811–3815. [CrossRef]
11. Wang, S.; Basson, M.D. Integrin-Linked Kinase: A Multi-functional Regulator Modulating Extracellular Pressure-Stimulated Cancer Cell Adhesion through Focal Adhesion Kinase and AKT. *Cell. Oncol.* **2009**, *31*, 273–289. [CrossRef]
12. Assi, K.; Mills, J.; Owen, D.; Ong, C.; St-Arnaud, R.; Dedhar, S.; Salh, B. Integrin-linked kinase regulates cell proliferation and tumour growth in murine colitis-associated carcinogenesis. *Gut* **2008**, *57*, 931–940. [CrossRef] [PubMed]
13. Bruney, L.; Liu, Y.; Grisoli, A.; Ravosa, M.J.; Stack, M.S. Integrin-linked kinase activity modulates the pro-metastatic behavior of ovarian cancer cells. *Oncotarget* **2016**, *7*, 21968–21981. [CrossRef] [PubMed]

14. Nagy, Á.; Lánczky, A.; Menyhárt, O.; Győrffy, B. Validation of miRNA prognostic power in hepatocellular carcinoma using expression data of independent datasets. *Sci. Rep.* **2018**, *8*, 1–9. [CrossRef]
15. Győrffy, B.; Lánczky, A.; Szállási, Z. Implementing an online tool for genome-wide validation of survival-associated biomarkers in ovarian-cancer using microarray data from 1287 patients. *Endocrine-Relat. Cancer* **2012**, *19*, 197–208. [CrossRef]
16. Ponnusamy, S.; Asemota, S.; Schwartzberg, L.S.; Guestini, F.; McNamara, K.M.; Pierobon, M.; Font-Tello, A.; Qiu, X.; Xie, Y.; Rao, P.K.; et al. Androgen Receptor Is a Non-canonical Inhibitor of Wild-Type and Mutant Estrogen Receptors in Hormone Receptor-Positive Breast Cancers. *Iscience* **2019**, *21*, 341–358. [CrossRef]
17. Ponnusamy, S.; He, Y.; Hwang, D.-J.; Thiyagarajan, T.; Houtman, R.; Bocharova, V.; Sumpter, B.G.; Fernandez, E.; Johnson, D.L.; Du, Z.; et al. Orally Bioavailable Androgen Receptor Degrader, Potential Next-Generation Therapeutic for Enzalutamide-Resistant Prostate Cancer. *Clin. Cancer Res.* **2019**, *25*, 6764–6780. [CrossRef]
18. Yue, J.; Sheng, Y.; Ren, A.; Penmatsa, S. A miR-21 hairpin structure-based gene knockdown vector. *Biochem. Biophys. Res. Commun.* **2010**, *394*, 667–672. [CrossRef]
19. Oliveira-Ferrer, L.; Rößler, K.; Haustein, V.; Schröder, C.; Wicklein, D.; Maltseva, D.; Khaustova, N.; Samatov, T.; Tonevitsky, A.; Mahner, S.; et al. c-FOS suppresses ovarian cancer progression by changing adhesion. *Br. J. Cancer* **2013**, *110*, 753–763. [CrossRef] [PubMed]
20. Nie, M.; Pan, X.; Tao, H.; Xu, M.; Liu, S.; Sun, W.; Wu, J.; Zou, X. Clinical and prognostic significance of MYH11 in lung cancer. *Oncol. Lett.* **2020**, *19*, 3899–3906. [CrossRef]
21. Gurbuz, I.; Chiquet-Ehrismann, R. CCN4/WISP1 (WNT1 inducible signaling pathway protein 1): A focus on its role in cancer. *Int. J. Biochem. Cell Biol.* **2015**, *62*, 142–146. [CrossRef] [PubMed]
22. Hu, H.; Liu, Z.; Liu, C. Correlation of OPN gene expression with proliferation and apoptosis of ovarian cancer cells and prognosis of patients. *Oncol. Lett.* **2019**, *17*, 2788–2794. [CrossRef] [PubMed]
23. Ganguly, D.; Cai, C.; Sims, M.; Yang, C.H.; Thomas, M.; Cheng, J.; Saad, A.; Pfeffer, L.M. APELA Expression in Glioma, and Its Association with Patient Survival and Tumor Grade. *Pharmaceuticals* **2019**, *12*, 45. [CrossRef]
24. Lee, S.-L.; Hsu, E.-C.; Chou, C.-C.; Chuang, H.-C.; Bai, L.-Y.; Kulp, S.K.; Chen, C.-S. Identification and Characterization of a Novel Integrin-Linked Kinase Inhibitor. *J. Med. Chem.* **2011**, *54*, 6364–6374. [CrossRef] [PubMed]
25. Kohn, E.C.; Romano, S.; Lee, J.-M. Clinical implications of using molecular diagnostics for ovarian cancers. *Ann. Oncol.* **2013**, *24*, x22–x26. [CrossRef]
26. Ulm, M.; Ramesh, A.V.; McNamara, K.M.; Ponnusamy, S.; Sasano, H.; Narayanan, R. Therapeutic advances in hormone-dependent cancers: Focus on prostate, breast and ovarian cancers. *Endocr. Connect.* **2019**, *8*, R10–R26. [CrossRef] [PubMed]
27. Vetter, M.H.; Hays, J.L. Use of Targeted Therapeutics in Epithelial Ovarian Cancer: A Review of Current Literature and Future Directions. *Clin. Ther.* **2018**, *40*, 361–371. [CrossRef] [PubMed]
28. Mabuchi, S.; Kuroda, H.; Takahashi, R.; Sasano, T. The PI3K/AKT/mTOR pathway as a therapeutic target in ovarian cancer. *Gynecol. Oncol.* **2015**, *137*, 173–179. [CrossRef]
29. Ahmed, N.; Riley, C.; Oliva, K.; Stutt, E.; Rice, G.E.; A Quinn, M. Integrin-linked kinase expression increases with ovarian tumour grade and is sustained by peritoneal tumour fluid. *J. Pathol.* **2003**, *201*, 229–237. [CrossRef]
30. Yang, X.; Xu, L.; Yang, Y.-E.; Xiong, C.; Yu, J.; Wang, Y.; Lin, Y. Knockdown of ribosomal protein S6 suppresses proliferation, migration, and invasion in epithelial ovarian cancer. *J. Ovarian Res.* **2020**, *13*, 1–11. [CrossRef]
31. Ghahremani, H.; Nabati, S.; Tahmori, H.; Peirouvi, T.; Sirati-Sabet, M.; Salami, S. Long-Term Glucose Restriction with or without β-Hydroxybutyrate Enrichment Distinctively Alters Epithelial-Mesenchymal Transition-Related Signalings in Ovarian Cancer Cells. *Nutr. Cancer* **2020**, *2020*, 1–19. [CrossRef] [PubMed]
32. Yuan, D.; Zhao, Y.; Wang, Y.; Che, J.; Tan, W.; Jin, Y.; Wang, F.; Wenliang, Z.; Fu, S.; Liu, Q.; et al. Effect of integrin-linked kinase gene silencing on microRNA expression in ovarian cancer. *Mol. Med. Rep.* **2017**, *16*, 7267–7276. [CrossRef] [PubMed]
33. Kalra, J.; Warburton, C.; Fang, K.; Edwards, L.; Daynard, T.; Waterhouse, D.; Dragowska, W.; Sutherland, B.W.; Dedhar, S.; Gelmon, K.; et al. QLT0267, a small molecule inhibitor targeting integrin-linked kinase (ILK), and docetaxel can combine to produce synergistic interactions linked to enhanced cytotoxicity, reductions in P-AKT levels, altered F-actin architecture and improved treatment outcomes in an orthotopic breast cancer model. *Breast Cancer Res.* **2009**, *11*, R25. [CrossRef] [PubMed]

34. Eke, I.; Leonhardt, F.; Storch, K.; Hehlgans, S.; Cordes, N. The Small Molecule Inhibitor QLT0267 Radiosensitizes Squamous Cell Carcinoma Cells of the Head and Neck. *PLoS ONE* **2009**, *4*, e6434. [CrossRef]
35. Tiwari, S.; Patel, A.; Prasad, S.M. Phytohormone up-regulates the biochemical constituent, exopolysaccharide and nitrogen metabolism in paddy-field cyanobacteria exposed to chromium stress. *BMC Microbiol.* **2020**, *20*. [CrossRef]
36. Li, Q.; Li, C.; Zhang, Y.; Chen, W.; Lv, J.-L.; Sun, J.; You, Q.-S. Silencing of integrin-linked kinase suppresses in vivo tumorigenesis of human ovarian carcinoma cells. *Mol. Med. Rep.* **2013**, *7*, 1050–1054. [CrossRef] [PubMed]
37. Ye, F.; Chen, C.; Qin, J.; Liu, J.; Zheng, C. Genetic profiling reveals an alarming rate of cross-contamination among human cell lines used in China. *FASEB J.* **2015**, *29*, 4268–4272. [CrossRef] [PubMed]
38. Carlson, J.W.; Miron, A.; Jarboe, E.A.; Parast, M.M.; Hirsch, M.S.; Lee, Y.; Muto, M.G.; Kindelberger, D.; Crum, C.P. Serous Tubal Intraepithelial Carcinoma: Its Potential Role in Primary Peritoneal Serous Carcinoma and Serous Cancer Prevention. *J. Clin. Oncol.* **2008**, *26*, 4160–4165. [CrossRef] [PubMed]
39. Liu, J.F.; Konstantinopoulos, P.A.; Matulonis, U.A. PARP inhibitors in ovarian cancer: Current status and future promise. *Gynecol. Oncol.* **2014**, *133*, 362–369. [CrossRef] [PubMed]

Publisher's Note: MDPI stays neutral with regard to jurisdictional claims in published maps and institutional affiliations.

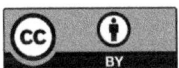

© 2020 by the authors. Licensee MDPI, Basel, Switzerland. This article is an open access article distributed under the terms and conditions of the Creative Commons Attribution (CC BY) license (http://creativecommons.org/licenses/by/4.0/).

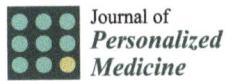

Review

Biomarker Development for Metastatic Renal Cell Carcinoma: Omics, Antigens, T-cells, and Beyond

Benjamin Miron, David Xu and Matthew Zibelman *

Department of Hematology/Oncology, Fox Chase Cancer Center, Philadelphia, PA 19111, USA; benjamin.miron@tuhs.temple.edu (B.M.); david.xu@tuhs.temple.edu (D.X.)
* Correspondence: Matthew.Zibelman@fccc.edu; Tel.: +1-215-728-3889

Received: 28 October 2020; Accepted: 10 November 2020; Published: 13 November 2020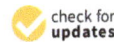

Abstract: The treatment of metastatic renal cell carcinoma has evolved quickly over the last few years from a disease managed primarily with sequential oral tyrosine kinase inhibitors (TKIs) targeting the vascular endothelial growth factor (VEGF) pathway, to now with a combination of therapies incorporating immune checkpoint blockade (ICB). Patient outcomes have improved with these innovations, however, controversy persists regarding optimal sequence and patient selection amongst the available combinations. Ideally, predictive biomarkers would aid in guiding treatment decisions and personalizing care. However, clinically-actionable biomarkers have remained elusive. We aim to review the available evidence regarding biomarkers for both TKIs and ICB and will present where the field may be headed in the years to come.

Keywords: biomarkers; renal cell carcinoma; clear cell; VEGF; immunotherapy; PD-L1; immune checkpoint inhibitors; immune checkpoint blockade; tyrosine-kinase inhibitors

1. Introduction

Renal cell carcinoma (RCC) is traditionally classified according to its histology. Clear cell (ccRCC) is the most common subtype, accounting for 75–85% of all RCCs. Current first-line standard of care therapies for metastatic ccRCC involve the use of vascular endothelial growth factor (VEGF) inhibitors, checkpoint inhibitors, anti-CTLA4 agents, or a combination of these drugs. Choice of therapy is guided by whether the patient's disease falls under favorite or intermediate/poor risk based on validated prognostic models. Within each risk category, there are several acceptable alternatives, including VEGF inhibitor monotherapy, combination immunotherapy (e.g., ipilimumab/nivolumab), or a combination of a VEGF inhibitor and a checkpoint inhibitor (e.g., axitinib/pembrolizumab). Given the increasing number of available treatment options for mRCC there is also a growing need for predictive biomarkers to help guide clinicians (Figure 1). We aim to review the literature regarding the evidence for selecting one type of regimen over another and determining who would benefit more from either angiogenesis antagonism or immune checkpoint blockade (ICB).

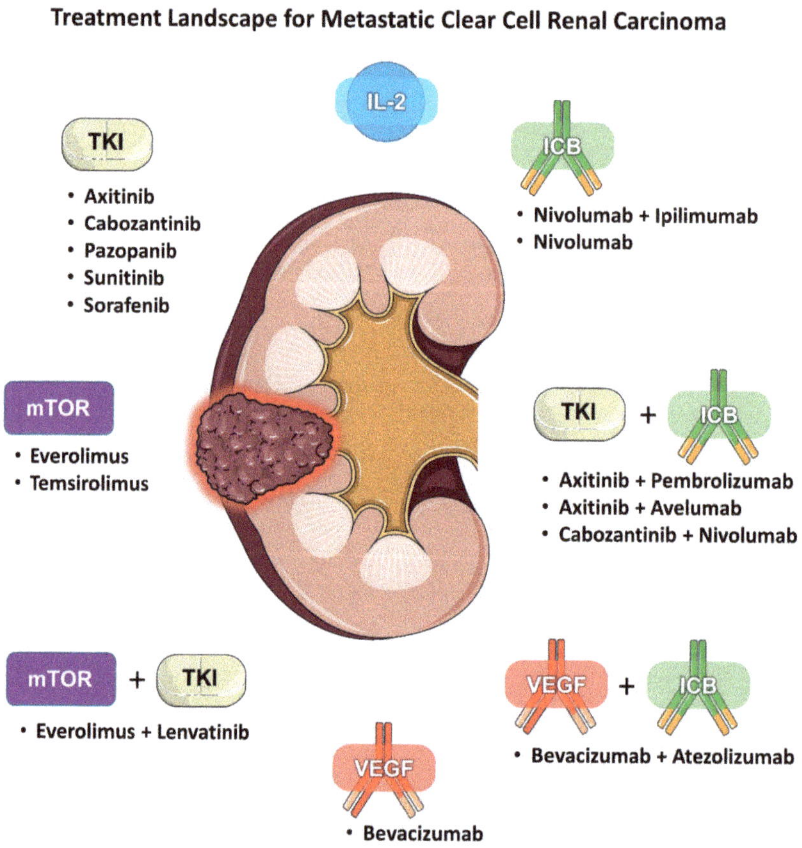

Figure 1. Treatment landscape for metastatic clear cell renal carcinoma.

2. Biomarkers for Angiogenesis Inhibitors

2.1. International Metastatic Renal Cell Carcinoma Database Consortium Score

Past attempts to create clinical prognostication tools to risk stratify patients treated with molecularly-targeted agents include the International Metastatic Renal Cell Carcinoma Database Consortium (IMDC) score. This was a model based on a multicenter study of 645 patients with metastatic RCC (mRCC) who were treated with VEGF pathway-targeted therapies, such as sunitinib, sorafenib, or bevacizumab (plus interferon-alfa) for mRCC [1]. Six factors were noted to be associated with worse survival: Karnofsky Performance Status (KPS) score < 80, time from diagnosis to initiation of targeted therapy < 1 year, hemoglobin less than lower limit of normal, corrected calcium greater than the upper limit of normal, absolute neutrophil count greater than upper limit of normal, and platelet count greater than the upper limit of normal. Scoring was binary with each factor assigned a score of 0 or 1, and a total sum was taken. A total score of 0 corresponded to a favorable risk group with a median overall survival (mOS) of 43.2 months; a score of 1–2 indicated intermediate risk with a mOS of 22.5 months; and a score ≥ 3 represented a poor risk group with a mOS of 7.8 months. This clinical prediction tool was subsequently externally validated in a study of 849 patients with mRCC who were treated with first-line anti-VEGF therapies [2]. Another study found that the IMDC score can be applied to patients who progressed after first-line anti-VEGF therapy [3]. Although there have been other risk models that have been developed, including the MSKCC model, Cleveland Clinic

Foundation model, French model, and International Kidney Cancer Working Group, the IMDC model has become the one most widely utilized in contemporary clinical trials.

While clinical tools such as the IMDC score were originally developed to estimate patients' prognoses regardless of the treatment early in the era of VEGF-targeted therapy, there has been a gradual evolution toward assuming a role in predicting response to therapy. The IMDC criteria has been used to retrospectively risk stratify patients who underwent ICB combination therapies (e.g., ipilimumab/nivolumab vs. axitinib + pembrolizumab/avelumab) or anti-VEGF agents in first-line or second-line settings [4]. There is growing evidence that using the risk score may be useful in guiding the selection of a particular therapy. For example, in KEYNOTE-426, there was a benefit for pembrolizumab/axitinib over sunitinib in the first-line treatment of advanced ccRCC in an updated analysis [5]. However, this effect was less pronounced for patients who fell into the IMDC favorable risk category. Similarly, a prospective trial comparing ipilimumab/nivolumab (ipi/nivo) combination vs. sunitinib in untreated advanced ccRCC showed that patients who were at intermediate or poor risk and treated with ipi/nivo had superior 18-month OS, progression free survival (PFS), overall response rate (ORR), and complete response (CR) rates as compared to patients treated with sunitinib alone [6]. However, an exploratory analysis of favorable risk patients, who were found to have a lower baseline PD-L1 expression level when compared to higher risk groups, failed to demonstrate the same benefits of ipi/nivo over sunitinib. In fact, the 18-month OS trended higher for sunitinib, and the ORR was lower and mPFS shorter for the ipi/nivo group in a statistically significant manner, although there was no OS advantage for sunitinib. Given such a disparate therapeutic response to ICB vs. sunitinib based on the risk profile, it is conceivable that IMDC scoring can be used to predict treatment response in addition to estimating the prognosis. That higher risk group patients with advanced ccRCC responded better to ICB-based therapies suggests that there may be differences in the underlying tumor and/or microenvironment biology that influence response to the current available treatments.

2.2. Genomic Alterations

Earlier studies on biomarkers focused on driver mutations, epigenetic modifications, or chromosomal aberrations associated with ccRCC to evaluate their potential in clinical prognostication. An obvious candidate was the *von Hippel-Lindau (VHL)* gene, which is inactivated in RCC via a point mutation or through epigenetic silencing. This mutation is present in about 60–90% of cases of ccRCC. Inactivation of the protein product of *VHL* leads to abnormal stabilization of hypoxia-inducible factor (HIF), which drives oncogene transcription. However, no clear relationship between *VHL* abnormalities and patient outcome exists [7]. A meta-analysis from 2017 revealed that *VHL* was not a predictive marker in patients treated with anti-VEGF-targeted agents, as abnormal *VHL* failed to show a relationship with ORR, PFS, or OS [8]. *Polybromo 1, (PBRM1)*, also known as BAF180, is encoded in a gene locus near *VHL* and is a component of the PBAF complex, a mammalian SWItch/Sucrose Non-Fermentable (SWI/SNF) complex, which is a tumor suppressor protein that is thought to become mutated early in RCC pathogenesis [9]. Older studies evaluating its role as a prognostic marker did not include targeted agents and failed to predict cancer-specific survival [9,10]. However, a study published in 2016 showed that among 31 metastatic ccRCC patients, the vast majority of whom received anti-VEGF therapy, those who were maintained for longer durations of therapy were more likely to harbor a *PBRM1* mutation [11]. A separate study found that a group of so-called "extreme responders," defined as partial response (PR) or complete response (CR) for ≥3 years in mRCC on either first-line sunitinib or pazopanib, was enriched for *PBRM1* mutations [12]. A third biomarker that has been studied is *SETD2*, which is sometimes co-mutated with *PBRM1*. It encodes for a histone-lysine N-methyltransferase and acts as a chromatin regulator. It does not appear to have a definite correlation with survival but is associated with higher risk of disease recurrence after surgery for localized disease. Its mutation status did not seem to correlate with PFS in mRCC patients treated with sunitinib [13].

2.3. Targets of Tumor-Driven Angiogenesis

With growing evidence that tumor and microenvironmental biology could impact clinical factors and lead to differential outcomes depending on the type of systemic therapy, identifying predictive biomarkers became an increasing focus. Earlier studies acknowledged the hyperangiogenic state of ccRCC and the mechanism of action of VEGF-targeted tyrosine kinase inhibitors (TKIs) as a rationale for studying the components of the VEGF signaling cascade. One study looked at whether VEGF expression in tumor and endothelial cells was predictive and/or prognostic in 41 patients with metastatic RCC (mRCC) treated with radical nephrectomy and sunitinib [14]. In this study, higher VEGF expression within the tumor cells correlated with the MSKCC group and was associated with higher tumor stage and inferior OS. There was no correlation between intratumoral VEGF expression and PFS or OS on first-line sunitinib, suggesting that the VEGF level may be prognostic but not predictive. A different study evaluated the role of serum VEGF levels in predicting treatment response to sunitinib in 85 patients with advanced RCC (mostly clear cell) who overwhelmingly fell into the favorable or intermediate categories based on the MSKCC model; these patients were undergoing systemic treatment in the second line and beyond [15]. The patients who had serum VEGF levels higher than reference value of 707 pg/mL had a longer PFS by about six months. A third small, single-institution study of 23 mRCC patients attempted to associate tumor expression of 16 selected biomarkers with treatment response to second-line sunitinib after the failure of first-line interferon-α. They quantified biomarker expression using qRT-PCR and categorized tumor response using the RECIST criteria. The authors noted that specific soluble VEGF isoforms, $VEGF_{121}$ and $VEGF_{165}$ in particular, were associated with partial response, and they proposed that a ratio of $VEGF_{121}/VEGF_{165}$ of <1.25 predicted superior OS [16]. Despite these studies, neither peritumoral nor serum VEGF is routinely measured in clinical practice.

2.4. Gene Expression Signatures

More recent studies have investigated gene expression signatures as potential guides for the tailoring of therapy. A study published in 2013 found that tumor upregulation of the so-called VEGF-dependent vascular gene profile appeared to predict improved PFS when bevacizumab was added to standard oxaliplatin-based systemic therapy for treatment-naïve metastatic colorectal cancer [17]. To see if such a phenomenon was also applicable to mRCC, an exploratory analysis of the IMmotion150 study looked at tumor mutation burden as well as angiogenesis and immune gene expression signatures in previously untreated mRCC patients who were treated with sunitinib vs. atezolizumab with or without bevacizumab [18]. The Angio gene signature consisted of the following genes: *VEGFA, KDR, ESM1, PECAM1, ANGPTL4,* and *CD34*. In the IMmotion150 study, increased the expression of the Angio signature correlated with a higher ORR and longer PFS among the group of patients treated with sunitinib, including a 7% CR rate as compared to 0% in the low Angio expression group. If the Angio expression level was low, the combination arm had better PFS as compared to that of sunitinib monotherapy. Although the angiogenesis gene signature tended to have upregulation of *VHL* and *PBRM1* mutants, *VHL* status itself was not associated with differences in PFS [18]. Although these results were intriguing, they remain hypothesis-generating.

2.5. Association of Angiogenesis Signatures with Traditional Biomarkers

One group analyzed data from the phase III COMPARZ trial to associate tumor gene expression profiling with clinical endpoints in untreated metastatic ccRCC [19]. This trial randomized untreated mRCC patients to receive either pazopanib or sunitinib to assess for differences in efficacy, toxicity, and quality of life. In patients treated with an anti-VEGF TKI, such as sunitinib or pazopanib, increased expression of angiogenesis genes significantly correlated with better ORR, PFS, and OS as compared to those with lower expression. However, this benefit appeared to be abrogated in the group of patients that was enriched for *TP53* and *BAP1* mutations. The group of patients with higher frequency of *TP53* and *BAP1* mutations tended to have high immune infiltration and higher PD-L1 expression. Ultimately, there was no significant difference in the angiogenesis gene profile among the three different IMDC risk groups, suggesting that the prediction of enhanced response to TKIs was independent of previously established clinical prognostic markers. As was the case in IMmotion150 study, in the COMPARZ trial, mRCC tumors with *PBRM1* mutations were noted to have upregulated angiogenesis gene expression in contrast to tumors harboring *BAP1* mutations, which were associated with decreased expression of angiogenesis-related genes. There was no association between the angiogenesis gene signature expression level and *SETD2* mutation.

2.6. Pure VEGF Antagonism vs. Combination Anti-VEGF/ICB Therapy

Combination therapy with anti-angiogenic agents and ICB has become the standard of care for the majority of patients with mRCC. It would be clinically actionable to understand whether angiogenic or immune biomarkers could help predict the therapeutic response in order to better stratify patients to combination therapy versus a single agent strategy to minimize toxicity while optimizing efficacy. A study evaluated association between angiogenesis signatures and outcomes in the phase 3 JAVELIN Renal trial that enrolled patients with untreated mRCC and randomized them to avelumab/axitinib or sunitinib. High levels of expression of angiogenesis-related genes were associated with better PFS in patients treated with sunitinib. In patients whose tumors had low expression of an angiogenesis signature, there was improved PFS in patients treated with avelumab/axitinib in comparison to sunitinib [20]. All in all, several studies have shown evidence that upregulation of a set of angiogenesis-related genes seemed to help predict a better response to anti-VEGF therapy, which would be important information in guiding selection of therapy. Those who registered low in angiogenesis gene expression predictably did not benefit as much, and there is a suggestion that mRCC patients harboring low tumor angiogenesis gene expression signatures represent an immune-enriched subtype that is less likely to respond to anti-VEGF therapy alone and may benefit more from strategies involving ICB.

2.7. Predictive Value of Trends in Angiogenesis-Related Biomarkers during Treatment

A retrospective analysis of tumor samples or blood samples obtained from 52 mRCC patients treated with first-line axitinib/pembrolizumab in a phase Ib trial was assessed for angiogenesis-related biomarkers [21]. Angiopoietin-1 and 2 (Ang-1; Ang-2), VEGF, VEGFR-1, VEGFR-2, and VEGFR-3 were chosen for evaluation as serum biomarkers given their known roles in angiogenesis [22]. The study authors found that serum concentrations of Ang-1, Ang-2, VEGF, VEGFR2, and VEGFR3 at baseline had no correlation with PFS as a continuous variable. However, when patients were divided into two categories of PFS (<9 months vs. >20 months), the median Ang-2 protein level on treatment was lower in the PFS > 20 month group as compared to PFS < 9 months. The Ang-1 protein level was lower in patients with PFS > 20 months at the end of the treatment. The ratio of VEGF at the end of treatment to VEGF at baseline was also lower for patients who experienced PFS > 20 months [21]. This study suggested the potential that these biomarkers may have in assessing whether a patient on treatment is a responder, enabling earlier escalation of therapy for those with a lower chance of response. These results require prospective validation, however (Table 1).

Table 1. Summary of biomarkers for angiogenesis inhibitors.

Biomarker	Key Findings as a Predictive or Prognostic Biomarker
von Hippel-Lindau (VHL) [7]	- No correlation with patient outcome in general - No correlation with ORR, PFS, or OS in patients treated with anti-VEGF therapy
Polybromo-1 (PBRM1) [11,12]	- Associated with a longer duration of response to anti-VEGF therapy
SET domain containing 2, histone lysine methyltransferase (SETD2) [13]	- No definite association with overall survival - Does not predict response to sunitinib
BRCA1 Associated Protein 1 (BAP1) [19]	- Associated with lower expression of angiogenesis-related genes - Possibly blunts response to anti-VEGF therapy
Vascular Endothelial Growth Factor (VEGF) [14–16,21]	- Intratumoral overexpression associated with worse OS but does not predict response to first-line sunitinib - Lower ratio of soluble isoforms 121–165 (<1.25) may help to predict response to second-line sunitinib after progression on interferon-α - Lower ratio of serum levels at the end of treatment to baseline level associated with longer PFS with first-line axitinib/pembrolizumab

Angiopoietins (Ang-1, Ang-2) [21]	- Associated with longer PFS when treated with first-line axitinib/pembrolizumab when either of the following were observed:
	  ○ Decrease in Ang-1 protein level at the end of treatment
	  ○ Decrease in Ang-2 protein level mid-treatment

Angio gene signature (VEGFA, KDR, ESM1, PECAM1, ANGPTL4, and CD34) [18–20]	- More often upregulated in VHL and PBRM1 mutants - Increased expression correlated with higher ORR, PFS, and/or OS in patients treated with first-line sunitinib or pazopanib except when TP53 or BAP1 mutations were present - Improved PFS with first-line avelumab/axitinib as compared to sunitinib monotherapy if the Angio expression level was low

3. Biomarkers for Immunotherapy

Renal cell carcinoma is often considered an immunogenic tumor. This has been evidenced from pathologic examination of RCC tumor tissue showing significant infiltration by both T-cells and natural killer cells [23]. In addition, efficacy of early immunotherapy agents, like interleukin-2 (IL-2) and Interferon alpha (IFN-α), and more recently ICB in the treatment of RCC support this notion pragmatically [24–26]. ICB targeting the programmed death 1 (PD-1) and cytotoxic T-lymphocyte associated protein 4 (CTLA-4) pathways have demonstrated favorable outcomes, with ORRs of 25% for anti-PD-1 targeted single-agent therapy and up to 39% and 59% when combined with CTLA-4 or vascular endothelial growth factor (VEGF) inhibitors, respectively [5,6,27]. Consequently, combination strategies with ICB have become the standard of care for most eligible mRCC patients.

However, since both combination ICB/ICB and ICB/TKI regimens are approved as first-line therapy for mRCC, it would be beneficial to have clinical biomarkers to understand which tumors are more likely to benefit from an immunotherapy based regimen versus a combination regimen with VEGF inhibition.

3.1. PD-L1 Expression

The programmed death-ligand 1 (PD-L1), also known as B7 homolog 1 (B7-H1), is found on tumor and immune cells in the TME, and its receptor PD-1 on T-cells are the primary targets for this form of ICB. In the era of ICB, expression of PD-L1 by immunohistochemistry (IHC) has been a focus of much of biomarker research across tumor types but in the case of mRCC it has not borne out to be a very useful predictive biomarker.

When focusing specifically on registration studies for ICB in mRCC, patients without any measurable PD-L1 expression have benefited from these drugs. In a meta-analysis of six randomized controlled trials of ICB in mRCC an association was observed between PD-L1 expression and PFS, but the analysis failed to show significant correlation with OS [28]. The authors concluded from this data that the role of PD-L1 expression in selecting treatment for RCC was not well established, in line with FDA drug approvals and the NCCN guidelines which do not include or require PD-L1 expression [29,30]. This difference is likely multifactorial and could be due to the unique biology of RCC, related to the non-standardized testing utilized in for PD-L1 expression as a biomarker in earlier trials, including the use of different antibodies for various IHC assays and inconsistent cutoffs for positivity, tumor heterogeneity and the dynamic nature of PD-L1 expression on tumor cells [31].

Furthermore, prior to the era of immunotherapy, PD-L1 expression by IHC was studied in mRCC and was shown to be associated with poor prognosis [32]. The observation that PD-L1 positivity is linked to poor prognosis was again reported more recently in a post-hoc analysis of the COMPARZ trial (pazopinib vs. sunitinib) which showed that patients who were PD-L1 positive had significantly worse OS and PFS compared to the PD-L1 negative population. This is also supported by an analysis of CHECKMATE-214 study (nivolumab+ipilumimab vs. sunitinib) which demonstrated that PD-L1 positivity was more common in patients with intermediate and poor risk disease as defined by IMDC criteria compared to those with favorable risk disease [6]. It is possible that the prognostic implications of PD-L1 positivity in mRCC also have a negative impact on its usefulness as a predictive biomarker.

3.2. Genomic Markers

3.2.1. PBRM1 Mutations

Differences in the genomic landscape of RCC have also been the subject of much study in the search for clinical biomarkers for ICB treatment PBRM1 and PBAF complex mutations have drawn much attention in this regard and, as discussed above, have also been investigated as both a prognostic and predictive markers for VEGF TKIs. In relation to ICB, PBRM1 was first identified by Miao et al. in a set of 35 patients with mRCC who participated in a prospective clinical study of nivolumab. Whole-exome sequencing was performed on tissue samples and identified PBRM1 as being strongly enriched in the group who derived clinical benefit. This finding was then validated in a separate 63 patient cohort treated with PD-1 or PD-L1 inhibitions alone or in combination with anti-CTLA-4 therapies and replicated findings of association with clinical benefit [33].

However, after this initial publication, PBRM1 mutations were subsequently studied in several additional patient cohorts. An analysis by McDermott et al. of a first-line clinical trial of atezolizumab alone or in combination with bevacizumab vs. sunitinib failed to demonstrate an association with clinical benefit in patients with PBRM1 mutations in the atezolizumab monotherapy arm but instead favored benefit in the sunitinib arm [18]. A subsequent analysis from the Checkmate-025 study of patients with mRCC treated in the second-line or beyond and randomized to nivolumab or everolimus showed that there was enrichment of clinical benefit in the PBRM1 mutant group in nivolumab-treated patients, though this trial did not include a VEGF-targeted therapy. The effect of PBRM1 mutations on response and survival in this study was modest, with median PFS 5.6 vs. 2.9 months (HR, 0.67; 95% CI, 0.47–0.96; $p = 0.03$) and median OS 27.9 vs. 20.9 months (HR, 0.65; 95% CI, 0.44–0.96; $p = 0.03$) [34].

Finally, a large retrospective analysis ($n = 2936$) explored the interaction between PBRM1 mutations and immunotherapy across cancer types and failed to show a statistically significant association with

OS (HR 0.9, $p = 0.7$). Interestingly, this trial included 189 patients with mRCC treated with ICB and this subgroup did demonstrate an association with OS (HR 1.24, $p = 0.47$). It was previously hypothesized in the initial discovery study by Miao et al. that PBRM1 mutations increased interferon-gamma (IFNγ) gene expression and thereby modulated the immune response. However, this analysis explored the impact of IFNγ signaling in both the cohort studied by McDermott et al. and a cohort from the previously mentioned COMPARZ trial and showed unchanged or decreased IFNγ signaling in PBRM1 mutants compared to the wild-type, which conflicted with the hypothesized mechanism of action [35]. Due to the conflicting nature of these results, doubt has been cast on the potential use of PBRM1 as a biomarker for ICB [36].

3.2.2. TERT Promoter Mutations

Although much focus is in finding mutations associated with response, it is also useful to examine the opposite phenomenon and identify mutations that are associated with resistance to immunotherapy. This would help route patients to therapies more likely to be beneficial and avoid unnecessary toxicity. For example, in non-small cell lung cancer mutations in STK11 have been identified as predictors of poor responses to ICBs [37]. STK11 is not a useful biomarker for RCC since it is very rarely found in RCC on the order of 0.2% of patients based on data from cBioPortal [38]. A retrospective study of patients with mRCC ($n = 75$), the majority with clear cell histology (~80%), who received comprehensive genomic profiling (whole exome and RNA sequencing) as part of routine care, including both immunotherapy and targeted therapy, attempted to identify genomic and transcriptomic correlates of clinical benefit. The authors found that mutations in the TERT promoter were specifically associated with a lack of benefit from ICB. In this subgroup of TERT promoter mutated tumors the authors also found enrichment of transcription factor targets of MYC and KATA2, and kinase targets of CDK4, ATM, and MAPK14 [39].

3.2.3. Multi-gene Expression Signatures

Similar to approaches in VEGF TKI treated patients, researchers have investigated potential tumor genomic signatures that might serve as predictive biomarkers for ICB. In an exploratory analysis of the IMmotion150 study, the authors used gene signatures previously defined and representing angiogenesis, immune response (T-effector/IFNγ), and myeloid inflammatory gene expression to perform a subgroup analysis and investigate associations with response. They found that tumors with high expression of a T-effector gene signature (T_{eff}^{High}) was positively associated with expression of PD-L1 and CD8 T-cell infiltration. They also showed that within this group there was increased expression of the myeloid inflammation genes. The T_{eff}^{High} gene signature was also associated with improved ORR and PFS when compared to the T_{eff}^{Low} group within the atezolizumab/bevacizumab arm. They also showed that T_{eff}^{High} was associated with improved PFS when compared across groups to the sunitinib arm. High myeloid inflammation gene signature expression ($Myeloid^{High}$), which had previously been shown to be associated with suppressed T-cell responses, was shown to be associated with worse PFS in both the atezolizumab monotherapy and atezolizumab/bevacizumab arms [18].

A separate group utilized machine learning techniques to build upon the prior IMmotion150 gene signatures to define a specific 66-gene signature created for mRCC using RNA sequencing data from The Cancer Genome Atlas (TCGA) dataset in cBioPortal. They identified that the genes in the IMmotion150 gene signature were selected by analysis of the literature and citations which defined the three biological axes explored in the study and not based on an empirical analysis of the data, which they considered to be a limitation of the previous approach. To develop their signature, they first leveraged the gene signatures defined by the IMmotion150 study to perform unsupervised clustering to categorize patients into three groups and confirmed they separated into the same three categories; angiogenesis, T-effector and myeloid inflammation. They then utilized a separate featured selection machine learning technique to analyze the global gene expression profile of the sub-classified patients and selected the top 500 ranked and subsequently refined them using several different techniques to investigate the underlying biology and came up with their 66-gene signature. Using training and validation cohorts, they were able to show that this signature performed better with regards to association with OS and DFS than the original IMmotion150 signature. However, interpretation of this signature thus far is limited since annotation of treatments record and outcome are not available in the TCGA data and survival data was calculated prior to the approval of ICBs. The signature does, however, hold promise to be tested in cohorts who did receive ICB to test what they hypothesize as an improvement in the clustering of patients into unique groups defined by tumor biology [40].

In an analysis of the results of KEYNOTE-427 (pembrolizumab monotherapy) 11 separate gene signatures were analyzed for associations with response. They identified one signature, a T-cell inflamed gene expression profile (GEP), which stood out demonstrating a strong association with ORR to pembrolizumab. The same T-cell inflamed GEP signature, however, was not associated with longer PFS or OS in the same study and thus remains hypothesis generating [41] (Table 2).

3.2.4. DNA Damage Repair Mutations, Microsatellite Instability, and Tumor Mutational Burden

Although less common in some other tumor types, RCC can harbor alterations in DNA damage repair (DDR) pathways, including defects in DNA mismatch repair (dMMR). Loss of function of certain genes related to dMMR defects can lead to lead to high levels of microsatellite instability (MSI), which has been established as a biomarker for response to immunotherapy irrespective of tumor type [42]. MSI-Hi tumors are not a common finding in RCC and are estimated to be present in only 1–2% of cases [43]. As a result, MSI is not a practical biomarker in a broad sense for ICB in RCC since many non-MSI RCC tumors respond to immunotherapy.

Looking more broadly, mutations in genes involved in the various DDR pathways, which do not necessarily result in MSI, are relatively prevalent in RCC. In one cohort published by Ged et al., about 19% of patients (43/229) with mRCC harbor DDR mutations, with CHEK2 and ATM being the most frequently mutated. In this cohort, they were able to demonstrate a correlation between DDR mutation status and superior OS (HR 0.41; 95% CI: 0.14–1.14; $p = 0.09$) in patients treated with ICB [44]. This finding was also reported in a smaller cohort ($n = 34$) by Labriola et al. who showed that patients with DDR mutant tumors had improved disease control (defined as CR, PR, or SD) with ICB [45].

Table 2. Summary of gene expression signatures.

Gene Signature	Dataset	Genes		Key Findings
IMmotion150 Signature [18]	Sample size: 263 patients Study Type: Randomized phase 2 study of atezolizumab alone or combined with bevacizumab (anti-VEGF) versus sunitinib	**Angiogenesis (Angio)** • VEGFA • PECAM1 • ANGPLT4 • ESM1 **Myeloid Inflammation** • CXCL1 • CXCL2 • CXCL3 **T-effector (T_{eff})** • CD8A • CD27 • IFNG • GZMA • GZMB • PRF1 • EOMES • CXCL9 • CXCL10 • CXCL11	• FLT1 • CD34 • KDR • CXCL8 • IL6 • PTGS2 • CD274 • CTLA4 • FOXP3 • TIGIT • IDO1 • PSMB8 • PSMB9 • TAP1 • TAP2	• T_{eff}^{High} associated with PD-L1 expression and CD8 T-cell infiltration • T_{eff}^{High} vs. T_{eff}^{Low} in atezolizumab + bevacizumab associated with improved ORR (49% vs. 16%) and improved PFS (HR 0.50; CI 0.30–0.86) • T_{eff}^{High} atezolizumab + bevacizumab vs. sunitinib improved PFS (HR 0.55; CI 0.32–0.95) • Myeloid^{High} associated with worse PFS in immunotherapy arms • Distinct population of Myeloid^{High} tumors within the T_{eff}^{High} group • T_{eff}^{High}Myeloid^{High} vs. T_{eff}^{High}Myeloid^{low} associated with worse activity of atezolizumab (HR 3.82; CI 1.70–8.60)

Table 2. Cont.

Gene Signature	Dataset	Genes		Key Findings
66 Gene Signature [40]	**Sample Size:** *Training cohort* 469 patients *Validation cohort* 64 patients **Study Type:** Retrospective analysis of ccRCC patients from The Cancer Genome Atlas (TCGA)	**Angiogenesis** • VEGFA • KDR • EDNRB • PECAM1 • ANGPLT4 • NOTCH1 **T-effector** • PSMB9 • PSMB8 • LTA • SLA2 • PYHIN1 • PDCD1 • EOMES **Ca2+-flux** • CD2 • CCL5 • CCL4 • GK2 • LCK • LAT **Invasion** • XCL2 • FOXP3 • FERMT3 • SLC9A3R2 • FASLG • NFATC1 • CD72 • WAS • PTK2B • CXCR3 • CORO1A • CCR5 • PDE2A • TBCA2R	• EDN1 • FLT1 • CD34 • STIM2 • ESM1 • CTLA4 • CD8A • GZMB • GZMA • TIGIT • PREF1 • LCP1 • CD38 • LAX1 • CD7 • CD3E • ITK • FYB1 • NES • S1PR1 • TCF4 • HEY1 • ETS1 • PTPRB • PPM1F • MCF2L • GJA1 • VWF • MYCT1 • NOS3 • IL16	• T-effector genes clustered with Ca2+-flux • Subclasified patients into 3 categories: Angio, T$_{eff}$, and Mixed • Mixed cohort expressed genes from all four pathways • Angio cohort had improved survival compared to T$_{eff}$ and Mixed (median OS 90.4 vs. 62.8 vs. 62.8 months) • Angio cohort had better DFS as compared to T$_{eff}$ (HR = 2.2091, p = 0.0201) and Mixed (HR = 1.7433, p = 0.0386) • Not yet tested or validated in a cohort who was homogenously treated • Developed on data prior to ICB
T-cell Inflamed GEP [41]	**Sample Size:** 78 patients **Study Type:** Open-label, single-arm phase 2 study of first-line pembrolizumab	**T-cell Inflamed** • CXCR6 • TIGIT • CD27 • LAG3 • NKG7 • STAT1 • CD8A • IDO1 • CCL5	• PSMB10 • CMKLR1 • CD274 (PD-L1) • PDCD1LG2 (PD-L2) • CXCL9 • HLA.DQA1 • CD276 • HLA.DRB1 • HLA.E	• T-cell-inflamed GEP associated with higher ORR • No association with PFS or OS

Another measure of disruption of genomic integrity is tumor mutational burden (TMB). TMB is defined by the total number of non-synonymous alterations (single-nucleotide variants or insertions/deletions) and is typically calculated from next-generation sequencing (NGS) data of either the whole exome or large targeted panels. A high TMB is thought to be integral in promoting increases in the expression of tumor neoantigens which promote T-cell mediated immune responses against tumors [46,47]. TMB, similarly to MSI, has been investigated independent of tumor histology and has been shown to enrich response to ICB [48,49]. This also led to an FDA approval on 16 June 2020 of pembrolizumab for all TMB-high tumors (defined as >10 mutations per megabase) regardless of histology.

However, this approval has been met with controversy because of concerns that cutoffs for TMB and its performance as a biomarker may differ between tumor types. This skepticism is supported in RCC based on some of the available data. For example, in the study discussed above by Labriola et al., which focused solely on RCC, there was no observed association between TMB and disease control in patients treated with ICB [45]. This was also seen in a separate and larger cohort of 592 patients treated with nivolumab (pooled analysis of checkmate 009, 010, and 025) showed no association with response to PD-1 blockade. Paradoxically, it also has been shown that high-TMB is actually associated with inhibition of immune cell infiltrates in RCC tumors, which supports and possibly explains these unexpected clinical observations on a cellular level [50].

Another interesting observation that may help explain why RCC is such an immunogenic tumor but has a characteristically low TMB is the distribution of mutations that comprise its TMB [51,52]. TMB high tumors traditionally have a predominance of many single nucleotide variants (SNVs) making up the majority of mutations, while RCC on the other hand has a uniquely high proportion of insertions and deletions (indels) relative to other tumors. This phenomenon was identified as part of an analysis of the Cancer Genome Atlas study of 5777 solid tumors which identified RCC tumors as having more than double the median proportion of indels to SNVs. The authors then hypothesized that indels are more efficient in the formation of immunogenic peptides serving as neoantigens and using in silico prediction models they were able to show an enrichment of high-affinity neoantigens from indels that was three times that of SNV [53]. This suggests that RCC may be a case of quality over quantity in regards to immunogenic mutations.

Another approach to improving performance of TMB as a biomarker is incorporating HLA correction. HLA correction is a computational method by which incorporation of loss of heterozygosity of HLA alleles is thought to improve upon TMB by predicting the proportion of functional neoantigens present. This has been studied in non-small cell lung cancer and shown to identify and reclassify tumors previously characterized as TMB-high and, in doing so, improve the association with the response to ICB, but has yet to be studied in RCC [54].

3.3. Analysis of Immune Cells

In the search for biomarkers predicting a response to ICB, the investigation has necessarily expanded beyond clinical- and tumor-dependent factors, such as performance status or genomics, and additionally focused on host-dependent components of the immune system. In order to study the cellular components of the immune system, including T-cells, neutrophils, NK cells, and antigen-presenting cells, a variety of techniques have been approached, ranging from simple analytes (like a complete blood count with differential) to more complex methods like flow cytometry and advanced staining techniques, like multiplex IHC.

3.3.1. Neutrophil Lymphocyte Ratio

One of the first biomarkers developed to attempt to quantify the immunologic milieu in patients with cancer is the neutrophil lymphocyte ratio (NLR). The biologic rationale for this biomarker is that it is a representation of cancer-related inflammation indicating more aggressive disease. Calculated simply by dividing the absolute neutrophil count by the absolute lymphocyte count on a complete blood count, this biomarker is essentially free and readily available for all patients. The NLR has been studied specifically in mRCC and a high pre-treatment NLR has been shown to have both prognostic and predictive implications. However, data in the specific context of treatment with ICB is limited [55–59]. One retrospective study of NLR in 42 patients with mRCC treated with ICB demonstrated that a pre-therapy NLR < 3 was associated with longer PFS (HR, 2.937; 95% CI, 1.44 to 5.97; $p = 0.003$) and OS (pre-therapy: HR, 3.977; 95% CI, 1.23 to 12.89; $p = 0.014$) [60]. A subsequent and larger study of 142 patients with mRCC treated with ICB showed that lower baseline NLR was only associated with a trend toward lower ORR, shorter PFS, and shorter OS. In this study they also looked at NLR at six weeks and showed that it was a significantly stronger predictor of all three outcomes than baseline NLR. They also, interestingly, showed that a > 25% decrease in NLR from baseline to six weeks was associated with significantly improved outcomes in mRCC patients treated with ICB [61]. Both of these were relatively small studies and larger prospective trials are needed to validate these findings before they could be incorporated more commonly into clinical practice.

3.3.2. Tumor Infiltrating Lymphocytes and Immune Microenvironment

Tumor infiltrating lymphocytes (TILs) and their role in the immune response against cancer has been investigated for decades and it is now understood that cytotoxic CD8+ T-cells, otherwise known as "T-killer cells," are essential components of a robust anti-tumor immune response. TILs are activated when presented an antigen via the class I major histocompatibility complex and release cytotoxins to kill the targeted cells [62]. RCC has long been understood to be one of the most immune-infiltrated tumors, as suggested as long as 30 years ago in a study characterizing samples from 120 different tumor histologies [63]. However, mere infiltration of a tumor with TILs does not prove that these immune cells have been properly activated to mount an anti-tumor response. The presence of PD-1 positive immune cells has been associated with worse outcomes as these tumors with large populations of PD-1-positive immune cells have evolved to promote quiescence of the immune system, which allows tumors to avoid detection and explains their more aggressive prognosis [64]. It has also been shown that changes in PD-1-positive immune cells were observed in response to surgical resection in a study of peripheral blood mononuclear cells (PBMC) from 90 patients with RCC before and after nephrectomy. This study showed that increased PD-1 expression on CD14 bright myelomonocytic cells, effector T cells, and natural killer (NK) cells correlated to disease stage, and expression was significantly reduced on all cell types soon after surgical resection of the primary tumor. This further suggests the association between PD-1 positivity of immune cells and the pathophysiology of this disease [65].

This phenomenon was further investigated with the incorporation of various known immune cell surface markers to better characterize the specific phenotype of ineffective TILs and the associated immune microenvironment. Giraldo et al. classified tumors into three basic categories defined by the phenotypic characteristics of their immune cells: immune-regulated, immune-activated, and immune silent. They showed in their study of 40 patients with mRCC that the immune-regulated tumors displayed aggressive histologic features and a high risk of disease progression in the year following nephrectomy for localized disease. The immune-regulated phenotype in this study was defined by CD8+PD-1+TIM-3+Lag-3+ TILs and CD4+ICOS+ helper T-cells in the presence of CD25+CD127-Foxp3+/Helios+GITR+ Tregs [66].

Understanding the importance of the immune infiltrate and microenvironment, new research has focused on the relationship between immune cell surface markers and response to immunotherapy. In an analysis of Checkmate-025 by Braun et al., they confirmed that RCC tumors tend to be heavily infiltrated with CD8+ TILs, but did not show an association between highly infiltrated tumors and ICB response. Interestingly, they noted that highly infiltrated tumors were less likely to carry PBRM1 mutations, which may help explain the association between PBRM1 mutations and favorable prognosis in RCC [67]. In a subsequent analysis of Checkmate-025 by the same group, subsets of the immune infiltrate were classified with methods similar to those used by Giraldo et al. They were able to show that having high levels of CD8+PD1+TIM3-LAG3- TILs was associated with benefit from nivolumab. They also showed that there was a linear association with the increased density of these cells and improvement in ORR, PFS, and OS. Furthermore, these observations were not seen in everolimus-treated patients suggesting a specific relationship to ICB response [68]. This data suggests specifically that TIM3 and LAG3 are important additional checkpoints, since their presence on TILs is associated with reduced benefit from ICB targeting the PD-1 pathway only. There are several inhibitors in development for both LAG3 and TIM3, including a bispecific antibody which targets both PD-L1 and LAG-3 and may be able to improve responses in these patients who express resistant immune phenotypes [69,70].

Lastly, there has been new research exploring the role of cancer-associated fibroblasts (CAFs) and their role in modulating the microenvironment in several tumor types, including mRCC. In mRCC models, CAFs have been shown to recruit macrophages leading to remodeling of the tumor microenvironment and, via signaling through fibroblast activation protein-a (FAP), may promote more aggressive tumor behavior [71]. FAP expression has also been shown to be associated with sarcomatoid features in mRCC, which have been shown, in a subgroup analysis of IMmotion151, to benefit from ICB in the first-line setting with atezolizumab and bevacizumab as compared to the VEGF TKI, sunitinib [18,72]. Finally, in lung cancer models CAFs have been shown to induce PD-L1 expression which further implies a specific role in modulating the immune response [73]. While they are not implicated directly as potential biomarkers for immunotherapy, the importance of CAFs in the immune milieu suggests they may have importance in biomarker development or become a potential target for future immunotherapy strategies.

4. Conclusions

Much progress has been made in the treatment of metastatic RCC since the early 2000s, first with the development of targeted therapies, and even more so with the addition of immunotherapy. Now, for the first time, clinicians are fortunate to have a dilemma of choice between equally efficacious first-line treatment for patients with this disease. Despite these advances, there is still ample room for improvement both in overcoming primary resistance and also in selecting the optimal treatment for each individual patient. Our review summarizes years of work and progress in both of these avenues but still few are validated for treatment selection with proven clinical utility. As a result, and in contrast to many other tumor types, there are still no biomarker-driven approvals for mRCC. However, we anticipate that as our understanding of the biology of mRCC and the molecular mechanisms that drive its evolution expands from studies like TRACERx Renal and large datasets, such as the TCGA, we will identify new biomarker-driven approaches to treatment [74]. Furthermore, as the treatment landscape of mRCC continues to evolve and more treatment options become available, the importance and need for clinically useful biomarkers will only increase. Given this growing need, we envision that a paradigm will be needed to guide clinicians to the best choice available to personalize treatment.

Author Contributions: B.M., D.X. and M.Z. performed data research, wrote, and edited this review. All authors have read and agreed to the published version of the manuscript.

Funding: This research received no external funding.

Conflicts of Interest: Benjamin Miron and David Xu declare no conflict of interest. Matthew Zibelman reports: Research funding: BMS, Exelixis, Pfizer, Horizon Pharma. Ad Board: Jannsen, EMD Serono.

References

1. Heng, D.Y.C.; Xie, W.; Regan, M.M.; Warren, M.A.; Golshayan, A.R.; Sahi, C.; Eigl, B.J.; Ruether, J.D.; Cheng, T.; North, S.; et al. Prognostic factors for overall survival in patients with metastatic renal cell carcinoma treated with vascular endothelial growth factor-targeted agents: Results from a large, multicenter study. *J. Clin. Oncol.* **2009**, *27*, 5794–5799. [CrossRef]
2. Heng, D.Y.C.; Xie, W.; Regan, M.M.; Harshman, L.C.; Bjarnason, G.A.; Vaishampayan, U.N.; Mackenzie, M.; Wood, L.; Donskov, F.; Tan, M.H.; et al. External validation and comparison with other models of the International Metastatic Renal-Cell Carcinoma Database Consortium prognostic model: A population-based study. *Lancet Oncol.* **2013**, *14*, 141–148. [CrossRef]
3. Ko, J.J.; Xie, W.; Kroeger, N.; Lee, J.; Rini, B.I.; Knox, J.J.; Bjarnason, G.A.; Srinivas, S.; Pal, S.K.; Yuasa, T.; et al. The International Metastatic Renal Cell Carcinoma Database Consortium model as a prognostic tool in patients with metastatic renal cell carcinoma previously treated with first-line targeted therapy: A population-based study. *Lancet Oncol.* **2015**, *16*, 293–300. [CrossRef]
4. Dudani, S.; Gan, C.L.; Wells, C.; Bakouny, Z.; Dizman, N.; Pal, S.K.; Wood, L.; Kollmannsberger, C.K.; Szabados, B.; Powles, T.; et al. Application of IMDC criteria across first-line (1L) and second-line (2L) therapies in metastatic renal-cell carcinoma (mRCC): New and updated benchmarks of clinical outcomes. *J. Clin. Oncol.* **2020**, *38*, 5063. [CrossRef]
5. Plimack, E.R.; Rini, B.I.; Stus, V.; Gafanov, R.; Waddell, T.; Nosov, D.; Pouliot, F.; Soulieres, D.; Melichar, B.; Vynnychenko, I.; et al. Pembrolizumab plus axitinib versus sunitinib as first-line therapy for advanced renal cell carcinoma (RCC): Updated analysis of KEYNOTE-426. *J. Clin. Oncol.* **2020**, *38*, 5001. [CrossRef]

6. Motzer, R.J.; Tannir, N.M.; McDermott, D.F.; Arén Frontera, O.; Melichar, B.; Choueiri, T.K.; Plimack, E.R.; Barthélémy, P.; Porta, C.; George, S.; et al. Nivolumab plus Ipilimumab versus Sunitinib in advanced renal-cell carcinoma. *N. Engl. J. Med.* **2018**, *378*, 1277–1290. [CrossRef]
7. Kondo, K.; Yao, M.; Yoshida, M.; Kishida, T.; Shuin, T.; Miura, T.; Moriyama, M.; Kobayashi, K.; Sakai, N.; Kaneko, S.; et al. Comprehensive mutational analysis of the VHL gene in sporadic renal cell carcinoma: Relationship to clinicopathological parameters. *Genes Chromosom. Cancer* **2002**, *34*, 58–68. [CrossRef]
8. Kim, B.J.; Kim, J.H.; Kim, H.S.; Zang, D.Y. Prognostic and predictive value of VHL gene alteration in renal cell carcinoma: A meta-analysis and review. *Oncotarget* **2017**, *8*, 13979–13985. [CrossRef]
9. Ricketts, C.J.; De Cubas, A.A.; Fan, H.; Smith, C.C.; Lang, M.; Reznik, E.; Bowlby, R.; Gibb, E.A.; Akbani, R.; Beroukhim, R.; et al. The Cancer Genome Atlas Comprehensive Molecular Characterization of Renal Cell Carcinoma. *Cell Rep.* **2018**, *23*, 313–326. [CrossRef]
10. Hakimi, A.A.; Chen, Y.B.; Wren, J.; Gonen, M.; Abdel-Wahab, O.; Heguy, A.; Liu, H.; Takeda, S.; Tickoo, S.K.; Reuter, V.E.; et al. Clinical and pathologic impact of select chromatin-modulating tumor suppressors in clear cell renal cell carcinoma. *Eur. Urol.* **2013**, *63*, 848–854. [CrossRef]
11. Ho, T.H.; Choueiri, T.K.; Wang, K.; Karam, J.A.; Chalmers, Z.; Frampton, G.; Elvin, J.A.; Johnson, A.; Liu, X.; Lin, Y.; et al. Correlation between Molecular Subclassifications of Clear Cell Renal Cell Carcinoma and Targeted Therapy Response. *Eur. Urol. Focus* **2016**, *2*, 204–209. [CrossRef]
12. Fay, A.P.; De Velasco, G.; Ho, T.H.; Van Allen, M.; Murray, B.; Albiges, L.; Signoretti, S.; Hakimi, A.A.; Stanton, M.L.; Bellmunt, J.; et al. Whole-exome sequencing in two extreme phenotypes of response to VEGF-targeted therapies in patients with metastatic clear cell renal cell carcinoma. *J. Natl. Compr. Cancer Netw.* **2016**, *14*, 820–824. [CrossRef]
13. Voss, M.H.; Reising, A.; Cheng, Y.; Patel, P.; Marker, M.; Kuo, F.; Chan, T.A.; Choueiri, T.K.; Hsieh, J.J.; Hakimi, A.A.; et al. Genomically annotated risk model for advanced renal-cell carcinoma: A retrospective cohort study. *Lancet Oncol.* **2018**, *19*, 1688–1698. [CrossRef]
14. Minardi, D.; Lucarini, G.; Santoni, M.; Mazzucchelli, R.; Burattini, L.; Pistelli, M.; Bianconi, M.; Di Primio, R.; Scartozzi, M.; Montironi, R.; et al. VEGF expression and response to sunitinib in patients with metastatic clear cell renal cell carcinoma. *Anticancer Res.* **2013**, *33*, 5017–5022. [PubMed]
15. Porta, C.; Paglino, C.; De Amici, M.; Quaglini, S.; Sacchi, L.; Imarisio, I.; Canipari, C. Predictive value of baseline serum vascular endothelial growth factor and neutrophil gelatinase-associated lipocalin in advanced kidney cancer patients receiving sunitinib. *Kidney Int.* **2010**, *77*, 809–815. [CrossRef] [PubMed]
16. Paule, B.; Bastien, L.; Deslandes, E.; Cussenot, O.; Podgorniak, M.P.; Allory, Y.; Naïmi, B.; Porcher, R.; de la Taille, A.; Menashi, S.; et al. Soluble isoforms of vascular endothelial growth factor are predictors of response to sunitinib in metastatic renal cell carcinomas. *PLoS ONE* **2010**, *5*, e10715. [CrossRef] [PubMed]
17. Brauer, M.J.; Zhuang, G.; Schmidt, M.; Yao, J.; Wu, X.; Kaminker, J.S.; Jurinka, S.S.; Kolumam, G.; Chung, A.S.; Jubb, A.; et al. Identification and analysis of in vivo VEGF downstream markers link VEGF pathway activity with efficacy of anti-VEGF therapies. *Clin. Cancer Res.* **2013**, *19*, 3681–3692. [CrossRef] [PubMed]
18. McDermott, D.F.; Huseni, M.A.; Atkins, M.B.; Motzer, R.J.; Rini, B.I.; Escudier, B.; Fong, L.; Joseph, R.W.; Pal, S.K.; Reeves, J.A.; et al. Clinical activity and molecular correlates of response to atezolizumab alone or in combination with bevacizumab versus sunitinib in renal cell carcinoma. *Nat. Med.* **2018**, *24*, 749–757. [CrossRef]
19. Hakimi, A.A.; Voss, M.H.; Kuo, F.; Sanchez, A.; Liu, M.; Nixon, B.G.; Vuong, L.; Ostrovnaya, I.; Chen, Y.B.; Reuter, V.; et al. Transcriptomic profiling of the tumor microenvironment reveals distinct subgroups of clear cell renal cell cancer: Data from a randomized phase III trial. *Cancer Discov.* **2019**, *9*, 510–525. [CrossRef] [PubMed]
20. Choueiri, T.K.; Albiges, L.; Haanen, J.B.A.G.; Larkin, J.M.G.; Uemura, M.; Pal, S.K.; Gravis, G.; Campbell, M.T.; Penkov, K.; Lee, J.-L.; et al. Biomarker analyses from JAVELIN Renal 101: Avelumab + axitinib (A+Ax) versus sunitinib (S) in advanced renal cell carcinoma (aRCC). *J. Clin. Oncol.* **2019**, *37*, 101. [CrossRef]
21. Martini, J.-F.; Plimack, E.R.; Choueiri, T.K.; McDermott, D.F.; Puzanov, I.; Fishman, M.N.; Cho, D.C.; Vaishampayan, U.; Rosbrook, B.; Fernandez, K.C.; et al. Angiogenic and immune-related biomarkers and outcomes following axitinib/pembrolizumab treatment in patients with advanced renal cell carcinoma. *Clin. Cancer Res.* **2020**, *26*, 5598–5608. [CrossRef] [PubMed]
22. Brindle, N.P.J.; Saharinen, P.; Alitalo, K. Signaling and functions of angiopoietin-1 in vascular protection. *Circ. Res.* **2006**, *98*, 1014–1023. [CrossRef]

23. Attig, S.; Hennenlotter, J.; Pawelec, G.; Klein, G.; Koch, S.D.; Pircher, H.; Feyerabend, S.; Wernet, D.; Stenzl, A.; Rammensee, H.G.; et al. Simultaneous infiltration of polyfunctional effector and suppressor T cells into renal cell carcinomas. *Cancer Res.* **2009**, *69*, 8412–8419. [CrossRef] [PubMed]
24. McDermott, D.F.; Regan, M.M.; Clark, J.I.; Flaherty, L.E.; Weiss, G.R.; Logan, T.F.; Kirkwood, J.M.; Gordon, M.S.; Sosman, J.A.; Ernstoff, M.S.; et al. Randomized phase III trial of high-dose interleukin-2 versus subcutaneous interleukin-2 and interferon in patients with metastatic renal cell carcinoma. *J. Clin. Oncol. Off. J. Am. Soc. Clin. Oncol.* **2005**, *23*, 133–141. [CrossRef] [PubMed]
25. Fyfe, G.; Fisher, R.I.; Rosenberg, S.A.; Sznol, M.; Parkinson, D.R.; Louie, A.C. Results of treatment of 255 patients with metastatic renal cell carcinoma who received high-dose recombinant interleukin-2 therapy. *J. Clin. Oncol. Off. J. Am. Soc. Clin. Oncol.* **1995**, *13*, 688–696. [CrossRef]
26. Negrier, S.; Escudier, B.; Lasset, C.; Douillard, J.Y.; Savary, J.; Chevreau, C.; Ravaud, A.; Mercatello, A.; Peny, J.; Mousseau, M.; et al. Recombinant human interleukin-2, recombinant human interferon alfa-2a, or both in metastatic renal-cell carcinoma. *N. Engl. J. Med.* **1998**, *338*, 1272–1278. [CrossRef]
27. Motzer, R.J.; Escudier, B.; McDermott, D.F.; George, S.; Hammers, H.J.; Srinivas, S.; Tykodi, S.S.; Sosman, J.A.; Procopio, G.; Plimack, E.R.; et al. Nivolumab versus Everolimus in Advanced Renal-Cell Carcinoma. *N. Engl. J. Med.* **2015**, *373*, 1803–1813. [CrossRef]
28. Carretero-González, A.; Lora, D.; Martín Sobrino, I.; Sáez Sanz, I.; Bourlon, M.T.; Anido Herranz, U.; Martínez Chanzá, N.; Castellano, D.; de Velasco, G. The Value of PD-L1 Expression as Predictive Biomarker in Metastatic Renal Cell Carcinoma Patients: A Meta-Analysis of Randomized Clinical Trials. *Cancers (Basel)* **2020**, *12*, 1945. [CrossRef]
29. National Comprehensive Cancer Network Kidney Cancer (Version 2.2020). Available online: https://www.nccn.org/professionals/physician_gls/pdf/kidney.pdf (accessed on 10 October 2020).
30. Nunes-Xavier, C.E.; Angulo, J.C.; Pulido, R.; López, J.I. A Critical Insight into the Clinical Translation of PD-1/PD-L1 Blockade Therapy in Clear Cell Renal Cell Carcinoma. *Curr. Urol. Rep.* **2019**, *20*, 1. [CrossRef]
31. López, J.I.; Pulido, R.; Cortés, J.M.; Angulo, J.C.; Lawrie, C.H. Potential impact of PD-L1 (SP-142) immunohistochemical heterogeneity in clear cell renal cell carcinoma immunotherapy. *Pathol. Res. Pract.* **2018**, *214*, 1110–1114. [CrossRef]
32. Thompson, R.H.; Kuntz, S.M.; Leibovich, B.C.; Dong, H.; Lohse, C.M.; Webster, W.S.; Sengupta, S.; Frank, I.; Parker, A.S.; Zincke, H.; et al. Tumor B7-H1 is associated with poor prognosis in renal cell carcinoma patients with long-term follow-up. *Cancer Res.* **2006**, *66*, 3381–3385. [CrossRef] [PubMed]
33. Miao, D.; Margolis, C.A.; Gao, W.; Voss, M.H.; Li, W.; Martini, D.J.; Norton, C.; Bossé, D.; Wankowicz, S.M.; Cullen, D.; et al. Genomic correlates of response to immune checkpoint therapies in clear cell renal cell carcinoma. *Science (80-)* **2018**, *359*, 801–806. [CrossRef] [PubMed]
34. Braun, D.A.; Ishii, Y.; Walsh, A.M.; Van Allen, E.M.; Wu, C.J.; Shukla, S.A.; Choueiri, T.K. Clinical Validation of PBRM1 Alterations as a Marker of Immune Checkpoint Inhibitor Response in Renal Cell Carcinoma. *JAMA Oncol.* **2019**, *5*, 1631. [CrossRef] [PubMed]
35. Hakimi, A.A.; Attalla, K.; DiNatale, R.G.; Ostrovnaya, I.; Flynn, J.; Blum, K.A.; Ged, Y.; Hoen, D.; Kendall, S.M.; Reznik, E.; et al. A pan-cancer analysis of PBAF complex mutations and their association with immunotherapy response. *Nat. Commun.* **2020**, *11*, 4168. [CrossRef]
36. Mizuno, R.; Oya, M. Biomarkers Towards New Era of Therapeutics for Metastatic Renal Cell Carcinoma. *Kidney Cancer* **2020**, *4*, 61–69. [CrossRef]
37. Skoulidis, F.; Goldberg, M.E.; Greenawalt, D.M.; Hellmann, M.D.; Awad, M.M.; Gainor, J.F.; Schrock, A.B.; Hartmaier, R.J.; Trabucco, S.E.; Gay, L.; et al. STK11/LKB1 mutations and PD-1 inhibitor resistance in KRAS-mutant lung adenocarcinoma. *Cancer Discov.* **2018**, *8*, 822–835. [CrossRef]
38. Cerami, E.; Gao, J.; Dogrusoz, U.; Gross, B.E.; Sumer, S.O.; Aksoy, B.A.; Jacobsen, A.; Byrne, C.J.; Heuer, M.L.; Larsson, E.; et al. The cBio Cancer Genomics Portal: An open platform for exploring multidimensional cancer genomics data. *Cancer Discov.* **2012**, *2*, 401–404. [CrossRef]
39. Salgia, N.; Dizman, N.; Lyou, Y.; Bergerot, P.G.; Hsu, J.; Byron, S.A.; Trent, J.M.; Pal, S.K. Genomic and transcriptomic correlates of clinical benefit from immunotherapy and targeted therapy among patients with metastatic renal cell carcinoma (mRCC). *J. Clin. Oncol.* **2020**, *38*, 5076. [CrossRef]
40. D'Costa, N.M.; Cina, D.; Shrestha, R.; Bell, R.H.; Lin, Y.Y.; Asghari, H.; Monjaras-Avila, C.U.; Kollmannsberger, C.; Hach, F.; Chavez-Munoz, C.I.; et al. Identification of gene signature for treatment response to guide precision oncology in clear-cell renal cell carcinoma. *Sci. Rep.* **2020**, *10*, 2026. [CrossRef]

41. McDermott, D.F.; Lee, J.-L.; Donskov, F.; Tykodi, S.S.; Bjarnason, G.A.; Larkin, J.M.G.; Gafanov, R.; Kochenderfer, M.D.; Malik, J.; Poprach, A.; et al. Association of gene expression with clinical outcomes in patients with renal cell carcinoma treated with pembrolizumab in KEYNOTE-427. *J. Clin. Oncol.* **2020**, *38*, 5024. [CrossRef]
42. Brahmer, J.R.; Tykodi, S.S.; Chow, L.Q.M.; Hwu, W.J.; Topalian, S.L.; Hwu, P.; Drake, C.G.; Camacho, L.H.; Kauh, J.; Odunsi, K.; et al. Safety and activity of anti-PD-L1 antibody in patients with advanced cancer. *N. Engl. J. Med.* **2012**, *366*, 2455–2465. [CrossRef] [PubMed]
43. Bonneville, R.; Krook, M.A.; Kautto, E.A.; Miya, J.; Wing, M.R.; Chen, H.-Z.; Reeser, J.W.; Yu, L.; Roychowdhury, S. Landscape of Microsatellite Instability Across 39 Cancer Types. *JCO Precis. Oncol.* **2017**, *1*, 1–15. [CrossRef] [PubMed]
44. Ged, Y.; Chaim, J.L.; DInatale, R.G.; Knezevic, A.; Kotecha, R.R.; Carlo, M.I.; Lee, C.H.; Foster, A.; Feldman, D.R.; Teo, M.Y.; et al. DNA damage repair pathway alterations in metastatic clear cell renal cell carcinoma and implications on systemic therapy. *J. Immunother. Cancer* **2020**, *8*, e000230. [CrossRef] [PubMed]
45. Labriola, M.K.; Zhu, J.; Gupta, R.; McCall, S.; Jackson, J.; Kong, E.F.; White, J.R.; Cerqueira, G.; Gerding, K.; Simmons, J.K.; et al. Characterization of tumor mutation burden, PD-L1 and DNA repair genes to assess relationship to immune checkpoint inhibitors response in metastatic renal cell carcinoma. *J. Immunother. Cancer* **2020**, *8*, 1–10. [CrossRef] [PubMed]
46. Chen, L.; Flies, D.B. Molecular mechanisms of T cell co-stimulation and co-inhibition. *Nat. Rev. Immunol.* **2013**, *13*, 227–242. [CrossRef]
47. Gubin, M.M.; Artyomov, M.N.; Mardis, E.R.; Schreiber, R.D. Tumor neoantigens: Building a framework for personalized cancer immunotherapy. *J. Clin. Investig.* **2015**, *125*, 3413–3421. [CrossRef]
48. Goodman, A.M.; Kato, S.; Bazhenova, L.; Patel, S.P.; Frampton, G.M.; Miller, V.; Stephens, P.J.; Daniels, G.A.; Kurzrock, R. Tumor mutational burden as an independent predictor of response to immunotherapy in diverse cancers. *Mol. Cancer Ther.* **2017**, *16*, 2598–2608. [CrossRef]
49. Marabelle, A.; Fakih, M.G.; Lopez, J.; Shah, M.; Shapira-Frommer, R.; Nakagawa, K.; Chung, H.C.; Kindler, H.L.; Lopez-Martin, J.A.; Miller, W.; et al. Association of tumour mutational burden with outcomes in patients with select advanced solid tumours treated with pembrolizumab in KEYNOTE-158. *Ann. Oncol.* **2019**, *30*, v477–v478. [CrossRef]
50. Zhang, C.; Li, Z.; Qi, F.; Hu, X.; Luo, J. Exploration of the relationships between tumor mutation burden with immune infiltrates in clear cell renal cell carcinoma. *Ann. Transl. Med.* **2019**, *7*, 648. [CrossRef]
51. Havel, J.J.; Chowell, D.; Chan, T.A. The evolving landscape of biomarkers for checkpoint inhibitor immunotherapy. *Nat. Rev. Cancer* **2019**, *19*, 133–150. [CrossRef]
52. McGrail, D.J.; Federico, L.; Li, Y.; Dai, H.; Lu, Y.; Mills, G.B.; Yi, S.; Lin, S.Y.; Sahni, N. Multi-omics analysis reveals neoantigen-independent immune cell infiltration in copy-number driven cancers. *Nat. Commun.* **2018**, *9*, 1–13. [CrossRef]
53. Turajlic, S.; Litchfield, K.; Xu, H.; Rosenthal, R.; McGranahan, N.; Reading, J.L.; Wong, Y.N.S.; Rowan, A.; Kanu, N.; Al Bakir, M.; et al. Insertion-and-deletion-derived tumour-specific neoantigens and the immunogenic phenotype: A pan-cancer analysis. *Lancet Oncol.* **2017**, *18*, 1009–1021. [CrossRef] [PubMed]
54. Shim, J.H.; Kim, H.S.; Cha, H.; Kim, S.; Kim, T.M.; Anagnostou, V.; Choi, Y.L.; Jung, H.A.; Sun, J.M.; Ahn, J.S.; et al. HLA-corrected tumor mutation burden and homologous recombination deficiency for the prediction of response to PD-(L)1 blockade in advanced non-small-cell lung cancer patients. *Ann. Oncol.* **2020**, *31*, 902–911. [CrossRef] [PubMed]
55. Hu, K.; Lou, L.; Ye, J.; Zhang, S. Prognostic role of the neutrophil-lymphocyte ratio in renal cell carcinoma: A meta-analysis. *BMJ Open* **2015**, *5*, e006404. [CrossRef]
56. Baum, Y.S.; Patil, D.; Huang, J.H.; Spetka, S.; Torlak, M.; Nieh, P.T.; Alemozaffar, M.; Ogan, K.; Master, V.A. Elevated preoperative neutrophil-tolymphocyte ratio may be associated with decreased overall survival in patients with metastatic clear cell renal cell carcinoma undergoing cytoreductive nephrectomy. *Asian J. Urol.* **2016**, *3*, 20–25. [CrossRef]
57. Pichler, M.; Hutterer, G.C.; Stoeckigt, C.; Chromecki, T.F.; Stojakovic, T.; Golbeck, S.; Eberhard, K.; Gerger, A.; Mannweiler, S.; Pummer, K.; et al. Validation of the pre-treatment neutrophil-lymphocyte ratio as a prognostic factor in a large European cohort of renal cell carcinoma patients. *Br. J. Cancer* **2013**, *108*, 901–907. [CrossRef]

58. Park, Y.H.; Ku, J.H.; Kwak, C.; Kim, H.H. Post-treatment neutrophil-to-lymphocyte ratio in predicting prognosis in patients with metastatic clear cell renal cell carcinoma receiving sunitinib as first line therapy. *Springerplus* **2014**, *3*, 1–6. [CrossRef]
59. Keizman, D.; Ish-Shalom, M.; Huang, P.; Eisenberger, M.A.; Pili, R.; Hammers, H.; Carducci, M.A. The association of pre-treatment neutrophil to lymphocyte ratio with response rate, progression free survival and overall survival of patients treated with sunitinib for metastatic renal cell carcinoma. *Eur. J. Cancer* **2012**, *48*, 202–208. [CrossRef]
60. Jeyakumar, G.; Kim, S.; Bumma, N.; Landry, C.; Silski, C.; Suisham, S.; Dickow, B.; Heath, E.; Fontana, J.; Vaishampayan, U. Neutrophil lymphocyte ratio and duration of prior anti-angiogenic therapy as biomarkers in metastatic RCC receiving immune checkpoint inhibitor therapy. *J. Immunother. Cancer* **2017**, *5*, 1–8. [CrossRef]
61. Lalani, A.K.A.; Xie, W.; Martini, D.J.; Steinharter, J.A.; Norton, C.K.; Krajewski, K.M.; Duquette, A.; Bossé, D.; Bellmunt, J.; Van Allen, E.M.; et al. Change in Neutrophil-to-lymphocyte ratio (NLR) in response to immune checkpoint blockade for metastatic renal cell carcinoma. *J. Immunother. Cancer* **2018**, *6*, 1–9. [CrossRef]
62. Lanzavecchla, A. Licence to kill. *Nature* **1998**, *393*, 413–414. [CrossRef]
63. Balch, C.M.; Riley, L.B.; Bae, Y.J.; Salmeron, M.A.; Platsoucas, C.D.; Von Eschenbach, A.; Itoh, K. Patterns of Human Tumor-Infiltrating Lymphocytes in 120 Human Cancers. *Arch. Surg.* **1990**, *125*, 200–205. [CrossRef] [PubMed]
64. Thompson, R.H.; Dong, H.; Lohse, C.M.; Leibovich, B.C.; Blute, M.L.; Cheville, J.C.; Kwon, E.D. PD-1 is expressed by tumor-infiltrating immune cells and is associated with poor outcome for patients with renal cell carcinoma. *Clin. Cancer Res.* **2007**, *13*, 1757–1761. [CrossRef] [PubMed]
65. MacFarlane, A.W.; Jillab, M.; Plimack, E.R.; Hudes, G.R.; Uzzo, R.G.; Litwin, S.; Dulaimi, E.; Al-Saleem, T.; Campbell, K.S. PD-1 expression on peripheral blood cells increases with stage in renal cell carcinoma patients and is rapidly reduced after surgical tumor resection. *Cancer Immunol. Res.* **2014**, *2*, 320–331. [CrossRef] [PubMed]
66. Giraldo, N.A.; Becht, E.; Vano, Y.; Petitprez, F.; Lacroix, L.; Validire, P.; Sanchez-Salas, R.; Ingels, A.; Oudard, S.; Moatti, A.; et al. Tumor-infiltrating and peripheral blood T-cell immunophenotypes predict early relapse in localized clear cell renal cell carcinoma. *Clin. Cancer Res.* **2017**, *23*, 4416–4428. [CrossRef] [PubMed]
67. Braun, D.A.; Hou, Y.; Bakouny, Z.; Ficial, M.; Sant' Angelo, M.; Forman, J.; Ross-Macdonald, P.; Berger, A.C.; Jegede, O.A.; Elagina, L.; et al. Interplay of somatic alterations and immune infiltration modulates response to PD-1 blockade in advanced clear cell renal cell carcinoma. *Nat. Med.* **2020**, *26*. [CrossRef] [PubMed]
68. Ficial, M.; Jegede, O.; Sant'Angelo, M.; Moreno, S.; Braun, D.A.; Wind-Rotolo, M.; Pignon, J.-C.; Catalano, P.J.; Sun, M.; Van Allen, E.M.; et al. Evaluation of predictive biomarkers for nivolumab in patients (pts) with metastatic clear cell renal cell carcinoma (mccRCC) from the CheckMate-025 (CM-025) trial. *J. Clin. Oncol.* **2020**, *38*, 5023. [CrossRef]
69. Kraman, M.; Faroudi, M.; Allen, N.L.; Kmiecik, K.; Gliddon, D.; Seal, C.; Koers, A.; Wydro, M.M.; Batey, S.; Winnewisser, J.; et al. FS118, a Bispecific Antibody Targeting LAG-3 and PD-L1, Enhances T-Cell Activation Resulting in Potent Antitumor Activity. *Clin. Cancer Res.* **2020**, *26*, 3333–3344. [CrossRef]
70. Long, L.; Zhang, X.; Chen, F.; Pan, Q.; Phiphatwatchara, P.; Zeng, Y.; Chen, H. The promising immune checkpoint LAG-3: From tumor microenvironment to cancer immunotherapy. *Genes Cancer* **2018**, *9*, 176–189. [CrossRef]
71. Errarte, P.; Larrinaga, G.; López, J.I. The role of cancer-associated fibroblasts in renal cell carcinoma. An example of tumor modulation through tumor/non-tumor cell interactions. *J. Adv. Res.* **2020**, *21*, 103–108. [CrossRef]
72. Errarte, P.; Guarch, R.; Pulido, R.; Blanco, L.; Nunes-Xavier, C.E.; Beitia, M.; Gil, J.; Angulo, J.C.; Lopez, J.I.; Larrinaga, G. The expression of fibroblast activation protein in clear cell renal cell carcinomas is associated with synchronous lymph node metastases. *PLoS ONE* **2016**, *11*, e169105. [CrossRef] [PubMed]
73. Inoue, C.; Miki, Y.; Saito, R.; Hata, S.; Abe, J.; Sato, I.; Okada, Y.; Sasano, H. PD-L1 induction by cancer-associated fibroblast-derived factors in lung adenocarcinoma cells. *Cancers (Basel)* **2019**, *11*, 1257. [CrossRef] [PubMed]

74. Turajlic, S.; Xu, H.; Litchfield, K.; Rowan, A.; Horswell, S.; Chambers, T.; O'Brien, T.; Lopez, J.I.; Watkins, T.B.K.; Nicol, D.; et al. Deterministic Evolutionary Trajectories Influence Primary Tumor Growth: TRACERx Renal. *Cell* **2018**, *173*, 595–610. [CrossRef] [PubMed]

Publisher's Note: MDPI stays neutral with regard to jurisdictional claims in published maps and institutional affiliations.

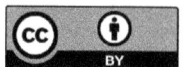 © 2020 by the authors. Licensee MDPI, Basel, Switzerland. This article is an open access article distributed under the terms and conditions of the Creative Commons Attribution (CC BY) license (http://creativecommons.org/licenses/by/4.0/).

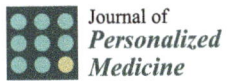

Review

Imaging Biomarkers of Tumour Proliferation and Invasion for Personalised Lung Cancer Therapy

Loredana G. Marcu [1,2]

1. Faculty of Informatics and Science, University of Oradea, 410087 Oradea, Romania; loredana@marcunet.com
2. Cancer Research Institute, University of South Australia, Adelaide, SA 5001, Australia

Received: 7 October 2020; Accepted: 10 November 2020; Published: 12 November 2020

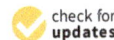

Abstract: Personalised treatment in oncology has seen great developments over the last decade, due to both technological advances and more in-depth knowledge of radiobiological processes occurring in tumours. Lung cancer therapy is no exception, as new molecular targets have been identified to further increase treatment specificity and sensitivity. Yet, tumour resistance to treatment is still one of the main reasons for treatment failure. This is due to a number of factors, among which tumour proliferation, the presence of cancer stem cells and the metastatic potential of the primary tumour are key features that require better controlling to further improve cancer management in general, and lung cancer treatment in particular. Imaging biomarkers play a key role in the identification of biological particularities within tumours and therefore are an important component of treatment personalisation in radiotherapy. Imaging techniques such as PET, SPECT, MRI that employ tumour-specific biomarkers already play a critical role in patient stratification towards individualized treatment. The aim of the current paper is to describe the radiobiological challenges of lung cancer treatment in relation to the latest imaging biomarkers that can aid in the identification of hostile cellular features for further treatment adaptation and tailoring to the individual patient's needs.

Keywords: biomarkers; molecular imaging; non-small cell lung cancer; proliferation; cancer stem cells; circulating tumour cells; personalised treatment

---

1. Introduction

According to the latest Global Cancer Statistics, lung cancer is the most commonly diagnosed cancer worldwide, in both males and females (11.6% of the total cases) and the leading cause of cancer death (18.4%) [1]. Non-small cell lung cancers (as opposed to small cell lung cancers) account for about 85% of lung cancer cases and encompass adenocarcinomas, squamous cell carcinomas and large-cell undifferentiated carcinomas. Conventional therapies (surgery, chemo-radiotherapy) are being improved with new drugs and targeted agents.

While the latest technological and pharmaceutical developments have increased the therapeutic index in lung cancer, research over the last decade reveals an imperative need to include radiobiological characteristics of cellular and subcellular structures as well as the tumour microenvironment into the big picture of personalised medicine [2]. Hypoxia, proliferation, intrinsic radioresistance, and the presence of cancer stem cells are only a few, but probably the most critical features that require better management to further improve cancer treatment outcomes in general, and lung cancer treatment in particular. However, the primary tumour is not the only entity to confront. Cancer invasion and metastasis poses a therapeutic challenge by broadening the curative needs from local to systemic disease management. In this context, the identification and quantification of circulating tumour cells represent an important undertaking.

Although most of aforementioned tumour characteristics and their impact on tumour control are well known, there is still no clear-cut solution to manage treatment resistance due to high proliferative potential, the presence of cancer stem cells or circulating tumour cells that are indicative of tumour aggressiveness.

In order to tackle the above challenges, one should first identify the hostile features and then target them with the best currently available techniques. In this respect, biomarkers play a key role, as their specific design allows the identification of tumour areas that are prone to treatment resistance, thus leading the way towards personalised, targeted therapies.

The current paper focuses on the (radio) biological challenges described above applied to non-small cell lung cancer (NSCLC) and the latest imaging biomarkers that can aid in their identification, targeting and treatment outcome prediction. The main features discussed in the paper are related to tumour kinetics, via tumour proliferation and the presence of cancer stem cells, and tumour dynamics, via progression, invasion and distant metastasis through circulating tumour cells.

2. Tumour Proliferation and Imaging Biomarkers

2.1. Tumour Proliferation

Cellular proliferation is a prerequisite for tissue growth and development. Uncontrolled proliferation is characteristic of cancer cells and represents one of the hallmarks of neoplastic growth. The rate of tumour proliferation differentiates slowly proliferating from rapidly proliferating tumours, a feature that dictates the type of treatment required for tumour control. The evaluation of a tumour's proliferative ability and of its growth kinetics are therefore critical aspects of cancer management.

Cell proliferation rate is commonly assessed through the presence in the cell nucleus of the Ki-67 monoclonal antibody, during the active phases of the cell cycle. The Ki-67 antibody labels nuclei of proliferating cells, enabling the quantification of the proliferating cell fraction within a tumour [3]. Clinical research over the years has proved Ki-67 proliferation index (or labeling index) to be a biomarker with important prognostic and predictive value in a number of cancers, including lung. The retrospective analysis of three NSCLC cohorts involving about 1500 patients showed that Ki-67 proliferation index is a highly significant and independent predictor of survival in these cancers [4]. An important aspect of the study was the individual assessment of Ki-67 correlation with each histological type of NSCLC. In this respect, the high proliferation index (PI) in adenocarcinomas was significantly associated with a worse prognosis for disease-free survival, whereas in squamous cell carcinomas the high PI was associated with better overall survival rates (cut-off value for PI of 50%). Treatment outcome among adenocarcinoma patients was further influenced by the administration of adjuvant chemo-radiotherapy, showing that patients with high PI may benefit to a higher extent from adjuvant treatment than those with low PI (cut-off value for PI of 25%).

This study showed the importance of data analysis based on histological characteristics (rather than NSCLC as a group) and the definition/validation of a Ki-67 cut-off value for each histological type of NSCLC. Furthermore, it was suggested that the predictive power of Ki-67 labeling could be enhanced by the concurrent employment of other clinical/pathological parameters as well as imaging biomarkers, which would eventually lead to better patient stratification and treatment optimisation.

Another important factor that controls cellular proliferation in lung cancers (and not only) is the epidermal growth factor receptor (EGFR). The EGFR is a transmembrane glycoprotein receptor of the ErbB family of cell surface tyrosine kinases with a role in regulating cell proliferation and apoptosis through signal transduction pathways [5]. Mutations and truncations of its extracellular matrix leads to upregulation of EGFR in several cancers, including NSCLC. Malignant as well as premalignant lesions can overexpress EGFR, with 40–80% of NSCLC patients being identified with abnormal expressions of EGFR (increased gene copy number per cell), with the highest rates seen in squamous cell carcinomas [6,7]. EGFR expression was found to be a poor prognostic factor in NSCLC, requiring efficient anti-EGFR therapies [6]. To date, EGFR-targeted therapies based on tyrosine kinase inhibitors (gefitinib, erlotinib) and monoclonal antibodies (cetuximab) have been developed with limited success, due to acquired or inherent resistance to EGFR inhibition [8]. Next to EGFR,

ALK (anaplastic lymphoma kinase) translocations are known to be oncogenic drivers in NSCLC [9]. ALK translocation is associated with high sensitivity to ALK inhibitors such as crizotinib, ceritinib and alectinib [10]. Moreover, the set of mutations in these cancers is much wider. Regarding targeting avenues, ROS1 translocation is associated with a positive response to crizotinib therapy, while for BRAF mutations the combined administration of dabrafenib and trametinib, as well as the low molecular weight tyrosine kinase inhibitors vemurafenib and dabrafenib, were shown to be effective. MET mutations in lung cancer are considered to be predictors of susceptibility to the MET inhibitor crizotinib, whereas RET translocations are correlated with a positive response to targeted therapy with RET inhibitors such as cabozatinib, vandetinib, and alectinib [10]. All these mutations are important therapeutic targets, which can be identified not only in biopsy samples (given that 30% of tumour biopsies yield inadequate tissue for molecular subtyping) but also in cell-free circulating tumour DNA [11].

More recently, research into tumour proliferation has been linked to microRNAs, owing to their role in multiple biological processes, including gene regulation [12]. MicroRNAs (miRNA) are short noncoding RNAs consisting of 21–25 nucleotides that can inhibit translation of messenger RNA (mRNA) and promote mRNA degradation, thus functioning as endogenous negative gene regulators. Through posttranscriptional regulation of gene expression, miRNAs have a great impact on a number of oncogenic pathways. Recent studies demonstrated a relationship between the EGFR signaling pathway and miRNAs, showing a direct regulatory effect on EGFR [13]. Studies in NSCLC revealed the potential of miRNAs to serve in patient stratification (by risk and histology) while also predicting prognosis in early-stage NSCLC [14].

2.2. Imaging Biomarkers for Proliferation

Cellular kinetic parameters are important indicators of tumour proliferation before, during and after therapy, thus their quantification warrants special consideration. As shown above, the most studied proliferation markers and, consequently, the most targeted molecules related to cellular proliferation in lung cancer imaging are EGFR and Ki-67. In this regard, numerous tracers have been developed and trialed with various results [15].

2.2.1. Positron Emission Tomography (PET) Imaging Biomarkers

Fluorodeoxyglucose-F18 (18F-FDG) is the most commonly used PET imaging radiotracer, being an indicator of tumour activity via glucose metabolism, and has an established role in tumour staging and treatment response monitoring. Its role in the assessment of tumour proliferation was also researched, with a considerable number of studies examining the potential of 18F-FDG in predicting EGFR mutation status in NSCLC patients. In a retrospective clinical study involving 109 NSCLC patients, Chen et al. showed that EGFR mutation decreases cellular accumulation of FDG via the NOX4/ROS/GLUT1 axis [16]. The SUVmax values in the cohort with EGFR mutations were significantly lower (6.52 mean value) than in the wild-type EGFR cohort (9.37 mean value, $p < 0.001$). Similarly, in a study of 102 NSCLC patients with EGFR mutation (22%), KRAS mutation (27%) and wild-type profiles (51%), it was observed that 18F-FDG uptake was significantly higher in those harbouring KRAS mutations as compared to EGFR+ or wild-type (SUVmean 9.5 vs. 5.7 vs. 6.6, $p < 0.001$) [17]. These findings are corroborated by a much larger study, encompassing 849 NSCLC patients with 45.9% identified with EGFR mutation, that also showed low SUVmax association with EGFR mutation status [18]. This result could be combined with other clinical factors to improve patient stratification, particularly when EGFR testing is not available [18,19].

A recent study reported on the development of a new PET tracer with high specificity to activating EGFR mutant kinase showing significant correlation between tracer uptake and the EGFR mutation status in both preclinical animal models and in patients with NSCLC [20]. The study aimed to identify, via a new imaging tracer—18F-MPG (N-(3-chloro-4-fluorophenyl)-7-(2-(2-(2-(2-^{18}F-fluoroethoxy) ethoxy) ethoxy) ethoxy)-6-methoxyquinazolin-4-amine)—, those patients that are sensitive to

EGFR-TKIs and to monitor the efficiency of EGFR-TKI therapy. The cut-off value for SUVmax was set at 2.23, showing a greater response to EGFR-TKI in those presenting with SUVmax ≥2.23 as compared to patients with values <2.23 (81.58% vs. 6.06%). Furthermore, 18F-MPG uptake positively correlated with median progression-free survival [20].

While 18F-FDG has its own merits in the functional imaging of lung cancer, it is not the optimal indicator of proliferation, showing poorer correlation with cellular proliferation markers than other PET tracers. Fluoro-3′-deoxythymidine-F18 (18F-FLT), a successfully used imaging marker of cellular proliferation, is a radiolabeled structural analog of a DNA nucleoside—thymidine—and its uptake relates to the activity of thymidine kinase 1 (TK1) that is expressed during DNA synthesis in the S-phase of the cell cycle [21]. The uptake of 18F-FLT in tumour cells is lower as compared to 18F-FDG, as it only accumulates in cells during the S-phase [15]. Yet, several studies demonstrated the superior correlation of 18F-FLT with cellular proliferation markers when compared to the traditional 18F-FDG [22,23]. In one of the first comparative studies that involved a cohort of 26 lung cancer patients, Buck et al. showed high correlation between 18F-FLT uptake and Ki-67 index ($p < 0.0001$; $r = 0.92$), and concluded that 18F-FLT may be a better imaging marker than FDG for response assessment and outcome prediction [22]. These observations are supported by a recent meta-analysis that assessed 1213 patients from 22 imaging studies that correlated the Ki-67 labeling index with FDG and FLT uptake, respectively, showing that the latter is a more robust marker of tumour proliferation in lung cancer [23].

In a recent pilot study, Kairemo et al. demonstrated the feasibility of 18F-FLT PET in monitoring treatment response by early signal activity in NSCLC patients receiving targeted therapies (c-MET inhibitors) [24]. Several others have confirmed the potential of 18F-FLT PET imaging to monitor and guide molecular targeted therapies in NSCLC [25–27].

Next to the most common Fluor-based radiotracers employed in PET for tumour proliferation imaging, copper is another successful candidate. Functional imaging with PET employing 64Cu-ATSM (Cu-labeled diacetyl-bis(N(4)-methylthiosemicarbazone) and 18F-FDG was undertaken for the intratumoral distribution assessment of the two radionuclides in Lewis lung carcinoma tumour cells implanted in mice [28]. Both proliferation markers (Ki-67 and BrdU-bromodeoxyuridine) and the hypoxic marker, pimonidazole, were used to compare radionuclide uptake with immunohistochemical staining patterns. The association of staining with radionuclide accumulation revealed an increase in Ki-67 positive areas with 18F-FDG uptake increase and, at the same time, a decrease with 64Cu-ATSM accumulation. Conversely, the other proliferation marker, BrdU, showed an opposite behaviour, with the number of BrdU-positive cells being positively correlated with 64Cu-ATSM uptake and negatively related to 18F-FDG accumulation. Given that BrdU is a marker for proliferation by way of DNA synthesis, the fact that cells with high 64Cu-ATSM uptake positively correlated with the number of BrdU cells indicates that they are able to undergo DNA synthesis, though not during the proliferation process (denoted by the low Ki-67 levels which are specific to G1 and early S phase). This result suggests that cells in regions with high 64Cu-ATSM uptake were quiescent, yet sustained DNA synthesis and were sensitive to progression factors, just like quiescent cancer stem cells. Clonogenic assays within the same study have proven the stem-like properties of cells originating from high 64Cu-ATSM uptake tumour areas [28]. Furthermore, pimonidazole-positive areas were specific to regions with low 64Cu-ATSM accumulation, suggestive of mild hypoxic conditions, still optimal for the thriving of clonogenic tumour cells.

This study is a clear illustration of the complexity of the tumour microenvironment and of the many factors that influence tumour development and response to therapy (hypoxia, proliferation, cancer stem cells). Based on the above results, 64Cu-ATSM could potentially serve as a complex imaging biomarker to supply prognostic information for treatment adaptation and optimisation.

2.2.2. Single Photon Emission Computed Tomography (SPECT) Imaging Biomarkers

Beside PET tracers, a number of researchers attempted to develop SPECT radioisotopes for novel insights into EGFR targeting. The capacity of 99mTc-HYNIC-MPG ((2-(2-(2-(2-(4-(3-chloro-4-

fluorophenylamino)-6-methoxyquinazolin-7-yloxy)ethoxy)ethoxy)ethoxy)ethyl-6-hydrazinylnicotinate hydrochloride) was evaluated in detecting EGFR-activating mutations both in vitro and in vivo, using human NSCLC cell lines [29]. The study showed that of the four cell lines (EGFR+, EGFR− and wild-type), 99mTc-HYNIC-MPG uptake was the highest in the cell line with exon 19 deletion (PC9), probably due to the activating mutations in EGFR tyrosine kinase domain. The results could serve to further stratify NSCLC patients by identifying the subgroup that would benefit the most from targeted therapies with EGFR-TKIs [29].

Table 1 is a compilation of different functional imaging agents tested as markers for tumour proliferation in NSCLC.

Table 1. Functional imaging biomarkers for tumour proliferation in non-small cell lung cancer (NSCLC).

Study Aim [Ref]	Study Type	Proliferation Marker/ Targeting Agent	Comments
Positron Emission Tomography			
Proliferation imaging with ^{18}F-FLT vs. ^{18}F-FDG [Buck et al. (2003)] [22]	Prospective study (26 patients with pulmonary nodules)	Proliferation marker: Ki-67 Targeting agent: ^{18}F-FLT ^{18}F-FDG	A highly significant correlation ($p < 0.0001$) and a high correlation coefficient ($r = 0.92$) was observed between ^{18}F-FLT uptake and Ki-67 index, while the correlation coefficient between Ki-67 and ^{18}F-FDG was weak ($r = 0.59$). No FLT uptake was detected in non-proliferating tumours.
PET imaging for EGFR mutation evaluation and response to treatment [Sun et al. (2018)] [20]	Preclinical rodent model; Clinical NSCLC study	Proliferation marker: EGFR Targeting agent: ^{18}F-MPG	A greater response to EGFR-TKI was found in patients with SUV$_{max}$ ≥ 2.23 (81.58% vs. 6.06%). Median progression-free survival was also longer (348 days) in the cohort with SUV$_{max}$ ≥ 2.23 than in SUV$_{max}$ < 2.23 (183 days). ^{18}F-MPG PET for quantification of EGFR-activating mutation status could identify patients sensitive to EGFR-TKIs.
Evaluation of the role of ^{64}Cu-ATSM in PET imaging [Oh et al. (2009)] [28]	In vivo mice study (Lewis lung carcinoma tumour cells implanted in mice)	Proliferation markers: Ki-67 BrdU Targeting agent: ^{64}Cu-ATSM ^{18}F-FDG	Tumour regions with high ^{18}F-FDG but low ^{64}Cu-ATSM uptake correlated with increase in Ki-67. On the other hand, the number of BrdU-positive cells were positively correlated with ^{64}Cu-ATSM uptake and negatively related to ^{18}F-FDG accumulation. This suggests that cells in regions with high ^{64}Cu-ATSM uptake were quiescent, yet were sensitive to progression factors, like quiescent CSCs.
Single Photon Emission Computed Tomography			
Evaluation of ^{99m}Tc-HYNIC-MPG for detection of EGFR-activating mutations [Xiao et al. (2017)] [29]	In vitro cell line study (human NSCLC cell lines EGFR+/− and wild-type); In vivo animal xenograft model	Proliferation marker: EGFR Targeting agent: ^{99m}Tc-HYNIC-MPG	^{99m}Tc-HYNIC-MPG uptake was the highest in the cell line with exon 19 deletion (PC9), probably due to the activating mutations in EGFR tyrosine kinase domain. SPECT imaging with ^{99m}Tc-HYNIC-MPG could potentially identify NSCLC patients that would benefit the most from targeted therapies with EGFR-TKIs.

Table 1. Cont.

Study Aim [Ref]	Study Type	Proliferation Marker/ Targeting Agent	Comments
Magnetic Resonance Imaging			
EGFR targeting with active iron oxide NP for MRI [Wang et al. (2017)] [30]	H460 lung cancer cells (in vitro) and tumour-bearing rats (H460 lung xenografts) in vivo.	**Proliferation marker:** EGFR **Targeting agent:** Anti-EGFR-polyethylene glycol-superparamagnetic iron oxide (anti-EGFR-PEG-SPIO)	Both in vitro and in vivo MRI studies showed the potential of anti-EGFR-labeled iron oxide nanoparticles to identify and target lung cells that overexpress EGFR. The study had both imaging and therapeutic (theranostic) goals achieved with anti-EGFR targeting based on magnetic nanoparticles using MRI and focused ultrasound ablation.

Abbreviations: EGFR = epidermal growth factor receptor; PET = positron emission tomography; CSCs = cancer stem cells; MRI = magnetic resonance imaging; NPs = nanoparticles.

2.2.3. Magnetic Resonance Imaging (MRI) Biomarkers

The latest advances in biomaterials, specifically in nanomedicine, have greatly increased the sensitivity of imaging techniques using magnetic resonance to perform accurate and non-invasive functional imaging. In this regard, one of the recent developments is in the field of superparamagnetic iron oxide (SPIO) nanoparticles (40–50 nm), whereby polyethylene glycol-coated SPIO nanoparticles (PEG-SPIO) were synthesized and further labeled with high affinity anti-EGFR monoclonal antibody (cetuximab) for targeted delivery to lung cancer that overexpresses EGFR [30]. The targeting efficiency, MRI contrast enhancement and cytotoxicity of this nanocomposite was evaluated in both H460 lung cancer cells (in vitro) and tumour-bearing rats (H460 lung xenografts) in vivo. The uptake of the nanocomposite in the cell lines was evaluated by Prussian blue staining which showed an increased cellular uptake of anti-EGFR targeted NPs compared to non-targeting NPs at the same iron concentration, suggesting that the high cellular accumulation of anti-EFGR NPs is due to the EGFR receptor-mediated endocytosis pathway. This was also illustrated by TEM (transmission electron microscopy) imaging, where cells incubated with anti-EGFR targeting NPs showed the presence of electron-dense particles in the cell endosome, in contrast with those incubated with non-targeting NPs, which showed no such uptake. To further confirm these results, MRI-based investigation was undertaken by measuring the T2 weighted signal intensity of lung cells after incubation with NPs having various iron concentrations. It was observed that the T2 signal decreased with the increasing iron concentrations in the EGFR targeting NPs group. Furthermore, the signal intensity of lung cancer cells that overexpressed EGFR and were targeted with anti-EGFR-PEG-SPIO decreased more significantly than in the PEG-SPIO (non-targeting NPs) group. The study concluded that efficient identification and targeting of lung cells overexpressing EGFR can be achieved by means of anti-EGFR-PEG-SPIO nanocomposite, under MRI monitoring [30].

2.3. Summary of Current Status for Proliferation Biomarkers

While Ki-67 is a marker of proliferation that is well studied in lung cancer, EGFR has a less clear impact and its prognostic role is obscured by new therapies currently employed in clinical practice (such as EGFR-TKIs). To justify further developments in the field of new tracers for EGFR positive NSCLC, also considering the rapid pace of treatment evolution in this subset of patients, a cost–benefit analysis would help clinicians in their decision making. While there are some promising reports, neither the treatment response prediction nor the prognosis of EGFR tumours offered by these biomarkers are convincing enough to support wide clinical implementation.

3. Cancer Stem Cells and Imaging Biomarkers

3.1. Cancer Stem Cells

Statistics show that recurrence rates among NSCLC remain as high as 30–50%, with low overall 5-year survival rates [31]. One reason for this relatively poor response is the ability of lung cancer cells within the residual disease to regenerate and repopulate the tumour. The power of regeneration is owed to the small fraction of cells with stem-like properties which are phenotypically different from their non-stem counterparts and exhibit vital features for cell survival [32].

Cancer stem cells (CSCs) are a subpopulation of cancer cells that coexist within a tumour with other, non-stem like cells. CSCs have several well-established properties that confer upon them immortality and resistance to both chemo and radiotherapy. Resistance to treatment is multifactorial and is due to the ability of CSCs to efficiently repair DNA damage, to recreate themselves via symmetrical division thus contributing to tumour repopulation, to preferentially reside in specific microenvironmental niches in order to conserve their status, to be recruited into the cell cycle from the quiescent phase, and to exhibit cellular plasticity that enables transformation from CSC to non-CSC state and vice versa [33–35].

While the first indicators about the presence of CSCs in lung cancer originate from the early 80s [29], today there are several putative markers for CSCs, from cell surface markers such as CD (cluster of differentiation) molecules, which are surface proteins that enable the analysis of cell differentiation, to aldehyde dehydrogenase (ALDH), an intracellular enzyme and a subset of the CD44+ cells that exhibits high selectivity for CSCs [36]. Overexpression of the hyaluronic acid receptor CD44 was found in neoplasms of epithelial origin, including lung [37,38].

Other putative lung CSCs markers that present multipotent characteristics of stem cells are CD166+/CD44+ and CD166+/EpCAM+ (epithelial cell adhesion molecule). Using the above markers, Zakaria et al. showed that isolated lung CSCs exhibit molecular signatures of both normal and cancer stem cells, with biological functions related to angiogenesis, mesenchymal cell differentiation, and cell migration [39].

Another trialed CSC marker in solid tumours is CD133, with several studies demonstrating a link between CD133 expression and stem cell characteristics, including tumour aggressiveness [40,41]. A meta-analysis looking into the prognostic value of the expression of CSC marker CD133 revealed a strong correlation between this marker and prognostic factors among 1004 NSCLC patients [41]. The analysis showed a close correlation of CD133 expression with tumour stage, grade and poor prognosis. On the other hand, Salnikov et al. could not demonstrate any association between CD133 expression and survival of NSCLC patients, despite the indication of CD133 towards a resistant phenotype [42]. Due to such discrepant reports, the prognostic role of CD133 in lung cancer is not fully established, showing the need for the identification of more robust markers.

3.2. Imaging Biomarkers for Cancer Stem Cells

Owing to their unique tumour-promoting properties, cancer stem cells must be identified in order to be targeted and eradicated. The identification and targeting of CSCs are greatly dependent on specific markers and/or a combination of markers that are expressed on the surface of cancer stem cells. As CSCs are relatively newly studied descriptors of tumour development and response to therapy, in vivo imaging of CSCs is still in its infancy. Functional imaging studies using CSC-specific radiolabeled markers have been reported for a number of solid cancers, although the majority are reported in tumour-bearing mice [28,43–45].

Lewis lung carcinoma tumour cells implanted in mice were evaluated via PET imaging using 64Cu-ATSM and 18F-FDG for the assessment of intratumoral distributions of the radionuclides [28]. Radionuclide uptake was compared with immunohistochemical staining patterns using both proliferation markers (Ki-67 and BrdU) as well as the hypoxic marker, pimonidazole. Furthermore, the clonogenic potential was evaluated via clonogenic assay and compared with 64Cu-ATSM distribution. The study found a direct correlation between tumour regions with high 64Cu-ATSM accumulation and colony forming ability, as cells originating from high 64Cu-ATSM areas had greater colony-forming capacities than those from regions with low and intermediate radionuclide uptake. This shows that 64Cu-ATSM has the potential to serve as a CSC-affinic imaging biomarker, identifying radioresistant tumour areas that could preferentially be targeted with more aggressive agents/techniques.

Another imaging approach tested for CSC identification in NSCLC is MRI, via magnetic nanoparticles. Zhou et al. synthesized a multifunctional peptide–fluorescent–magnetic nanocomposite to be used for in vivo live fluorescence imaging and magnetic resonance imaging in lung tumour xenografts [45]. Owing to their great versatility and applicability, magnetic iron oxide (Fe_3O_4) nanoparticles (NPs) are widely studied and used from MRI to cancer therapy. One of the greatest advantages of these magnetic NPs is their flexibility to be designed and synthesized as multifunctional NPs, by adapting the surface ligands according to the intended application [45]. Specific binding peptides for lung cancer stem cells, named as HCBP-1, have been previously identified and validated by the same group, via flow cytometry and fluorescence microscopy [46], being now modified on the surface of fluorescent magnetic nanoparticles to be used for MR imaging of CSCs. The effectiveness of the NPs was tested on cultured human lung cancer cell line (H460) injected in nude mice. Flow cytometry results indicated the potential of NPs to isolate HCBP-1 positive cells in vitro, while in vivo live fluorescent imaging and MRI showed that the multifunctional nanocomposite could serve as an imaging marker for CSC identification [45].

While the number of imaging studies undertaken in lung tumours using biomarkers for CSCs is limited, they open new avenues towards personalised treatment and identify gaps that could promote further research in this field. Among imaging techniques, perhaps the most relevant for further human trials are functional imaging methods employing PET/CT, SPECT and MRI.

The field of functional imaging is continuously growing with new radionuclides (PET) and magnetic nanoparticles (MRI) that have affinity towards CSCs, which could assist in the quantitative assessment of these cancer stem cells within a tumour.

3.3. Summary of Current Status for CSC Biomarkers

Most of the current evidence on the value of CSC biomarkers is based on proof-of-concept studies. Since clinically applicable techniques for noninvasive CSC imaging in NSCLC are lacking, taking the existing pre-clinical research of CSC biomarkers to the next level is greatly desirable. To be clinically implementable, there is need for CSC markers with high sensitivity and specificity, which also allow for high-resolution monitoring. With well-designed biocompatible markers, identification and targeting of cancer stem cells using functional imaging techniques could be the next step towards personalised therapy in oncology.

4. Circulating Tumour Cells and Imaging Biomarkers

4.1. Circulating Tumour Cells and Distant Metastasis

Circulating tumour cells (CTC) are epithelial malignant cells detached from the primary tumour that underwent the epithelial–mesenchymal transition (EMT) and gained the ability to intravasate into the blood stream, migrate to distant anatomic regions and extravasate to favourable metastatic sites. The CTC population is heterogenous and consists of various cellular sub-populations with different phenotypes and functional features, including the capacity of clustering with other blood cells such as leukocytes and platelets. Owing to their ability to convert from one state to the other via EMT, the CTC population includes a subset of multipotent cells with stem-like properties, that were described above as cancer stem cells, and in this context of circulating tumour cells they are the ones responsible for cancer dissemination and formation of micrometastases [47]. Furthermore, CTC clusters, also known as circulating tumour microemboli, were shown to increase the metastatic potential in lung cancer patients [48].

While distant metastasis is known as a final-stage event during cancer progression, experimental studies have shown that cancer cells can actually spread to distant anatomic sites even at early stages of cancer development [49]. Furthermore, there are ways of detecting CTCs from the peripheral blood of patients (so called liquid biopsy) with early stage neoplasms, which might be indicative of tumour aggressiveness and treatment outcome [50]. Given that a number of studies showed a direct correlation between the quantity and types of CTCs detected in blood and patient survival, CTCs could offer an important insight into disease progression and treatment prediction [51].

More research into the role of CTCs reveals important insights into various correlations between factors influencing tumour development and treatment outcome prediction in NSCLC. As discussed above, the identification of EGFR mutations in advanced NSCLC patients is a critical aspect of patient stratification for optimal targeted therapies. While tumour tissue is the commonly preferred standard sample for the evaluation of EGFR mutations, for many patients such samples are not available, which is the reason why a study has been undertaken to search for a surrogate marker for EGFR status through a more accessible way [52]. Circulating-free tumour DNA from plasma/serum samples of NSCLC patients was found to correlate with EGFR mutation with high concordance rate (94.3%) and specificity (99.8%).

Isolation and detection of CTCs is not without challenges as the capturing technique of these cells from blood must be highly sensitive and specific, which is the reason why different methods of CTC isolation often provided conflicting results. Traditionally, the definition of circulating tumour cells encompasses three components; accordingly, a CTC is a cell that is (1) negative for the hematopoietic cell marker CD45; (2) positive for cytokeratin, a structural protein expressed by epithelial cells; and (3) positive for the epithelial cell adhesion molecule EpCAM, an epithelial cell surface marker [53]. Having these properties as a starting point, a number of techniques have been developed to isolate and quantify the CTC population from blood samples.

CTCs are currently detected in the peripheral blood at a single cell level, with the most commonly employed techniques in lung cancer being the CellSearch® system, the CTC chips or the Isolation by Size of Epithelial Tumour Cells (ISET) filter device. Both the CellSearch® system and the CTC chips employ the EpCAM (epithelial cell specific adhesion molecule) to capture CTCs. The detection rate varies as a function of lung cancer type (NSCLC or SCLC) and stage, with NSCLC patients presenting with lower counts of CTCs than those diagnosed with SCLC, even in late stages of the disease [54]. This observation was explained by the possibly higher fraction of CTCs in NSCLC patients that undergone the EMT, which in turn, led to downregulation of EpCAM expression. In these situations, a CTC detection technique that is independent of EpCAM—such as ISET or the CTChip®, which exploits size-based differences between CTCs and hematopoietic cells—could offer more reliable results [55,56].

Studies to date show the potential of circulating tumour markers (such as CTCs and circulating tumour DNA) to serve as surrogates or markers on their own to provide treatment response monitoring, prognosis prediction, detection of early recurrence, etc., which warrants further research in evaluating their role in NSCLC.

4.2. Circulating Tumour Cells as Biomarkers in NSCLC

Due to their highly heterogeneous nature, imaging of circulating tumour cells at a single time point might not be relevant for outcome prediction or treatment monitoring, which is the reason why established functional imaging techniques are not adequate for this task. Instead, to evaluate all steps involved in tumour metastasis, continuous monitoring of the primary tumour and of CTCs is recommended [57]. In support of this idea, Wyckoff et al. have transfected both metastatic and non-metastatic rat-derived mammary adenocarcinoma cell lines with green fluorescent protein to quantify tumour cell density in the blood, individual cells in the lung as well as lung metastases.

Cells were viewed minute-by-minute using time-laps confocal imaging and revealed the fact that both metastatic and non-metastatic cells display protrusive behaviour; however, metastatic cells showed greater intravasation potential and larger numbers originating from the primary tumour [57]. Over the years, in vivo flow cytometry was developed to increase the time resolution and to create a more dynamic picture of the metastatic process [58].

One of the latest technologies for real-time in vivo imaging of CTCs and CSCs employs multiphoton microscopy and antibody conjugated quantum dots [59]. The study has showed promising results in identifying CTCs with high metastatic potential in mice and concurrently measuring the number, velocity and trajectories of CTCs in the bloodstream. Due to the unique fluorescence signal exhibited by CTCs, this experiment allowed the study of a CTC subpopulation via antibody conjugated quantum dots using various wavelength emissions [59]. To enable direct imaging, tumours (human pancreatic cell line) were grown on the earlobes of mice, thus allowing visualization of blood vessels, of tumour growth over time and CTC detection in the blood vessels near the solid tumour 1 week after inoculation. Metastatic sites were detected in the stomach and intestines. Cancer stem cells in the blood, as a subpopulation of CTCs, were identified through labeling with monoclonal CD24 antibodies conjugated on quantum dots. CSCs were found both in the peripheral tumour tissue as well as on the solid tumour, accumulating specifically on one side of the solid tumour. This observation, whereby CSCs cluster in certain parts of the tumour, suggests the potential of better targeting.

High definition imaging of CTCs in NSCLC was undertaken by means of automated digital microscopy using fluorescent labeling, with the aim of quantifying the CTCs and evaluating their prognostic value in lung cancer patients [60]. For CTC detection, cells were incubated with anti-Cytokeratin antibodies and pre-conjugated anti-CD45 antibody. The detection method offered cytomorphologic evaluation of the cells, looking for Cytokeratin positive and at the same time CD45 negative cells, with a high nuclear cytoplasmic ratio and a large size (compared to other cells in the blood sample). The clinical study encompassed 28 NSCLC patients with evidence of distant metastasis, with all patients receiving chemotherapy or EGFR kinase inhibitor. For CTC evaluation, blood specimens were collected periodically (overall, 66 specimens at various time periods), over 12 months. CTCs were detected in 68% of samples and no differences in prevalence or quantity was found between adenocarcinomas and squamous cell carcinomas. During the time course of the study, an increase in CTC prevalence was observed, from 56% of specimens presenting CTCs in the first month of enrollment, to 63% after 3 months and a further increase to 94% at 6 months and afterwards. A cut-off value of 5 CTCs/mL was chosen to correlate the CTC count with outcome (survival). As such, patients with $\geq$ 5 CTCs/mL had a median survival of 244 days, while in those patients with < 5 CTCs/mL the median survival was not reached at a median follow-up of 304 days. Patients with high CTC counts had a hazard ratio for death of 4.0, relative to those with low counts ($p = 0.0084$) [60]. CTCs could, therefore, serve as potential biomarkers for patient stratification and risk assessment, contingent on the availability of high precision CTC detection and quantification assays.

Based on the premise that both CTC counts and metabolic parameters defined by 18F-FDG can be correlated with patient prognosis, a number of studies combined the two techniques (PET imaging and CTCs quantification) to find possible relationships between them. A multi-center study that included 71 NSCLC patients (all stages, predominantly early-stage) who underwent 18F-FDG PET imaging was designed to evaluate CTCs from samples within 90 days and prior to surgery or radio-chemotherapy [61]. CTCs were quantified by a non-EpCAM based method, using immunofluorescence (cytokeratins, CD45, DAPI-staining for nuclear quantitation). The results revealed that while FDG uptake via SUVmax was strongly dependent on tumour stage and histology, no such association was found for CTCs, suggesting that the two biomarkers may act in a complementary manner. Furthermore, the identification of many individual and clustered CTCs in early-stage disease (characterized by weak FDG uptake) may not be indicative of distant metastasis formation. The association between tumour glucose metabolism and CTCs could be influenced by the heterogeneity of CTCs and might depend on the CTC subpopulation type [61].

A prospective biomarker trial that enrolled 53 patients with advanced NSCLC found no correlation between circulating tumour DNA (cell-free DNA) and metabolic tumour volume or total lesion glycolysis based on FDG PET imaging, hypothesizing that cell-free DNA may be representative of more complex biological mechanisms [62]. In a similar study, Morbelli et al. evaluated the correlation between circulating tumour DNA counts and PET parameters, both locoregionally and at distant sites, showing a positive correlation between cell-free DNA base line levels and tumour metabolic activity [63]. As only SUVmax was associated with circulating DNA, the authors concluded that this biomarker may be more reflective of tumour metabolism and biologic behaviour than tumour burden in advanced NSCLC.

The association of CTCs with early relapse in resected NSCLC was analysed using PET images from 102 patients both before and 1 month after radical resection [64]. CTCs were detected in 39.2% of patients before surgery and in 27.5% after the resection, which was strongly correlated with SUVmax and pathological stage. The presence of CSCs post-surgery was also associated with a shorter recurrence free survival, irrespective of staging.

A recent study reported preliminary data on a cohort of 17 metastatic NSCLC patients that underwent 18F-FDG PET imaging with the aim of finding a correlation between CTC numbers (determined with the ISET method) and clinical/metabolic parameters. The results indicated a strong association of CTCs present in blood with tumour uptake characterized by SUVmean [65]. CTCs were detected in 59% of patients with a mean of 3 CTCs/mL (1–7 range), with a lower number of CTCs found in patients that underwent chemotherapy.

Based on the study findings, which are corroborated by data from previous reports, it was suggested that the combination between CTC quantification and FDG PET parameters could offer an improved prognostic stratification of NSCLC patients [65].

While to date the number of studies is limited, identification and quantification of CTCs in NSCLC could have an important impact on the evaluation of treatment response and overall prognosis. Studies have indicated that treatment of NSCLC can influence the CTC population both negatively and positively [66]. Mobilization of CTCs after radiotherapy, surgery or systemic treatment might either lead to cell eradication and improved tumour control, or may promote metastasis, in which case CTCs should be targeted and eliminated. Martin et al. showed that in patients with advanced NSCLC treated with palliative intent using large doses of radiation, CTC numbers increased after treatment. Many of these cells presented with high levels of DNA damage, as identified by γH2AX assay, suggesting that the damaged CTCs originated from the irradiated tumour [67]. CTCs isolated from post-irradiation blood samples showed viability through in vitro proliferation. This observation justifies the need for further studies into therapy-triggered CTC mobilization and the development of efficient systemic therapies to specifically target CTCs to overcome the formation of micrometastases.

4.3. Summary of Current Status for CTC Biomarkers

The role of CTCs as prognostic biomarkers is already well understood. Future developments in CTC detection in clinical practice will occur together with liquid biopsy studies of circulating tumour DNA (ctDNA). While CTCs correlation with PET parameters often show conflicting results (or weak correlations) among existing studies, further investigations are required in order to understand patient heterogeneity among NSCLC sufferers. Moreover, identification and biological characterization of CTCs could offer real-time monitoring of personalised targeted therapies in combination with functional imaging modalities.

5. Imaging Biomarkers for Apoptosis

Apoptosis, or programmed cell death, is a key physiological feature that ensures tissue homeostasis in normal conditions. Evasion of apoptosis is one of the hallmarks of cancer. It is acknowledged that numerous effects of radio- and chemotherapy are mediated by apoptosis, including resistance to treatment through altered apoptosis, upregulation of anti-apoptotic signals and downregulation of pro-apoptotic ones [68]. For instance, decrease in p53 signalling is an indicator of apoptosis evasion. As a tumour suppressor protein, p53 regulates cell cycle and has the potential to induce apoptosis as a response to various cellular signalling. Mutations in p53 signalling pathways lead to uncontrolled proliferation and inhibition of apoptosis. Similarly, proteins of the Bcl-2 family are important regulators of programmed cell death. Borner et al. examined the expression of the p53 and Bcl-2 family proteins in 49 specimens of patients with NSCLC via immunostaining, showing a negative influence of Bcl-2 expression on relapse-free survival ($p = 0.02$), while the expression of p53 and Bcl-2 was significantly associated with metastasis-free survival ($p < 0.01$) [69]. The authors concluded that Bcl-2 family proteins have no clear or direct impact on clinical outcome owing to their complex interaction with the apoptotic pathway.

The insulin-like growth factor 1 receptor (IGF-1R) is a transmembrane receptor tyrosine kinase overexpressed in neoplasms, having an anti-apoptotic effect through enhancement of survival and proliferation [70]. Furthermore, IGF-1R expression was shown to be activated in cancers that are resistant to EGFR inhibitors, including lung cancer [71]. High expressions of IGF-1R were associated with poor disease-free survival in NSCLC [72]. Being identified as a potential diagnostic and therapeutic biomarker, IGF-1R is currently assessed from a non-invasive imaging perspective. When labelled with 111In for SPECT imaging, IGF-1 showed good selectivity for tumour cells and strong correlation with IGF-1R expression in human breast cancer cells, suggesting potential application in the molecular imaging of other carcinomas [73].

Imaging of apoptotic pathway can serve for treatment response monitoring after radio/chemotherapy through the evaluation of apoptotic death rate. Imaging biomarkers developed for programmed cell death include annexin V labelled with common PET radionuclides such as 11C, 18F, 64Cu and 68Ga [74,75]. Most of these radio-compounds are in pre-clinical evaluation. Owing to activation of caspase-3 during apoptotic death, radiolabelled caspase-3 was tested as a substitute for annexin V. The first human study designed for apoptotic imaging involved eight subjects and employed an 18F-labelled PET tracer (18F-ML-10), demonstrating efficient binding to apoptotic sites, and favourable biodistribution as well as safety profile [76].

Summary of Current Status for Apoptosis Biomarkers

The role of apoptosis in cancer development and response to therapy is well established. Although apoptosis is acknowledged as a promising target for anticancer therapy, imaging biomarkers of apoptosis are still in their early days of development, as most radiolabelled markers have not seen clinical applications. As far as lung cancer is concerned, even pre-clinical studies on apoptotic cell death imaging are scarce, requiring translation from other anatomical sites that showed promising results.

6. Conclusions

There is no doubt that, nowadays, the field of oncology is strongly oriented towards personalised treatment, irrespective of the type of cancer. The latest insights into the biological and radiobiological properties of tumours and their cellular sub-populations have offered the possibility to develop and clinically implement specific tracers and markers, allowing for more accurate diagnosis, treatment planning and delivery [77]. NSCLC patients are also gaining from these advances, starting from the discovery of EGFR mutations which confer sensitivity to tyrosine kinase inhibitors. The refinement of lung cancer subtypes and their corresponding therapies have further improved patient outcome.

The world of new radiobiological tracers is greatly stimulating, owing to the possibility of studying the heterogeneity of lung cancers, of stratifying tumours by their prognostic characteristics and of overcoming the limit of biopsy that often does not allow a complete and exhaustive description of the biology of such tumours. The clinical management of tumour heterogeneity is a significant challenge as tumour response is dictated by the particular behaviour of each sub-group of cancer cells. Cellular heterogeneity given by proliferation kinetics, stemness, hypoxia or other factors calls for specific markers and targeting; therefore, the near future of biomarkers will rely on complementarity rather than a common solution valid for all (radio)biological particularities of a tumour [78].

This paper focused on three main factors influencing tumour kinetics (development and proliferation of primary tumour) and tumour dynamics (infiltration and distant metastases) in the context of NSCLC: tumour proliferation, cancer stem cells and circulating tumour cells. While advances in knowledge cover all these aspects, there is potential for improvement on the clinical side to better understand tumour resistance to chemotherapy, to augment the efficiency of immunotherapy for primary as well as metastatic cancers, and to design clinical trials that employ specific biomarkers to identify and tackle resistant tumour sub-populations. The near future will likely bring further developments in the emerging areas, such as cancer stem cell biomarkers, where research is still in pre-clinical stages, whereas in the more established fields—of proliferation and tumour progression—research has advanced into clinical phases, with the expectation of more refined utilization and wider implementation.

Funding: This research received no external funding.

Conflicts of Interest: The authors declare no conflict of interest.

References

1. Bray, F.; Ferlay, J.; Soerjomataram, I.; Siegel, R.L.; Torre, L.A.; Jemal, A. Global cancer statistics 2018: GLOBOCAN estimates of incidence and mortality worldwide for 36 cancers in 185 countries. *CA Cancer J. Clin.* **2018**, *68*, 394–424. [CrossRef] [PubMed]
2. European Society of Radiology (ESR). Medical imaging in personalised medicine: A white paper of the research committee of the European Society of Radiology (ESR). *Insights Imag.* **2015**, *6*, 141–155. [CrossRef]
3. Gerdes, J.; Schwab, U.; Lemke, H.; Stein, H. Production of a mouse monoclonal antibody reactive with a human nuclear antigen associated with cell proliferation. *Int. J. Cancer* **1983**, *31*, 13–20. [CrossRef] [PubMed]
4. Warth, A.; Cortis, J.; Soltermann, A.; Meister, M.; Budczies, J.; Stenzinger, A.; Goeppert, B.; Thomas, M.; Herth, F.J.; Schirmacher, P.; et al. Tumour cell proliferation (Ki-67) in non-small cell lung cancer: A critical reappraisal of its prognostic role. *Br. J. Cancer* **2014**, *111*, 1222–1229. [CrossRef] [PubMed]
5. Wee, P.; Wang, Z. Epidermal Growth Factor Receptor Cell Proliferation Signaling Pathways. *Cancers* **2017**, *9*, 52. [CrossRef]
6. Hirsch, F.R.; Varella-Garcia, M.; Bunn, P.A., Jr.; Di Maria, M.V.; Veve, R.; Bremmes, R.M.; Barón, A.E.; Zeng, C.; Franklin, W.A. Epidermal growth factor receptor in non-small-cell lung carcinomas: Correlation between gene copy number and protein expression and impact on prognosis. *J. Clin. Oncol.* **2003**, *21*, 3798–3807. [CrossRef]
7. Grandis, J.R.; Sok, J.C. Signaling through the epidermal growth factor receptor during the development of malignancy. *Pharmacol. Ther.* **2004**, *102*, 37–46. [CrossRef]
8. Vokes, E.E.; Chu, E. Anti-EGFR therapies: Clinical experience in colorectal, lung, and head and neck cancers. *Oncology* **2006**, *20* (Suppl. 2), 15–25.
9. Kris, M.G.; Johnson, B.E.; Berry, L.D.; Kwiatkowski, D.J.; Iafrate, A.J.; Wistuba, I.I.; Varella-Garcia, M.; Franklin, W.A.; Aronson, S.L.; Su, P.F.; et al. Using multiplexed assays of oncogenic drivers in lung cancers to select targeted drugs. *JAMA* **2014**, *311*, 1998–2006. [CrossRef]
10. Hoang, T.; Myung, S.K.; Pham, T.T.; Kim, J.; Ju, W. Comparative Efficacy of Targeted Therapies in Patients with Non-Small Cell Lung Cancer: A Network Meta-Analysis of Clinical Trials. *J. Clin. Med.* **2020**, *9*, 1063. [CrossRef]
11. Zugazagoitia, J.; Ramos, I.; Trigo, J.M.; Palka, M.; Gómez-Rueda, A.; Jantus-Lewintre, E.; Camps, C.; Isla, D.; Iranzo, P.; Ponce-Aix, S.; et al. Clinical utility of plasma-based digital next-generation sequencing in patients with advance-stage lung adenocarcinomas with insufficient tumor samples for tissue genotyping. *Ann. Oncol.* **2019**, *30*, 290–296. [CrossRef]
12. Nana-Sinkam, S.P.; Geraci, M.W. MicroRNA in lung cancer. *J. Thorac. Oncol.* **2006**, *1*, 929–931. [CrossRef]
13. Webster, R.J.; Giles, K.M.; Price, K.J.; Zhang, P.M.; Mattick, J.S.; Leedman, P.J. Regulation of epidermal growth factor receptor signaling in human cancer cells by microRNA-7. *J. Biol. Chem.* **2009**, *284*, 5731–5741. [CrossRef] [PubMed]

14. Lin, P.Y.; Yu, S.L.; Yang, P.C. MicroRNA in lung cancer. *Br. J. Cancer* **2010**, *103*, 1144–1148. [CrossRef]
15. Szyszko, T.A.; Yip, C.; Szlosarek, P.; Goh, V.; Cook, G.J. The role of new PET tracers for lung cancer. *Lung Cancer* **2016**, *94*, 7–14. [CrossRef] [PubMed]
16. Chen, L.; Zhou, Y.; Tang, X.; Yang, C.; Tian, Y.; Xie, R.; Chen, T.; Yang, J.; Jing, M.; Chen, F.; et al. EGFR mutation decreases FDG uptake in non-small cell lung cancer via the NOX4/ROS/GLUT1 axis. *Int. J. Oncol.* **2019**, *54*, 370–380. [CrossRef]
17. Caicedo, C.; Garcia-Velloso, M.J.; Lozano, M.D.; Labiano, T.; Vigil Diaz, C.; Lopez-Picazo, J.M.; Gurpide, A.; Zulueta, J.J.; Richter Echevarria, J.A.; Perez Gracia, J.L. Role of [^{18}F]FDG PET in prediction of KRAS and EGFR mutation status in patients with advanced non-small-cell lung cancer. *Eur. J. Nucl. Med. Mol. Imaging* **2014**, *41*, 2058–2065. [CrossRef] [PubMed]
18. Lv, Z.; Fan, J.; Xu, J.; Wu, F.; Huang, Q.; Guo, M.; Liao, T.; Liu, S.; Lan, X.; Liao, S.; et al. Value of ^{18}F-FDG PET/CT for predicting EGFR mutations and positive ALK expression in patients with non-small cell lung cancer: A retrospective analysis of 849 Chinese patients. *Eur. J. Nucl. Med. Mol. Imaging* **2018**, *45*, 735–750. [CrossRef]
19. Guan, J.; Xiao, N.J.; Chen, M.; Zhou, W.L.; Zhang, Y.W.; Wang, S.; Dai, Y.M.; Li, L.; Zhang, Y.; Li, Q.Y.; et al. 18F-FDG uptake for prediction EGFR mutation status in non-small cell lung cancer. *Medicine* **2016**, *95*, e4421. [CrossRef]
20. Sun, X.; Xiao, Z.; Chen, G.; Han, Z.; Liu, Y.; Zhang, C.; Sun, Y.; Song, Y.; Wang, K.; Fang, F.; et al. A PET imaging approach for determining EGFR mutation status for improved lung cancer patient management. *Sci. Transl. Med.* **2018**, *10*, eaan8840. [CrossRef]
21. Shields, A.F.; Grierson, J.R.; Dohmen, B.M.; Machulla, H.J.; Stayanoff, J.C.; Lawhorn-Crews, J.M.; Obradovich, J.E.; Muzik, O.; Mangner, T.J. Imaging proliferation in vivo with [F-18]FLT and positron emission tomography. *Nat. Med.* **1998**, *4*, 1334–1336. [CrossRef] [PubMed]
22. Buck, A.K.; Halter, G.; Schirrmeister, H.; Kotzerke, J.; Wurziger, I.; Glatting, G.; Mattfeldt, T.; Neumaier, B.; Reske, S.N.; Hetzel, M. Imaging proliferation in lung tumours with PET: 18F-FLT versus 18F-FDG. *J. Nucl. Med.* **2003**, *44*, 1426–1431. [PubMed]
23. Shen, G.; Ma, H.; Pang, F.; Ren, P.; Kuang, A. Correlations of 18F-FDG and 18F-FLT uptake on PET with Ki-67 expression in patients with lung cancer: A meta-analysis. *Acta Radiol.* **2018**, *59*, 188–195. [CrossRef] [PubMed]
24. Kairemo, K.; Santos, E.B.; Macapinlac, H.A.; Subbiah, V. Early Response Assessment to Targeted Therapy Using 3′-deoxy-3′[(18)F]-Fluorothymidine (^{18}F-FLT) PET/CT in Lung Cancer. *Diagnostics* **2020**, *10*, 26. [CrossRef]
25. Zannetti, A.; Iommelli, F.; Speranza, A.; Salvatore, M.; Del Vecchio, S. 3′-deoxy-3′-18F-fluorothymidine PET/CT to guide therapy with epidermal growth factor receptor antagonists and Bcl-xL inhibitors in non-small cell lung cancer. *J. Nucl. Med.* **2012**, *53*, 443–450. [CrossRef]
26. Iommelli, F.; De Rosa, V.; Gargiulo, S.; Panico, M.; Monti, M.; Greco, A.; Gramanzini, M.; Ortosecco, G.; Fonti, R.; Brunetti, A.; et al. Monitoring reversal of MET-mediated resistance to EGFR tyrosine kinase inhibitors in non-small cell lung cancer using 3′-deoxy-3′-[18F]-fluorothymidine positron emission tomography. *Clin. Cancer Res.* **2014**, *20*, 4806–4815. [CrossRef]
27. Iommelli, F.; De Rosa, V.; Terlizzi, C.; Monti, M.; Panico, M.; Fonti, R.; Del Vecchio, S. Inositol Trisphosphate Receptor Type 3-mediated Enhancement of EGFR and MET Cotargeting Efficacy in Non-Small Cell Lung Cancer Detected by ^{18}F-fluorothymidine. *Clin. Cancer Res.* **2018**, *24*, 3126–3136. [CrossRef]
28. Oh, M.; Tanaka, T.; Kobayashi, M.; Furukawa, T.; Mori, T.; Kudo, T.; Fujieda, S.; Fujibayashi, Y. Radio-copper-labeled Cu-ATSM: An indicator of quiescent but clonogenic cells under mild hypoxia in a Lewis lung carcinoma model. *Nucl. Med. Biol.* **2009**, *36*, 419–426. [CrossRef]
29. Xiao, Z.; Song, Y.; Kai, W.; Sun, X.; Shen, B. Evaluation of 99mTc-HYNIC-MPG as a novel SPECT radiotracer to detect EGFR-activating mutations in NSCLC. *Oncotarget* **2017**, *8*, 40732–40740. [CrossRef]
30. Wang, Z.; Qiao, R.; Tang, N.; Lu, Z.; Wang, H.; Zhang, Z.; Xue, X.; Huang, Z.; Zhang, S.; Zhang, G.; et al. Active targeting theranostic iron oxide nanoparticles for MRI and magnetic resonance-guided focused ultrasound ablation of lung cancer. *Biomaterials* **2017**, *127*, 25–35. [CrossRef]
31. Kelsey, C.R.; Marks, L.B.; Hollis, D.; Hubbs, J.L.; Ready, N.E.; D'Amico, T.A.; Boyd, J.A. Local recurrence after surgery for early stage lung cancer: An 11-year experience with 975 patients. *Cancer* **2009**, *115*, 5218–5227. [CrossRef] [PubMed]

32. Carney, D.N.; Gazdar, A.F.; Bunn, P.A., Jr.; Guccion, J.G. Demonstration of the stem cell nature of clonogenic tumor cells from lung cancer patients. *Stem Cells* **1982**, *1*, 149–164. [PubMed]
33. Moore, N.; Lyle, S. Quiescent, slow-cycling stem cell populations in cancer: A review of the evidence and discussion of significance. *J. Oncol.* **2011**. [CrossRef] [PubMed]
34. Peitzsch, C.; Perrin, R.; Hill, R.P.; Dubrovska, A.; Kurth, I. Hypoxia as a biomarker for radioresistant cancer stem cells. *Int. J. Radiat. Biol.* **2014**, *90*, 636–652. [CrossRef] [PubMed]
35. Cabrera, M.C. Hollingsworth RE, Hurt EM. Cancer stem cell plasticity and tumor hierarchy. *World J. Stem Cells* **2015**, *7*, 27–36. [CrossRef] [PubMed]
36. Jiang, F.; Qiu, Q.; Khanna, A.; Todd, N.W.; Deepak, J.; Xing, L.; Wang, H.; Liu, Z.; Su, Y.; Stass, S.A.; et al. Aldehyde dehydrogenase 1 is a tumor stem cell-associated marker in lung cancer. *Mol. Cancer Res.* **2009**, *7*, 330–338. [CrossRef] [PubMed]
37. Leung, E.L.; Fiscus, R.R.; Tung, J.W.; Tin, V.P.; Cheng, L.C.; Sihoe, A.D.; Fink, L.M.; Ma, Y.; Wong, M.P. Non-small cell lung cancer cells expressing CD44 are enriched for stem cell-like properties. *PLoS ONE* **2010**, *5*, e14062. [CrossRef]
38. Zöller, M. CD44: Can a cancer-initiating cell profit from an abundantly expressed molecule? *Nat. Rev. Cancer* **2011**, *11*, 254–267. [CrossRef]
39. Zakaria, N.; Yusoff, N.M.; Zakaria, Z.; Lim, M.N.; Baharuddin, P.J.; Fakiruddin, K.S.; Yahaya, B. Human non-small cell lung cancer expresses putative cancer stem cell markers and exhibits the transcriptomic profile of multipotent cells. *BMC Cancer* **2015**, *15*, 84. [CrossRef]
40. Eramo, A.; Lotti, F.; Sette, G.; Pilozzi, E.; Biffoni, M.; Di Virgilio, A.; Conticello, C.; Ruco, L.; Peschle, C.; De Maria, R. Identification and expansion of the tumorigenic lung cancer stem cell population. *Cell Death Differ.* **2008**, *15*, 504–514. [CrossRef]
41. Qu, H.; Li, R.; Liu, Z.; Zhang, J.; Luo, R. Prognostic value of cancer stem cell marker CD133 expression in non-small cell lung cancer: A systematic review. *Int. J. Clin. Exp. Pathol.* **2013**, *6*, 2644–2650. [PubMed]
42. Salnikov, A.V.; Gladkich, J.; Moldenhauer, G.; Volm, M.; Mattern, J.; Herr, I. CD133 is indicative for a resistance phenotype but does not represent a prognostic marker for survival of non-small cell lung cancer patients. *Int. J. Cancer* **2010**, *126*, 950–958. [CrossRef] [PubMed]
43. Yoshii, Y.; Furukawa, T.; Kiyono, Y.; Watanabe, R.; Waki, A.; Mori, T.; Yoshii, H.; Oh, M.; Asai, T.; Okazawa, H.; et al. Copper-64-diacetyl-bis (N4-methylthiosemicarbazone) accumulates in rich regions of CD133+ highly tumorigenic cells in mouse colon carcinoma. *Nucl. Med. Biol.* **2010**, *37*, 395–404. [CrossRef]
44. Yang, Y.; Hernandez, R.; Rao, J.; Yin, L.; Qu, Y.; Wu, J.; England, C.G.; Graves, S.A.; Lewis, C.M.; Wang, P.; et al. Targeting CD146 with a 64Cu-labeled antibody enables in vivo immunoPET imaging of high-grade gliomas. *Proc. Natl. Acad. Sci. USA* **2015**, *112*, E6525–E6534. [CrossRef] [PubMed]
45. Zhou, X.; Chen, L.; Wang, A.; Ma, Y.; Zhang, H.; Zhu, Y. Multifunctional fluorescent magnetic nanoparticles for lung cancer stem cells research. *Colloids Surf. B Biointerfaces* **2015**, *134*, 431–439. [CrossRef]
46. Wang, A.; Chen, L.; Pu, K.; Zhu, Y. Identification of stem-like cells in non-small cell lung cancer cells with specific peptides. *Cancer Lett.* **2014**, *351*, 100–107. [CrossRef]
47. Gomez-Casal, R.; Bhattacharya, C.; Ganesh, N.; Bailey, L.; Basse, P.; Gibson, M.; Epperly, M.; Levina, V. Non-small-cell lung cancer cells survived ionizing radiation treatment display cancer stem cell and epithelial–mesenchymal transition phenotypes. *Mol. Cancer* **2013**, *12*, 94. [CrossRef]
48. Hou, J.M.; Krebs, M.G.; Lancashire, L.; Sloane, R.; Backen, A.; Swain, R.K.; Priest, L.J.; Greystoke, A.; Zhou, C.; Morris, K.; et al. Clinical significance and molecular characteristics of circulating tumor cells and circulating tumor microemboli in patients with small-cell lung cancer. *J. Clin. Oncol.* **2012**, *30*, 525–532. [CrossRef]
49. Klein, C.A. Cancer. The metastasis cascade. *Science.* **2008**, *321*, 1785–1787. [CrossRef]
50. Alix-Panabières, C.; Riethdorf, S.; Pantel, K. Circulating tumor cells and bone marrow micrometastasis. *Clin. Cancer Res.* **2008**, *14*, 5013–5021. [CrossRef]
51. Krebs, M.G.; Hou, J.M.; Ward, T.H.; Blackhall, F.H.; Dive, C. Circulating tumour cells: Their utility in cancer management and predicting outcomes. *Ther. Adv. Med. Oncol.* **2010**, *2*, 351–365. [CrossRef] [PubMed]
52. Douillard, J.Y.; Ostoros, G.; Cobo, M.; Ciuleanu, T.; Cole, R.; McWalter, G.; Walker, J.; Dearden, S.; Webster, A.; Milenkova, T.; et al. Gefitinib treatment in EGFR mutated caucasian NSCLC: Circulating-free tumor DNA as a surrogate for determination of EGFR status. *J. Thorac. Oncol.* **2014**, *9*, 1345–1353. [CrossRef] [PubMed]
53. Van de Stolpe, A.; Pantel, K.; Sleijfer, S.; Terstappen, L.W.; den Toonder, J.M. Circulating tumor cell isolation and diagnostics: Toward routine clinical use. *Cancer Res.* **2011**, *71*, 5955–5960. [CrossRef] [PubMed]

54. Taenzer, A.; Alix-Panabières, C.; Wikman, H.; Pantel, K. Circulating tumor-derived biomarkers in lung cancer. *J. Thorac. Dis.* **2012**, *4*, 448–449. [CrossRef] [PubMed]
55. Krebs, M.G.; Hou, J.M.; Sloane, R.; Lancashire, L.; Priest, L.; Nonaka, D.; Ward, T.H.; Backen, A.; Clack, G.; Hughes, A.; et al. Analysis of circulating tumor cells in patients with non-small cell lung cancer using epithelial marker-dependent and -independent approaches. *J. Thorac. Oncol.* **2012**, *7*, 306–315. [CrossRef] [PubMed]
56. Kulasinghe, A.; Kapeleris, J.; Kimberley, R.; Mattarollo, S.R.; Thompson, E.W.; Thiery, J.P.; Kenny, L.; O'Byrne, K.; Punyadeera, C. The prognostic significance of circulating tumor cells in head and neck and non-small-cell lung cancer. *Cancer Med.* **2018**, *7*, 5910–5919. [CrossRef]
57. Wyckoff, J.B.; Jones, J.G.; Condeelis, J.S.; Segall, J.E. A critical step in metastasis: In vivo analysis of intravasation at the primary tumor. *Cancer Res.* **2000**, *60*, 2504–2511.
58. He, W.; Wang, H.; Hartmann, L.C.; Cheng, J.X.; Low, P.S. In vivo quantitation of rare circulating tumor cells by multiphoton intravital flow cytometry. *Proc. Natl. Acad. Sci. USA* **2007**, *104*, 11760–11765. [CrossRef]
59. Kuo, C.W.; Chueh, D.Y.; Chen, P. Real-time in vivo imaging of subpopulations of circulating tumor cells using antibody conjugated quantum dots. *J. Nanobiotechnol.* **2019**, *17*, 26. [CrossRef]
60. Nieva, J.; Wendel, M.; Luttgen, M.S.; Marrinucci, D.; Bazhenova, L.; Kolatkar, A.; Santala, R.; Whittenberger, B.; Burke, J.; Torrey, M.; et al. High-definition imaging of circulating tumor cells and associated cellular events in non-small cell lung cancer patients: A longitudinal analysis. *Phys. Biol.* **2012**, *9*, 016004. [CrossRef]
61. Nair, V.S.; Keu, K.V.; Luttgen, M.S.; Kolatkar, A.; Vasanawala, M.; Kuschner, W.; Bethel, K.; Iagaru, A.H.; Hoh, C.; Shrager, J.B.; et al. An observational study of circulating tumor cells and (18)F-FDG PET uptake in patients with treatment-naive non-small cell lung cancer. *PLoS ONE* **2013**, *8*, e67733. [CrossRef] [PubMed]
62. Nygaard, A.D.; Holdgaard, P.C.; Spindler, K.L.; Pallisgaard, N.; Jakobsen, A. The correlation between cell-free DNA and tumour burden was estimated by PET/CT in patients with advanced NSCLC. *Br. J. Cancer* **2014**, *110*, 363–368. [CrossRef] [PubMed]
63. Morbelli, S.; Alama, A.; Ferrarazzo, G.; Coco, S.; Genova, C.; Rijavec, E.; Bongioanni, F.; Biello, F.; Dal Bello, M.G.; Barletta, G.; et al. Circulating Tumor DNA Reflects Tumor Metabolism Rather Than Tumor Burden in Chemotherapy-Naive Patients with Advanced Non-Small Cell Lung Cancer: ^{18}F-FDG PET/CT Study. *J. Nucl. Med.* **2017**, *58*, 1764–1769. [CrossRef] [PubMed]
64. Bayarri-Lara, C.I.; de Miguel Pérez, D.; Cueto Ladrón de Guevara, A.; Rodriguez Fernández, A.; Puche, J.L.; Sánchez-Palencia Ramos, A.; Ruiz Zafra, J.; Giraldo Ospina, C.F.; Delgado-Rodríguez, M.; Expósito Ruiz, M.; et al. Association of circulating tumour cells with early relapse and 18F-fluorodeoxyglucose positron emission tomography uptake in resected non-small-cell lung cancers. *Eur. J. Cardio-Thorac. Surg.* **2017**, *52*, 55–62. [CrossRef] [PubMed]
65. Monterisi, S.; Castello, A.; Toschi, L.; Federico, D.; Rossi, S.; Veronesi, G.; Lopci, E. Preliminary data on circulating tumor cells in metastatic NSCLC patients candidate to immunotherapy. *Am. J. Nucl. Med. Mol. Imaging* **2019**, *9*, 282–295.
66. Mason, J.; Blyth, B.; MacManus, M.P.; Martin, O.A. Treatment for non-small-cell lung cancer and circulating tumor cells. *Lung Cancer Manag.* **2017**, *6*, 129–139. [CrossRef]
67. Martin, O.A.; Anderson, R.L.; Russell, P.A.; Cox, R.A.; Ivashkevich, A.; Swierczak, A.; Doherty, J.P.; Jacobs, D.H.; Smith, J.; Siva, S.; et al. Mobilization of viable tumor cells into the circulation during radiation therapy. *Int. J. Radiat. Oncol. Biol. Phys.* **2014**, *88*, 395–403. [CrossRef]
68. Brown, J.M.; Attardi, L.D. The role of apoptosis in cancer development and treatment response. *Nat. Rev. Cancer* **2005**, *5*, 231–237. [CrossRef]
69. Borner, M.M.; Brousset, P.; Pfanner-Meyer, B.; Bacchi, M.; Vonlanthen, S.; Hotz, M.A.; Altermatt, H.J.; Schlaifer, D.; Reed, J.C.; Betticher, D.C. Expression of apoptosis regulatory proteins of the Bcl-2 family and p53 in primary resected non-small-cell lung cancer. *Br. J. Cancer* **1999**, *79*, 952–958. [CrossRef]
70. Maki, R.G. Small is beautiful: Insulin-like growth factors and their role in growth, development, and cancer. *J. Clin. Oncol.* **2010**, *28*, 4985–4995. [CrossRef]
71. Yeo, C.D.; Park, K.H.; Park, C.K.; Lee, S.H.; Kim, S.J.; Yoon, H.K.; Lee, Y.S.; Lee, E.J.; Lee, K.Y.; Kim, T.J. Expression of insulin-like growth factor 1 receptor (IGF-1R) predicts poor responses to epidermal growth factor receptor (EGFR) tyrosine kinase inhibitors in non-small cell lung cancer patients harboring activating EGFR mutations. *Lung Cancer* **2015**, *87*, 311–317. [CrossRef] [PubMed]

72. Xu, J.; Bie, F.; Wang, Y.; Chen, X.; Yan, T.; Du, J. Prognostic value of IGF-1R in lung cancer: A PRISMA-compliant meta-analysis. *Medicine* **2019**, *98*, e15467. [CrossRef] [PubMed]
73. Cornelissen, B.; McLarty, K.; Kersemans, V.; Reilly, R.M. The level of insulin growth factor-1 receptor expression is directly correlated with the tumor uptake of (111)In-IGF-1(E3 R) in vivo and the clonogenic survival of breast cancer cells exposed in vitro to trastuzumab (Herceptin). *Nucl. Med. Biol.* **2008**, *35*, 645–653. [CrossRef] [PubMed]
74. Li, X.; Link, J.M.; Stekhova, S.; Yagle, K.J.; Smith, C.; Krohn, K.A.; Tait, J.F. Site-specific labeling of annexin V with F-18 for apoptosis imaging. *Bioconjug. Chem.* **2008**, *19*, 1684–1688. [CrossRef] [PubMed]
75. Lahorte, C.M.; Vanderheyden, J.L.; Steinmetz, N.; Van de Wiele, C.; Dierckx, R.A.; Slegers, G. Apoptosis-detecting radioligands: Current state of the art and future perspectives. *Eur. J. Nucl. Med. Mol. Imaging* **2004**, *31*, 887–919. [CrossRef] [PubMed]
76. Höglund, J.; Shirvan, A.; Antoni, G.; Gustavsson, S.Å.; Långström, B.; Ringheim, A.; Sörensen, J.; Ben-Ami, M.; Ziv, I. 18F-ML-10, a PET tracer for apoptosis: First human study. *J. Nucl. Med.* **2011**, *52*, 720–725. [CrossRef]
77. Marcu, L.G.; Moghaddasi, L.; Bezak, E. Imaging of Tumor Characteristics and Molecular Pathways with PET: Developments Over the Last Decade Toward Personalized Cancer Therapy. *Int. J. Radiat. Oncol. Biol. Phys.* **2018**, *102*, 1165–1182. [CrossRef]
78. Marcu, L.G.; Reid, P.; Bezak, E. The Promise of Novel Biomarkers for Head and Neck Cancer from an Imaging Perspective. *Int. J. Mol. Sci.* **2018**, *19*, 2511. [CrossRef]

Publisher's Note: MDPI stays neutral with regard to jurisdictional claims in published maps and institutional affiliations.

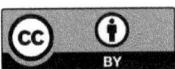

© 2020 by the author. Licensee MDPI, Basel, Switzerland. This article is an open access article distributed under the terms and conditions of the Creative Commons Attribution (CC BY) license (http://creativecommons.org/licenses/by/4.0/).

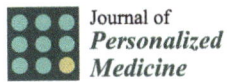

Article

Targeted Therapy Recommendations for Therapy Refractory Solid Tumors—Data from the Real-World Precision Medicine Platform MONDTI

Hossein Taghizadeh [1,2], Matthias Unseld [1,2], Martina Spalt [1,2], Robert M. Mader [1,2], Leonhard Müllauer [2,3], Thorsten Fuereder [1,2], Markus Raderer [1,2], Maria Sibilia [2,4], Mir Alireza Hoda [2,5], Stefanie Aust [2,6], Stephan Polterauer [2,6], Wolfgang Lamm [1,2], Rupert Bartsch [1,2], Matthias Preusser [1,2], Kautzky-Willer A. [7,8] and Gerald W. Prager [1,2,*]

1. Department of Medicine I, Division of Clinical Oncology, Medical University of Vienna, 1090 Vienna, Austria; seyed.taghizadehwaghefi@meduniwien.ac.at (H.T.); matthias.unseld@meduniwien.ac.at (M.U.); martina.spalt@akhwien.at (M.S.); robert.mader@meduniwien.ac.at (R.M.M.); thorsten.fuereder@meduniwien.ac.at (T.F.); markus.raderer@meduniwien.ac.at (M.R.); wolfgang.lamm@meduniwien.ac.at (W.L.); rupert.bartsch@meduniwien.ac.at (R.B.); matthias.preusser@meduniwien.ac.at (M.P.)
2. Comprehensive Cancer Center Vienna, 1090 Vienna, Austria; leonhard.muellauer@meduniwien.ac.at (L.M.); maria.sibilia@meduniwien.ac.at (M.S.); mir.hoda@meduniwien.ac.at (M.A.H.); stefanie.aust@meduniwien.ac.at (S.A.); stephan.polterauer@meduniwien.ac.at (S.P.)
3. Clinical Institute of Pathology, Medical University Vienna, 1090 Vienna, Austria
4. Department of Medicine I, Institute of Cancer Research, Medical University of Vienna, 1090 Vienna, Austria
5. Department of Surgery, Institute of Cancer Research, Medical University of Vienna, 1090 Vienna, Austria
6. Department of Obstetrics and Gynecology, Medical University of Vienna, 1090 Vienna, Austria
7. Department of Medicine III, Division of Endocrinology and Metabolism, Medical University of Vienna, 1090 Vienna, Austria; alexandra.kautzky-willer@meduniwien.ac.at
8. Department of Medicine III, Gender Medicine Unit, Medical University of Vienna, 1090 Vienna, Austria
* Correspondence: gerald.prager@meduniwien.ac.at; Tel.: +43-1-40400-44500

Received: 1 September 2020; Accepted: 21 October 2020; Published: 23 October 2020

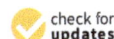

Abstract: Advanced therapy-refractory solid tumors bear a dismal prognosis and constitute a major challenge in offering effective treatment strategies. In this real-world retrospective analysis of our precision medicine platform MONDTI, we describe the molecular profile of 554 patients diagnosed with 17 different types of advanced solid tumors after failure of all standard treatment options. In 304 cases (54.9% of all patients), a molecular-driven targeted therapy approach could be recommended, with a recommendation rate above 50% in 12 tumor entities. The three highest rates for therapy recommendation per tumor classification were observed in urologic malignancies (90.0%), mesothelioma (78.6%), and male reproductive cancers (71.4%). Tumor type ($p = 0.46$), expression of p-mTOR ($p = 0.011$), expression of EGFR ($p = 0.046$), and expression of PD-L1 ($p = 0.023$) had a significant impact on the targeted therapy recommendation rate. Therapy recommendations were significantly more often issued for men ($p = 0.015$) due to gender-specific differences in the molecular profiles of patients with head and neck cancer and malignant mesothelioma. This analysis demonstrates that precision medicine was feasible and provided the basis for molecular-driven therapy recommendations in patients with advanced therapy refractory solid tumors.

Keywords: molecular profiling; immunohistochemistry; next-generation sequencing; precision medicine; targeted therapy; molecular oncology

1. Introduction

Many efforts were undertaken for a thorough and more profound understanding of cancer diseases to develop potent strategies in prevention, diagnosis, and therapy. Despite great scientific advances and major breakthroughs in cancer research, it still poses an enormous challenge to medicine.

Cancer-related mortality is the second leading cause of death worldwide after cardiovascular diseases, being responsible for around 1 in 6 deaths. In 2018, over 18 million people were diagnosed with cancer and over 9 million patients died of it. Thus, cancer globally constitutes a major health and socioeconomic challenge, accounting for roughly over 213 million disability-adjusted life years and with resulting annual costs of over USD 1 trillion to the global economy [1,2].

Currently, chemotherapeutic agents are still the mainstay in the therapy management of cancer.

In contrast to conventional systemic cytotoxic chemotherapy that inhibits DNA synthesis and mitosis and causes a broad range of significant treatment-adverse related events, targeted antitumoral agents—consisting mainly of antibodies and small molecular agents—interfere with and alter the signaling pathways of malignant cells to induce damage to the cancer cells.

In recent years, there has been an effort to develop targeted agents and thus to individualize and personalize therapy concepts in many cancer entities. This approach is known as precision medicine. The main rationale of precision medicine is to match a therapeutic agent to its corresponding molecular target, to allow a precise treatment tailored to a specific patient. It aims to achieve a better and more sustained response than more generic treatments, without damaging healthy cells and tissues.

Currently, in several cancer entities, tailored therapy attempts with immunotherapeutics or tyrosine kinase inhibitors are used, e.g., trastuzumab in HER2 positive breast cancer or gastric cancer [3,4]. Another important example is the combination of BRAF and MEK inhibition with dabrafenib and trametinib or vemurafenib and cobimetinib for the treatment of melanoma harboring a BRAF V600E mutation [5–7]. For the treatment of non-small cell lung cancer (NSCLC), molecularly targeted agents are already an integral part of therapeutic algorithms, including the inhibitors of the epidermal growth factor receptor (EGFR), including erlotinib, gefitinib, and osimertinib [8–10].

Recently, the FDA has also approved tissue-agnostic targeted drugs, including pembrolizumab for the treatment of microsatellite instability-high (MSI-H) tumors and larotrectinib and entrectinib for the therapeutic management of NTRK gene fusion-positive tumors.

Precision medicine is a rapidly evolving and highly dynamic field. Since 2010, several important large-scale prospective clinical trials have been conducted that herald the era of personalized medicine in the 21st century. These trials attempted to realize precision medicine in routine clinical practice and to eventually overcome the old habit to treat cancer entities with a "one size fits all" approach.

Several trials already demonstrated the clinical benefit of precision medicine by translating the concept of targeted therapies based on the molecular information of the cancer patients into longer overall survival (OS), higher overall response rate (ORR), and lower treatment-related adverse effects (TRAE) [11–13].

We conducted a single center retrospective cohort analysis of patients with 17 different types of advanced therapy refractory solid tumor that had been enrolled and profiled in our precision medicine platform MONDTI (molecular oncologic diagnostics and therapy) of the Medical University of Vienna. We sought to describe the potential, the likelihood, and the gender aspects of targeted therapy recommendations in patients with different types of advanced solid tumors without further standard treatment option.

2. Materials and Methods

2.1. Patients and Design of the Precision Medicine Platform

Patients with pretreated, advanced solid tumors who had progressed to all standard treatment options confirmed by response evaluation criteria in solid tumors 1.1 (RECIST 1.1) criteria were eligible for inclusion in our precision medicine platform, provided that tissue samples for molecular profiling were available. The specimens were either obtained by fresh tumor biopsy performed by physicians at the Department of Interventional Radiology or were provided by the archives of the Department of Pathology when tumor biopsy was not feasible. Patients had to have an Eastern Cooperative Oncology Group (ECOG) performance status of 0 or 1. Our precision medicine platform is not a clinical trial but intends to provide targeted therapy recommendations to patients where no standard anti-tumoral treatment is available. All patients in this analysis had to be at least 18 years old at the time of molecular analysis and had to provide informed consent before inclusion in our platform. This analysis was approved by the Institutional Ethics Committee of the Medical University of Vienna (Nr. 1039/2017).

In this single center, real-world, retrospective analysis of our precision cancer medicine platform MONDTI, we describe the molecular profile and the likelihood of targeted therapy recommendations for 554 patients diagnosed with 17 different types of advanced solid tumor, with at least 10 patients per tumor type. Tumor samples of the patients were examined using next-generation sequencing panels, immunohistochemistry, and fluorescence in situ hybridization, as described in detail below.

All profiles were reviewed by a multidisciplinary team for the evaluation of a targeted treatment recommendation in a molecular tumor board.

2.2. Tissue Samples

Formalin-fixed, paraffin-embedded tissue samples from patients with advanced solid tumors who had progressed to all standard therapy regimens were obtained from the archive of the Department of Pathology, Medical University of Vienna, Austria.

2.3. Cancer Gene Panel Sequencing

DNA was extracted from paraffin-embedded tissue blocks with a QIAamp Tissue KitTM (Qiagen, Hilden, Germany). In total, 10 ng DNA per tissue sample was provided for sequencing. The DNA library was created by multiplex polymerase chain reaction with the Ion AmpliSeq Cancer Hotspot Panel v2 (Thermo Fisher Scientific, Waltham, MA, USA) that covers mutation hotspots of 50 genes. The panel includes driver mutations, oncogenes, and tumor suppressor genes. By the middle of 2018, the gene panel was expanded using the 161-gene next-generation sequencing panel of Oncomine Comprehensive Assay v3 (Thermo Fisher Scientific, Waltham, MA, USA) that covers genetic alterations and gene fusions. All of the genes detected by the 50-gene panel and 87 genes detected by the 161-gene panel were hotspot alterations. See Supplementary Materials (Table S1) for a complete list of the gene panels. The Ampliseq cancer hotspot panel was sequenced with an Ion PGM (Thermo Fisher) and the Oncomine Comprehensive Assay v3 on an Ion S5 sequencer (Thermo Fisher Scientific, Waltham, MA, USA). The generated sequencing data were afterwards analyzed with the help of the Ion Reporter Software (Thermo Scientific Fisher). We referred to BRCA Exchange, ClinVar, COSMIC, dbSNP, OMIM, and 1000 genomes for variant calling and classification. The variants were classified according to a five-tier system comprising the modifiers pathogenic, likely pathogenic, uncertain significance, likely benign, or benign. This classification was based on the standards and guidelines for the interpretation of sequence variants of the American College of Medical Genetics and Genomics [14]. The variants pathogenic and likely pathogenic were taken into consideration for the recommendation of targeted therapy.

2.4. Immunohistochemistry

Immunohistochemistry (IHC) was performed using 2-µm-thin tissue sections read by a Ventana Benchmark Ultra stainer (Ventana Medical Systems, Tucson, AZ, USA). The following antibodies were applied: anaplastic lymphoma kinase (ALK) (clone 1A4; Zytomed, Berlin, Germany), CD20 (clone L26; Dako), CD30 (clone BerH2; Agilent Technologies, Vienna, Austria), DNA mismatch repair (MMR) proteins including MLH1 (clone M1, Ventana Medical Systems), PMS2 (clone EPR3947, Cell Marque, Rocklin, CA, USA), MSH2 (clone G219-1129, Cell Marque), and MSH6 (clone 44, Cell Marque), epidermal growth factor receptor (EGFR) (clone 3C6; Ventana), estrogen receptor (clone SP1; Ventana

Medical Systems), human epidermal growth factor receptor 2 (HER2) (clone 4B5; Ventana Medical Systems), HER3 (clone SP71; Abcam, Cambridge, UK), C-kit receptor (KIT) (clone 9.7; Ventana Medical Systems), MET (clone SP44; Ventana), NTRK (clone EPR17341, Abcam), phosphorylated mammalian target of rapamycin (p-mTOR) (clone 49F9; Cell Signaling Technology, Danvers, MA, USA), platelet-derived growth factor alpha (PDGFRA) (rabbit polyclonal; Thermo Fisher Scientific), PDGFRB (clone 28E1, Cell Signaling Technology), programmed death-ligand 1 (PD-L1) (clone E1L3N; Cell Signaling Technology till mid-2018; as of mid-2018, the clone BSR90 from Nordic Biosite, Stockholm, Sweden is used), progesteron receptor (clone 1E2; Ventana), phosphatase and tensin homolog (PTEN) (clone Y184; Abcam), and ROS1 (clone D4D6; Cell Signaling Technology).

To assess the immunostaining intensity for the antigens EGFR, p-mTOR, PDGFRA, PDGFRB, and PTEN, a combinative semiquantitative score for immunohistochemistry was used. The immunostaining intensity was graded from 0 to 3 (0 = negative, 1 = weak, 2 = moderate, 3 = strong). To calculate the score, the intensity grade was multiplied by the percentage of corresponding positive cells: (maximum 300) = (% negative × 0) + (% weak × 1) + (% moderate × 2) + (% strong × 3).

The immunohistochemical staining intensity for HER2 was scored from 0 to 3+ (0 = negative, 1+ = negative, 2+ = positive, 3+ = positive) pursuant to the scoring guidelines of the Dako HercepTestR from the company Agilent Technologies (Agilent Technologies, Vienna, Austria). In the case of HER2 2+, a further test with HER2 in situ hybridization was performed to verify the HER2 gene amplification.

Estrogen receptor and progesterone receptor stainings were graded according to the Allred scoring system from 0 to 8. MET staining was scored from 0 to 3 (0 = negative, 1 = weak, 2 = moderate, 3 = strong) based on a paper by Koeppen et al. [15]. For PD-L1 protein expression, the tumor proportion score was calculated, which is the percentage of viable malignant cells showing membrane staining. In addition, as of 2019, the expression is also determined by the combined positive score.

The intensity of immunostaining intensity of a specific biomarker, including p-mTOR, HER2, PDGFR, PD-L1, is associated with the efficacy of the respective targeted therapy [16–21].

ALK, CD30, CD20, and ROS1 staining were classified as positive or negative based on the percentage of reactive tumor cells, however without graduation of the staining intensity. In ALK or ROS1 positive cases, the presence of a possible gene translocation was evaluated by fluorescence in situ hybridization (FISH).

All antibodies used in this study were validated and approved at the Clinical Institute of Pathology of the Medical University of Vienna and are used in routine IHC staining for clinical purposes. The antibodies have been validated—by proper positive and negative tissue controls and by non-IHC methods such as immunoblotting and flow cytometry—to detect the respective epitope of the antigens. For the control, the use of the antibodies was optimized in terms of intensity, concentration, signal/noise ratio, incubation time, and blocking. The negative control was conducted by omitting the primary antibody and by substitution of isotype-specific antibody and serum at the exact same dilution and laboratory conditions as the primary antibody to preclude unspecific binding.

For the positive control, the antibodies were shown not to cross-react with closely related molecules of the target epitope.

The status of MSI was analyzed by the MSI Analysis System, Version 1.1 (Promega Corporation, Madison, WI, USA).

2.5. Fluorescence In Situ Hybridization (FISH)

FISH was applied only in selected cases to verify PTEN loss. FISH was performed with 4-µm-thick formalin-fixed, paraffin-embedded tissue sections. The following FISH probe was utilized: PTEN (10q23.31)/Centromere 10 (ZytoVision, Bremerhaven, Germany). Two hundred cell nuclei per tumor were evaluated. The PTEN FISH was considered positive for PTEN gene loss with ≥30% of cells with only one or no PTEN signals. A chromosome 10 centromere FISH probe served as a control for ploidy of chromosome 10.

2.6. Multidisciplinary Team for Precision Medicine

After thorough examination of the molecular profile of each tumor sample by a qualified and competent molecular pathologist, the results and findings were reviewed in a multidisciplinary team (MDT) meeting that was held every other week.

Members of the MDT included molecular pathologists, radiologists, clinical oncologists, surgical oncologists, and basic scientists. The MDT recommended the targeted therapy based on the specific molecular profile of each patient. The targeted therapies included tyrosine kinase inhibitors, checkpoint inhibitors (e.g., anti- PD-L1 monoclonal antibodies), and growth factor receptor antibodies with or without endocrine therapy. The treatment recommendations by the MDT were prioritized dependent on the level of evidence from high to low according to phase III to phase I trials. Recommendations based on phase III, phase II, and phase I were designated as high, intermediate, and low, respectively.

In cases where more than one druggable molecular aberration was identified, the MDT recommended a therapy regimen to target as many molecular aberrations as possible, with special consideration of the toxicity profile of each antitumoral agent and their potential interactions. Since all patients were given all available standard treatment options for their cancer disease prior to their inclusion in our precision medicine platform, nearly all targeted agents were suggested as off-label use. If the tumor profile and the clinical characteristics of a patient met the requirements of a clinical trial for targeted therapies that was open for inclusion in our cancer center, patients were preferentially asked if they wanted to participate in the respective trial.

2.7. Study Design and Statistics

This study is a retrospective single center cohort analysis of 17 different types of advanced solid tumors, with at least 10 patients per tumor type. The objective was to describe the molecular portrait and to evaluate the likelihood and the molecular and gender aspects of a targeted therapy recommendation for common tumor types. Rare tumor types with less than 10 patients per tumor type discussed in our MONDTI platform over this seven-year period were excluded. We also used the method of frequency distribution to delineate the characteristics of the cancer patients. We used the method of frequency distribution to delineate the characteristics of the cancer patients.

Since our study had an exploratory and hypothesis-generating design, no adjustment for multiple testing was used [22]. Binary logistic regression analysis was employed to assess the influence of various factors on the therapy recommendation rate. To evaluate whether our dataset has a normal distribution, Shapiro–Wilk test and Kolmogorov–Smirnov test were utilized. To examine gender-specific differences, Chi-squared test $\chi 2$ and Mann–Whitney U test were applied.

For statistical analysis, the software package IBM SPSS Statistics Version 26 was used.

3. Results

From June 2013 to January 2020, 554 patients diagnosed with 17 different types of advanced therapy refractory solid tumors, with at least 10 patients per tumor entity, were included in this retrospective cohort analysis. This analysis is from the total cohort of our platform MONDTI, which has so far profiled 580 patients with various advanced cancer types. In this analysis, all patients were Caucasians. The median age at initial diagnosis was 54.3 years, ranging from 18 to 81 years, and the median age at the time when the molecular profiling was performed was 57.4 years, ranging from 18 to 84 years (Table 1). The tumor tissue was obtained from biopsy or during surgical intervention.

The five most frequent tumor types were gynecologic malignancy (n = 90; 16.1%), colorectal cancer (n = 56; 10.0%), tumor of the central nervous system (n = 55; 9.9%), squamous cell carcinoma of the head and neck (n = 44; 8.4%), and neuroendocrine carcinoma (n = 41; 7.4%), with details provided in Table 2.

Table 1. Patient characteristics (N = 554).

Patient Characteristics	Number
Men	279
Women	275
Median age at initial diagnosis	54.3 (18–87)
Median age at molecular profiling	57.4 (18–89)
Caucasian	554
Types of advanced solid tumors	17
Prior lines of antitumoral therapy	1–5

Table 2. Number of patients and recommendation rate.

Type of Solid Tumor	Number of Patients	Number of Recommendations and Recommendation Rate; Evidence Level for Recommendation	Outcome of Patients Who Received the Targeted Therapy
Urologic malignancy	10	N = 9; 90.0%; intermediate: $n = 7$, low: $n = 2$	PD: $n = 3$
Mesothelioma	14	N = 11, 78.6%; intermediate: $n = 5$, low: $n = 6$	SD: $n = 1$; PD: $n = 3$; died prior to assessment: $n = 1$
Male reproductive cancer	14	N = 10; 71.4%; intermediate: $n = 5$, low: $n = 5$	PR: $n = 2$; PD: $n = 1$; died prior to assessment: $n = 2$
Tumor of the central nervous system	55	N = 37; 67.8%; low: $n = 37$	PR: $n = 2$; SD: $n = 4$; PD: $n = 3$; died prior to assessment: $n = 2$
Squamous cell carcinoma of the head and neck	44	N = 29; 65.9%; high: $n = 9$, intermediate: 8, low: $n = 12$	SD: $n = 3$; PD: $n = 4$; died prior to assessment: $n = 3$
Sarcoma	17	N = 11; 64.7%; intermediate: $n = 2$, low: $n = 9$	CR: $n = 1$
Gynecologic malignancy	90	N = 58; 64.4%; high: $n = 4$; intermediate: $n = 39$, low: 13	SD: $n = 4$; PD = 2; died prior to assessment: $n = 5$; trials: $n = 2$
Hepatocellular carcinoma	16	N = 9; 56.3%; high: $n = 1$, intermediate: $n = 1$, low: 7	SD: $n = 4$; PD: $n = 1$; died prior to assessment: $n = 2$
Colorectal cancer	56	N = 30; 53.6%; high: $n = 10$, intermediate: $n = 11$, low: 6	PR: $n = 2$; trials: $n = 3$; PD: $n = 1$; died prior to assessment: $n = 2$
Lung cancer (without small cell lung cancer)	15	N = 9; 52.9%; high: $n = 1$, intermediate: $n = 3$, low: $n = 5$	PD: $n = 3$
Biliary Tract cancer	37	N = 19; 51.4%; intermediate: $n = 6$, low: $n = 10$	PR: $n = 2$; PD: $n = 2$; trials: $n = 3$; died prior to assessment: $n = 2$
Cancer of unknown primary	35	N = 18; 51.4%; low: $n = 18$	SD: $n = 3$; PR: $n = 1$; CR: $n = 1$; PD: $n = 2$; died prior to assessment: $n = 1$
Esophagogastric cancer	21	N = 9; 42.9%; low: $n = 8$	SD: $n = 1$; trial: $n = 1$; died prior to assessment: $n = 1$
Neuroendocrine carcinoma	41	N = 16; 39.0%; intermediate: $n = 5$; low: 11	SD: $n = 1$, PD = 3
Breast cancer	21	N = 8; 38.1%; intermediate: $n = 5$, low: $n = 3$	PD: $n = 1$
Pancreatic cancer	38	N = 12; 31.6%; low: $n = 12$	SD: $n = 1$; died prior to assessment: $n = 2$

Table 2. Cont.

Type of Solid Tumor	Number of Patients	Number of Recommendations and Recommendation Rate; Evidence Level for Recommendation	Outcome of Patients Who Received the Targeted Therapy
Diffuse large B-cell lymphoma	30	N = 9; 30.0%; intermediate: n = 2, low: n = 7	SD: n = 1; PD: n = 1; died prior to assessment: n = 1
Total	554	N = 304, 54.9%	

At the time of molecular profiling, all patients had an advanced solid tumor which was refractory to therapy, all lines of standard treatment having been exhausted. Patients received between 1 and 5 lines of prior systemic chemotherapy; 287 patients had undergone a surgical intervention (51.8%).

In total, 397 tumor samples (71.7%) were tested with the 50-gene panel and 166 specimens (28.3%) were analyzed with the 161-gene panel.

In total, we identified 1143 genomic aberrations in 441 (79.6%) patients: the 10 most frequent were TP53 (n = 228; 19.9%), KRAS (n = 103; 9.0%), PIK3CA (n = 54; 4.7%), PTEN (n = 35; 3.2%), APC (n = 28; 2.4%), CDKN2A (n = 28; 2.4%), NOTCH1 (n = 26; 2.3%), ATM (n = 25; 2.2%), SMAD4 (n = 19; 1.7%), IDH1 (n = 17, 1.5%). In 113 (20.4%) patients, no genetic alterations were detected. The inter- and intratumoral genomic profile was heterogeneous and mutations were seen in 123 different genes tested with the 161-gene panel (see Figure 1 and Table 3). The median number of mutations was two in the whole cohort. The median numbers of mutations were one and two when tested with the 50-gene panel and 161-gene panel, respectively.

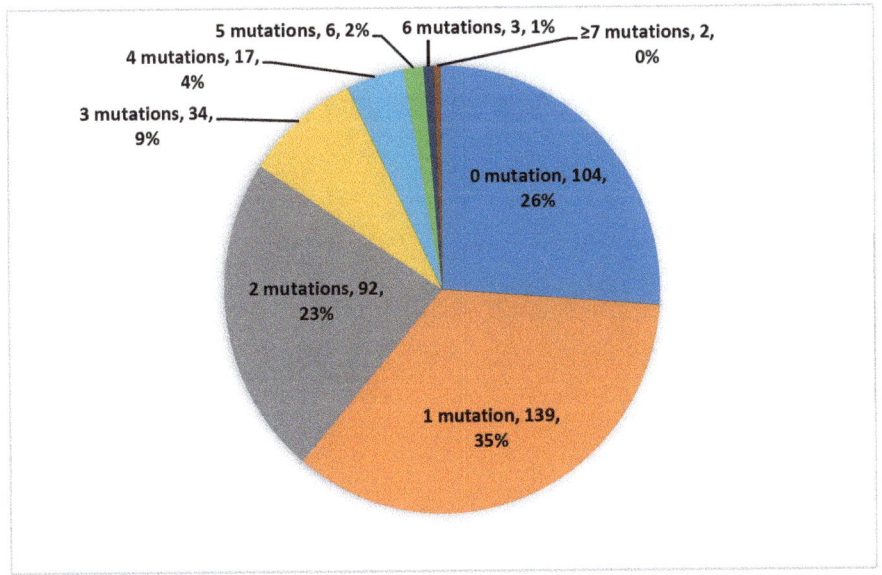

(a) Distribution of number of mutations among 397 patients tested with the 50-gene panel.

Figure 1. Cont.

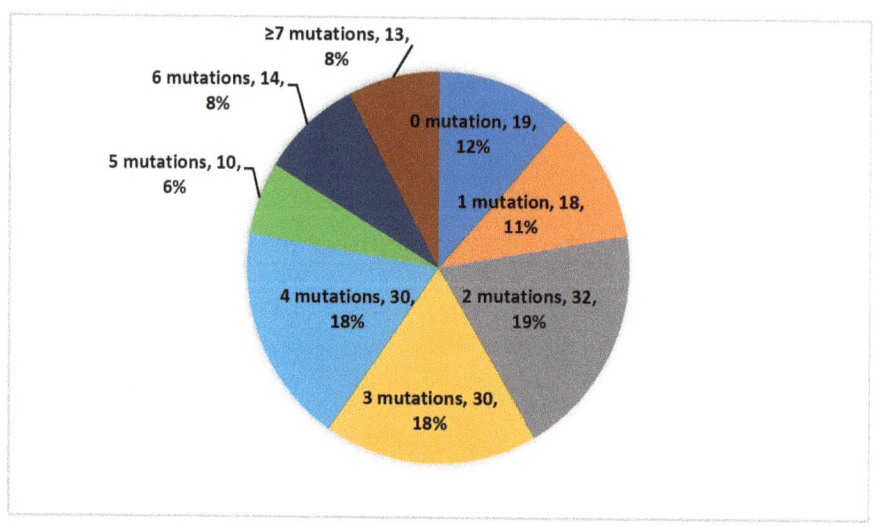

(**b**) Distribution of number of mutations among 166 patients tested with the 161-gene panel.

Figure 1. Distribution of number of mutations among the patients.

Table 3. Detected molecular alterations.

Genomic Alteration	Absolute Numbers	Frequency in %									
TP53	228	19.9%	MET	9	0.8%	VA65:C90HL	4	0.3%	RHOA	2	0.2%
KRAS	103	9.0%	PTCH1	9	0.8%	CCND1	3	0.3%	ROS1	2	0.2%
PIK3CA	54	4.7%	RAD50	9	0.8%	CDH1	3	0.3%	SF3B1	2	0.2%
PTEN	37	3.2%	AKT1	8	0.7%	DDR2	3	0.3%	SRC	2	0.2%
APC	28	2.4%	FGFR3	8	0.7%	ESR1	3	0.3%	TERT	2	0.2%
CDKN2A	28	2.4%	SMARCB1	8	0.7%	FGFR4	3	0.3%	RHOA	2	0.2%
NOTCH1	26	2.3%	BRCA1	7	0.6%	HRAS	3	0.3%	ROS1	2	0.2%
ATM	25	2.2%	IDH2	7	0.6%	MAP2K1	3	0.3%	SF3B1	2	0.2%
SMAD4	19	1.7%	MSH6	7	0.6%	MYCL	3	0.3%	AKT2	1	0.1%
IDH1	17	1.5%	PALB2	7	0.6%	NTRK1	3	0.3%	AR	1	0.1%
PIK3R1	17	1.5%	SMARCA4	7	0.6%	PDGFRA	3	0.3%	AXL	1	0.1%
CTNNB1	16	1.4%	TSC1	7	0.6%	RAD51B	3	0.3%	CBL	1	0.1%
BRCA2	15	1.3%	ALK	6	0.5%	RNF43	3	0.3%	CD274	1	0.1%
RB1	15	1.3%	BAP1	6	0.5%	CDK4	2	0.2%	CDK4	1	0.1%
EGFR	14	1.2%	FGFR2	6	0.5%	CCND2	2	0.2%	CHEK2	1	0.1%
FANCA	14	1.2%	NBN	6	0.5%	CDK2	2	0.2%	FANCI	1	0.1%
POLE	14	1.2%	NF2	6	0.5%	CHEK1	2	0.2%	IGF1R	1	0.1%
TSC2	14	1.2%	SMO	6	0.5%	ERBB3	2	0.2%	JAK1	1	0.1%
ATR	13	1.1%	CDK12	5	0.4%	EZH2	2	0.2%	JAK2	1	0.1%
BRAF	13	1.1%	ERBB4	5	0.4%	FANCD2	2	0.2%	MAPK1	1	0.1%
NF1	13	1.1%	FGFR1	5	0.4%	FLT3	2	0.2%	MCL1	1	0.1%
ARID1A	12	1.0%	MLH1	5	0.4%	GNAQ	2	0.2%	MDM2	1	0.1%
CREBBP	12	1.0%	PMS2	5	0.4%	JAK3	2	0.2%	MDM4	1	0.1%
KIT	12	1.0%	PTPN11	5	0.4%	MAF	2	0.2%	MSH	1	0.1%

Table 3. *Cont.*

Genomic Alteration	Absolute Numbers	Frequency in %									
FBXW7	11	1.0%	ABL1	4 0.3%	MAX	2 0.2%	NFE2L2	1 0.1%
RET	11	1.0%	ATRX	4 0.3%	MSH2	2 0.2%	NTRK3	1 0.1%
SLX4	11	1.0%	CCND3	4 0.3%	mTOR	2 0.2%	PPP2R1A	1 0.1%
STK11	11	1.0%	ERBB2	4 0.3%	MYCN	2 0.2%	RICTOR	1 0.1%
NOTCH2	10	0.9%	KDR	4 0.3%	NTRK2	2 0.2%	TET2	1 0.1%
NOTCH3	10	0.9%	MRE11A	4 0.3%	PDGFRB	2 0.2%	UTR3	1 0.1%
SETD2	10	0.9%	NRAS	4 0.3%	PIK3CB	2 0.2%	AKT2	1 0.1%
GNAS	9	0.8%	RAD51D	4 0.3%	RAD51C	2 0.2%		

The next generation sequencing (NGS) analysis rate was high at 98.0%. Only in 11/554 (1.9%) patients, the NGS run failed. In 31/554 (5.6%) cases, IHC could not be performed (see Figure 2, which shows the flow of patients).

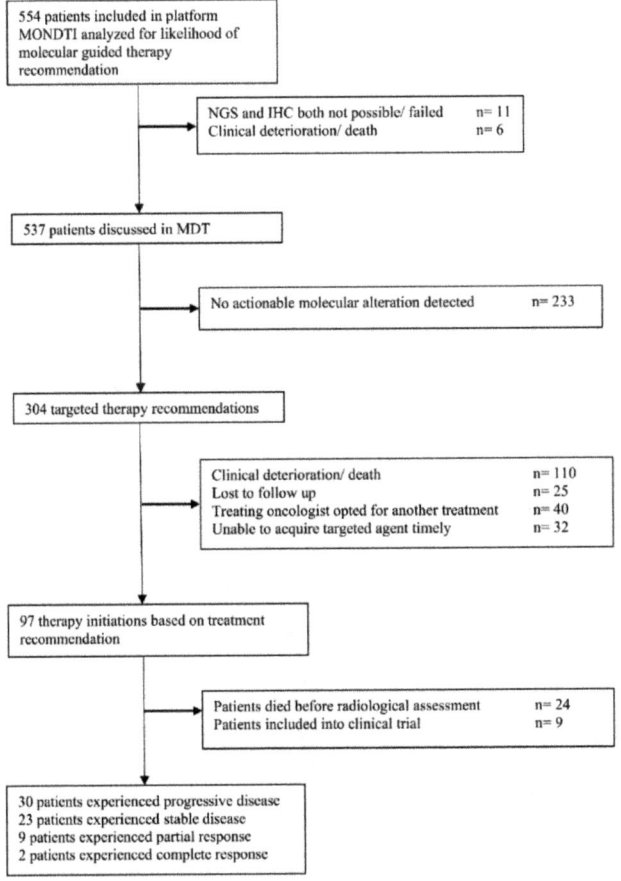

Figure 2. Flow of patients.

The studied population included 279 men and 275 women. The mutation rate was almost equal between the two genders: 48.9% in men versus 51.0% in women. The targeted recommendation rate, however, was slightly higher for men (53.6%, $n = 163$) when compared with women (46.4%, $n = 141$).

IHC revealed expression of p-mTOR ($n = 419$; 75.1%), EGFR ($n = 386$; 69.1%), PDGFRA ($n = 183$; 32.8%), PDGFRB ($n = 45$; 8.1%) MET ($n = 178$; 31.9 %), KIT ($n = 35$; 6.3%), HER2 ($n = 36$; 6.5%), HER3 ($n = 58$; 10.4%), PD-L1 ($n = 92$; 16.5%). In 57 cases (10.3%), loss of PTEN signal was reported. Seven patients (1.3%) had an MSI high status.

In total, we identified 33 gene fusions in our cohort (see Table 4).

Table 4. Detected gene fusions.

Tumor Entity	Number of Gene Fusions	Type of Gene Fusions
Colorectal cancer	7	FGFR3-TACC3 ($n = 2$) WHSC1L1-FGFR1 PTPRK-RSPO3 FNDC3B-PIK3CA SND1-BRAF EIF3E-RSPO2
Tumors of the central nervous system	6	EIF3E-RSPO2 ESR1-CCDC170 TPM3-NTRK1 FGFR3-TACC3 BRAF-MRPS33 ESR1-CCDC170
Squamous cell carcinoma of the head and neck	6	TBL1XR1-PIK3CA MYB-NFIB EIF3E-RSPO2 FNDC3B-PIK3CA EIF3E-RSPO2 FNDC3B-PIK3CA
Hepatocellular carcinoma	5	EIF3E-RSPO2 ($n = 2$) DNAJB1-PRKACA ($n = 3$)
Gynecologic malignancies	3	TBL1XR1-PIK3CA ($n = 2$) EIF3E-RSPO2 ($n = 2$) ESR1-CCDC170
Lung cancer	3	PCNX-RAD51B EIF3E-RSPO2 PTPRK-RSPO3
Pancreatic ductal adenocarcinoma	1	TBL1XR1-PIK3CA
Biliary tract cancer	1	FGFR2-OFD1
Sarcoma	1	EIF3E-RSPO2

In over half ($n = 304$, 54.9%) of the 554 patients, a targeted therapy was suggested, based on the identified molecular aberrations. The recommendation rate was over 50% in 12 different solid tumors. The five highest rates for therapy suggestion were observed in urologic malignancies (90.0%), mesothelioma (78.6%), male reproductive cancers (71.4%), tumors of the central nervous system (67.8%), and squamous cell carcinoma of the head and neck (SCCHN) (65.9%). In contrast, the three lowest rates were seen in breast cancer (38.1%), pancreatic ductal adenocarcinoma (31.6%), and diffuse large B-cell lymphoma (30.0%). We refer here to Table 2.

Of the 304 targeted treatment suggestions, 262 (86.2%) were mainly derived from the molecular information provided by IHC, while only in 39 cases (12.8%), the recommendation was mainly based on the genomic variations. In three cases (1%), the targeted therapy strategy was tailored based on the detection of FGFR fusion genes.

In total, 42 different antitumoral agents were recommended, either in combination or as a monotherapy. The three most frequently applied therapy regimens included the PD-1 inhibitors pembrolizumab and nivolumab ($n = 62$; 20.4%), the anti EGFR antibodies cetuximab and panitumumab ($n = 29$; 9.5%), and everolimus monotherapy ($n = 26$; 8.6%) (see Table 5).

The level of evidence was high, intermediate, and low in 25 (8.2%), 99 (32.6%), and 171 (56.3%) cases, respectively. Nine patients were enrolled in a clinical trial.

Eventually, 97 patients (17.5%) received the molecular guided treatment and thus experienced a change in clinical management because of the generated molecular information. Six out of 97 patients (6.2%) received on-label treatment. Nine of the 97 patients (9.3%) were treated in a clinical trial; 24 of 97 patients (24.7%) died before a radiological assessment could be performed; 30 patients (30.9%) did not respond and experienced a progressive disease. Stable disease was achieved in 23 patients (23.7%). Partial response and complete response were observed in nine (9.3%) and two (2.1%) patients, respectively. Thus, the disease control rate (DCR) was 35.1% and the overall response rate (ORR) was 11.3% in those patients who received the targeted therapy. Related to the whole cohort, the DCR was 6.1% (34/554) and the ORR was 2.0% (11/554).

The application of the Shapiro–Wilk test suggested that the distribution of age and genetic mutations was not normally distributed.

To detect possible gender-specific differences regarding the recommendation rate, we excluded gender-specific cancer diseases (breast cancers, gynecologic, and male reproductive malignancies) and used the Chi-squared test χ^2. The test revealed a significant difference regarding the recommendation rate in the total cohort in favor of the male patients ($p = 0.015$). On the level of tumor subtypes, the Chi-squared test χ^2 demonstrated a significant gender-specific difference in patients with SCCHN ($p = 0.0027$) and malignant mesothelioma ($p = 0.008$). Male patients with SCCHN had significantly more often PD-L1 expression than female patients (10/28 men versus 1/16 women; $p = 0.030$). Similarly, male patients with malignant mesothelioma had significantly more often PDGFRα expression than women (6/9 men versus 0/6 women; $p = 0.017$). After exclusion of these two tumor types, the gender-specific differences were not significant anymore ($p = 0.24$). These gender differences in the molecular profile of these two tumor entities are reflected by the type of targeted therapy recommendation.

In the next step, we investigated the effects of age, tumor type, and molecular profile on therapy recommendation using a binary logistic regression analysis, which showed that several of these factors had a significant impact on the recommendation rate: tumor type ($p = 0.46$), expression of p-mTOR ($p = 0.011$), expression of EGFR ($p = 0.046$), and expression of PD-L1 ($p = 0.023$).

Other parameters including age ($p = 0.855$), number of mutations ($p = 0.850$), expression of PDGFRα ($p = 0.097$), and expression of PDGFRβ ($p = 0.420$) were not significantly associated with therapy recommendation. The omnibus tests of model coefficients for the binary logistic regression were highly significant ($p < 0.0001$).

By using the Mann–Whitney U test, we could not find any gender-specific differences regarding age ($p = 0.250$) or number of mutations ($p = 0.390$). However, the Chi-squared test χ2 revealed, after exclusion of gender-specific cancer diseases, five different genetic mutations that are significantly more common in men than in women: CDKN2A ($p = 0.04$), CTNNB1 ($p = 0.002$), KIT ($p = 0.0005$), SLX4 ($p = 0.034$), and VHL ($p = 0.046$).

The median time interval between the failure of the last standard treatment line and the start of the molecularly targeted therapy was 63 days.

Table 5. Recommended agents in monotherapy and in combination therapies.

Type of Targeted Agent	Number of Recommendations in Monotherapy	Biomarkers for Targeted Therapy Recommendation	Type of Targeted Agents	Number of Recommendations in Combination Therapies	Biomarkers for Targeted Therapy Recommendation
PD-1 Inhibitor	62	PD-L1 expression, MSI-H status	Everolimus + Exemestane	21	p-mTOR expression and PTEN loss; estrogen receptor
EGFR inhibitor (Cetuximab/Panitumuab)	29	EGFR expression and RAS wildtype	Everolimus + Cetuximab	6	p-mTOR expression and PTEN loss; EGFR expression and RAS wildtype
Everolimus	26	p-mTOR expression and PTEN loss	Everolimus + Sorafenib	1	p-mTOR expression and PTEN loss; estrogen receptor
Imatinib	19	ABL, KIT, PDGFR	Everolimus + Carboplatin	1	p-mTOR expression and PTEN loss; ATM, BRCA1, BRCA2, PALB2
Crizotinib	14	ALK, ROS1	Trastuzumab + Pertuzumab	5	HER2
Sunitinib	14	FLT3, KIT, PDGFR	Trametinib + Dabrafenib	5	BRAF V600E
Afatinib	12	EGFR, HER2, HER3	Cetuximab + Irinotecan	5	EGFR expression and RAS wildtype
Regorafenib	9	ABL, FGFR, PDGFR, KIT,	Cetuximab + Vemurafenib	3	EGFR expression and RAS wildtype; BRAF V600E
Palbociclib	8	CDK4, CDK6	Cetuximab + Temsirolimus	2	EGFR expression and RAS wildtype; p-mTOR expression and PTEN loss
Cabozantinib	5	KIT, FLT-3, AXL, RET, MET	Lapatinib + Trastuzumab	2	EGFR and HER2
Ponatinib	4	ABL, FLT3, KIT, PDGFR, RET	Sunitinib + Anastrozol	1	FLT3, KIT, PDGFR; estrogen receptor
Olaparib	4	BRCA1, BRCA2	Idelalisib + Rituximab	1	PIK3CA; CD20
Pazopanib	3	PDGFR, FGFR3	Alpelisib + Fulvestrant	1	PIK3CA; estrogen receptor
Erlotinib	3	EGFR	Olaparib + platinum-based chemotherapy	1	BRCA1, BRCA2; ATM, BRCA1, BRCA2, PALB2

Table 5. Cont.

Type of Targeted Agent	Number of Recommendations in Monotherapy	Biomarkers for Targeted Therapy Recommendation	Type of Targeted Agents	Number of Recommendations in Combination Therapies	Biomarkers for Targeted Therapy Recommendation
Pemigatinib	3	FGFR2	Pembrolizumab + Bevacizumab	1	PD-L1 expression; VEGFA
Platinum based chemotherapy	2	ATM, BRCA1, BRCA2, PALB2	Imatinib + Everolimus	1	ABL, KIT, PDGFR; p-mTOR expression and PTEN loss
Enasidenib	2	IDH2	Imatinib + Letrozole	1	ABL, KIT, PDGFR; estrogen receptor
Fulvestrant	2	Estrogen receptor	Bevacizumab + Paclitaxel	1	VEGFA
Androgen receptor antagonists	2	Androgen receptor	Bevacizumab + Everolimus	1	VEGFA; p-mTOR expression and PTEN loss
Temsirolimus	2	p-mTOR expression and PTEN loss	Total	304	
Nintedanib	2	FLT3, FGFR, PDGFR			
Tamoxifen	2	Estrogen receptor			
Lapatinib	2	EGFR, HER2			
Idelalisib	1	PIK3CA, PIK3R1			
T-DM1	1	HER2			
Trametinib	1	BRAF V600E			
AKT inhibitor	1	AKT			
Foretinib	1	MET			
Capmatinib	1	MET exon 14 skipping			
Dasatinib	1	ABL KIT, PDGFR			
Alemtuzumab	1	CD52			
Brentuximab Vedotin	1	CD30			
Vismodegib	1	SMO			
Vemurafenib	1	BRAF V600E			
Exemestane	1	Estrogen receptor			
Bevacizumab	1	VEGFA			

4. Discussion

This comprehensive analysis presents data from a real-world precision medicine platform.

The MONDTI platform for precision medicine is an open, tissue-agnostic and molecular-driven platform that seeks to provide targeted therapy strategies to patients based on the respective molecular profile. In our platform, we could offer tailored therapy concepts in over 50% of our patients, with 19 different advanced solid tumors with recommendation rates well above 70% in selected entities. Our study demonstrates that precision medicine is implementable into clinical routine. Considering the clinical outcome of targeted therapies in this retrospective analysis, the outcome was relatively poor.

Related to the whole cohort, the DCR was 6.1% (34/554) and the ORR was 2.0% (11/554). There are several reasons that might explain this poor outcome.

Firstly, we observed a median turnaround time of more than two months between the failure of the last standard treatment line and the start of the targeted therapy. In this time interval, over 100 patients experienced clinical deterioration or died before the start of the targeted therapy. Nearly a quarter of the patients who eventually received the targeted therapy died prior to radiological assessment. One reason for the poor outcome of molecular-driven treatment approaches in this study is the relatively long turnaround time, during which patients do not receive effective therapy. Even if the targeted therapy is applied, it may not have enough time for the targeted therapy to unfold its full antitumorigenic potential.

Thus, time is a highly critical factor in the therapeutic management of therapy refractory solid tumors. Moreover, we detected a broad variety of mutations highlighting the well-known tumoral heterogeneity in cancer diseases [23,24].

Based on our data, the likelihood for rational identification of molecular-based treatment concepts was above 50% for 12 different solid tumors. However, the majority of these recommendations (88.8%) were not based on a high level of evidence.

Hence, the poor clinical outcome may be partly related to the long turnaround time, the extreme tumor heterogeneity, and the low level of evidence for therapy recommendations.

Thus, it is clinically relevant to consider these factors, particularly in patients for whom no guideline-based treatment is available anymore.

Interestingly, we observed in our cohort gender-specific differences in the molecular profile and therapy recommendations of SCCHN and mesothelioma patients.

The binary logistic regression analysis revealed that the expression of p-mTOR, EGFR, and PD-L1 significantly influenced therapy recommendations. This finding is reflected in the most common types of recommended targeted therapy: pembrolizumab and nivolumab, the anti EGFR antibodies cetuximab and panitumumab, as well as everolimus in monotherapy and in combination therapies.

Genomic profiling was performed in 98.0% patients, which is higher than or comparable to the rate reported by NEXT-1 (95%), MOSCATO 01 (89%), IMPACT/COMPACT (87%), SAFIR01 (70%), and SHIVA (67%) [13,25–28]. We detected 1143 genetic alterations and observed gender-specific differences regarding the distribution of the aberrations.

This study has several limitations. First, we acknowledge that our analysis was retrospective. Although all patients with advanced solid tumors with no further standard treatment options were included in this platform, this study is biased to a certain degree, since we included only patients with available tumor specimens for molecular profiling and a good ECOG status between 0 and 1.

Additionally, we did not consider the generally known dynamic of spatial and temporal intratumoral heterogeneity. We recommended the targeted therapy based on a molecular profile from one biopsy and from one timepoint, which was not necessarily close to molecular profiling. To overcome these limitations in future, liquid biopsy might be an additional practicable tool to monitor the dynamic molecular landscape of patients to revise and adapt the targeted therapy accordingly at any given timepoint. Particularly, early signs of treatment resistance may help to direct our therapy decisions using serial liquid biopsies. By reducing the turnaround time via liquid biopsy and by accelerating the creation of a molecular profile, the potential targeted agent could more likely be applied before the performance status of the patients deteriorates or before the molecular landscape changes and makes the therapy ineffective. Liquid biopsy would also be an interesting option for patients unfit to undergo a biopsy [29].

Another limitation of this study is that the found distribution of the mutations may be confounded by the employment of two different gene panels (50-gene panel versus 161-gene panel).

There are several burning issues to be addressed in future clinical trials and translational research. The first is to harmonize procedures and introduce international standards regarding the applied methods and treatment decision-making strategies, e.g., a standardized method for PD-L1 staining and scoring. International cut-offs in immunohistochemistry should be introduced and adhered to in order to achieve comparable results in clinical trials.

Several clinical trials have demonstrated the clinical benefit of tissue-agnostic molecular-guided treatment concepts and strategies in advanced stages of solid tumors. It would be important and interesting to introduce precision medicine at earlier stages of cancer disease to evaluate the efficacy of this treatment strategy. For instance, I-SPY 2 platform trial tests personalized treatment concepts for the neoadjuvant treatment of locally advanced breast cancer [30].

This analysis demonstrates that precision medicine was feasible and provided the basis for molecular-driven therapy recommendations in patients with advanced therapy refractory solid tumors. Studies are ongoing to define the clinical benefit of this approach in the real-life setting. Although the concept of molecular-guided therapy strategies is a relatively new concept, it has the potential to inform, shape, and enrich the antitumoral therapeutic armamentarium.

Supplementary Materials: The following are available online at http://www.mdpi.com/2075-4426/10/4/188/s1, Table S1: List of gene targets in Oncomine Comprehensive Assay v3 (Thermo Fisher Scientific, Waltham, MA, USA)—161 gene panel.

Author Contributions: H.T., M.U., R.M.M., G.W.P. conceived and designed the presented idea; L.M. performed the experiments; H.T., M.U., R.M.M., L.M., G.W.P. analyzed the data; All authors contributed to the interpretation of the results; G.W.P. supervised the work; H.T. wrote the paper. All authors provided critical feedback and helped shape the research, analysis and manuscript. All authors have read and agreed to the published version of the manuscript.

Funding: This research received no external funding.

Conflicts of Interest: M.P. has received honoraria for lectures, consultation, or advisory board participation from the following for-profit companies: Bayer, Bristol-Myers Squibb, Novartis, Gerson Lehrman Group (GLG), CMC Contrast, GlaxoSmithKline, Mundipharma, Roche, BMJ Journals, MedMedia, Astra Zeneca, AbbVie, Lilly, Medahead, Daiichi Sankyo, Sanofi, Merck Sharp & Dome, Tocagen. The following for-profit companies have supported clinical trials and contracted research conducted by M.P. with payments made to his institution: Böhringer-Ingelheim, Bristol-Myers Squibb, Roche, Daiichi Sankyo, Merck Sharp & Dome, Novocure, GlaxoSmithKline, AbbVie. R.B. has received honoraria from the following for-profit companies. Astra-Zeneca, Celgene, Daiichi, Eisai, Eli-Lilly, MSD, Novartis, Pfizer, Pierre-Fabre, Roche, Samsung, BMS, Sandoz. G.W.P. has received honoraria from the following for-profit companies: Merck Serono, Roche, Amgen, Sanofi, Lilly, Servier, Taiho, Bayer, Halozyme, BMS, Celgene, Pierre Fabre, Shire. The remaining authors have no conflicts of interest to declare.

References

1. Bray, F.; Ferlay, J.; Soerjomataram, I.; Siegel, R.L.; Torre, L.A.; Jemal, A. Global cancer statistics 2018: GLOBOCAN estimates of incidence and mortality worldwide for 36 cancers in 185 countries. *CA Cancer J. Clin.* **2018**, *68*, 394–424. [CrossRef] [PubMed]
2. Global Burden of Disease Cancer Collaboration; Fitzmaurice, C.; Akinyemiju, T.F.; Al Lami, F.H.; Alam, T.; Alizadeh-Navaei, R.; Allen, C.; Alsharif, U.; Alvis-Guzman, N.; Amini, E.; et al. Global, Regional, and National Cancer Incidence, Mortality, Years of Life Lost, Years Lived With Disability, and Disability-Adjusted Life-Years for 29 Cancer Groups, 1990 to 2016: A Systematic Analysis for the Global Burden of Disease Study. *JAMA Oncol.* **2018**, *4*, 1553–1568.
3. Slamon, D.; Eiermann, W.; Robert, N.; Pienkowski, T.; Martin, M.; Press, M.; Mackey, J.; Glaspy, J.; Chan, A.; Pawlicki, M.; et al. Adjuvant trastuzumab in HER2-positive breast cancer. *N. Engl. J. Med.* **2011**, *365*, 1273–1283. [CrossRef] [PubMed]

4. Bang, Y.J.; Van Cutsem, E.; Feyereislova, A.; Chung, H.C.; Shen, L.; Sawaki, A.; Lordick, F.; Ohtsu, A.; Omuro, Y.; Satoh, T.; et al. Trastuzumab in combination with chemotherapy versus chemotherapy alone for treatment of HER2-positive advanced gastric or gastro-oesophageal junction cancer (ToGA): A phase 3, open-label, randomised controlled trial. *Lancet* **2010**, *376*, 687–697. [CrossRef]
5. Long, G.V.; Stroyakovskiy, D.; Gogas, H.; Levchenko, E.; de Braud, F.; Larkin, J.; Garbe, C.; Jouary, T.; Hauschild, A.; Grob, J.J.; et al. Combined BRAF and MEK inhibition versus BRAF inhibition alone in melanoma. *N. Engl. J. Med.* **2014**, *371*, 1877–1888. [CrossRef]
6. Robert, C.; Karaszewska, B.; Schachter, J.; Rutkowski, P.; Mackiewicz, A.; Stroiakovski, D.; Lichinitser, M.; Dummer, R.; Grange, F.; Mortier, L.; et al. Improved overall survival in melanoma with combined dabrafenib and trametinib. *N. Engl. J. Med.* **2015**, *372*, 30–39. [CrossRef]
7. Larkin, J.; Ascierto, P.A.; Dreno, B.; Atkinson, V.; Liszkay, G.; Maio, M.; Mandala, M.; Demidov, L.; Stroyakovskiy, D.; Thomas, L.; et al. Combined vemurafenib and cobimetinib in BRAF-mutated melanoma. *N. Engl. J. Med.* **2014**, *371*, 1867–1876. [CrossRef]
8. Wang, Y.; Schmid-Bindert, G.; Zhou, C. Erlotinib in the treatment of advanced non-small cell lung cancer: An update for clinicians. *Ther. Adv. Med. Oncol.* **2012**, *4*, 19–29. [CrossRef]
9. Dhillon, S. Gefitinib: A review of its use in adults with advanced non-small cell lung cancer. *Target Oncol.* **2015**, *10*, 153–170. [CrossRef]
10. Ramalingam, S.S.; Vansteenkiste, J.; Planchard, D.; Cho, B.C.; Gray, J.E.; Ohe, Y.; Zhou, C.; Reungwetwattana, T.; Cheng, Y.; Chewaskulyong, B.; et al. Overall Survival with Osimertinib in Untreated, EGFR-Mutated Advanced NSCLC. *N. Engl. J. Med.* **2020**, *382*, 41–50. [CrossRef]
11. Von Hoff, D.D.; Stephenson, J.J., Jr.; Rosen, P.; Loesch, D.M.; Borad, M.J.; Anthony, S.; Jameson, G.; Brown, S.; Cantafio, N.; Richards, D.A.; et al. Pilot study using molecular profiling of patients' tumors to find potential targets and select treatments for their refractory cancers. *J. Clin. Oncol.* **2010**, *28*, 4877–4883. [CrossRef] [PubMed]
12. Prager, G.W.; Unseld, M.; Waneck, F.; Mader, R.; Wrba, F.; Raderer, M.; Fuereder, T.; Staber, P.; Jager, U.; Kieler, M.; et al. Results of the extended analysis for cancer treatment (EXACT) trial: A prospective translational study evaluating individualized treatment regimens in oncology. *Oncotarget* **2019**, *10*, 942–952. [CrossRef]
13. Massard, C.; Michiels, S.; Ferte, C.; Le Deley, M.C.; Lacroix, L.; Hollebecque, A.; Verlingue, L.; Ileana, E.; Rosellini, S.; Ammari, S.; et al. High-Throughput Genomics and Clinical Outcome in Hard-to-Treat Advanced Cancers: Results of the MOSCATO 01 Trial. *Cancer Discov.* **2017**, *7*, 586–595. [CrossRef]
14. Richards, S.; Aziz, N.; Bale, S.; Bick, D.; Das, S.; Gastier-Foster, J.; Grody, W.W.; Hegde, M.; Lyon, E.; Spector, E.; et al. Standards and guidelines for the interpretation of sequence variants: A joint consensus recommendation of the American College of Medical Genetics and Genomics and the Association for Molecular Pathology. *Genet Med.* **2015**, *17*, 405–424. [CrossRef]
15. Koeppen, H.; Yu, W.; Zha, J.; Pandita, A.; Penuel, E.; Rangell, L.; Raja, R.; Mohan, S.; Patel, R.; Desai, R.; et al. Biomarker analyses from a placebo-controlled phase II study evaluating erlotinib ± onartuzumab in advanced non-small cell lung cancer: MET expression levels are predictive of patient benefit. *Clin. Cancer Res.* **2014**, *20*, 4488–4498. [CrossRef] [PubMed]
16. Gelsomino, F.; Casadei-Gardini, A.; Caputo, F.; Rossi, G.; Bertolini, F.; Petrachi, T.; Spallanzani, A.; Pettorelli, E.; Kaleci, S.; Luppi, G. mTOR Pathway Expression as Potential Predictive Biomarker in Patients with Advanced Neuroendocrine Tumors Treated with Everolimus. *Cancers* **2020**, *12*, 1201. [CrossRef] [PubMed]
17. Li, S.; Kong, Y.; Si, L.; Chi, Z.; Cui, C.; Sheng, X.; Guo, J. Phosphorylation of mTOR and S6RP predicts the efficacy of everolimus in patients with metastatic renal cell carcinoma. *BMC Cancer* **2014**, *14*, 376. [CrossRef]
18. Baselga, J. Herceptin alone or in combination with chemotherapy in the treatment of HER2-positive metastatic breast cancer: Pivotal trials. *Oncology* **2001**, *61* (Suppl. 2), 14–21. [CrossRef]
19. Dawood, S.; Broglio, K.; Buzdar, A.U.; Hortobagyi, G.N.; Giordano, S.H. Prognosis of women with metastatic breast cancer by HER2 status and trastuzumab treatment: An institutional-based review. *J. Clin. Oncol.* **2010**, *28*, 92–98. [CrossRef] [PubMed]
20. Marty, M.; Cognetti, F.; Maraninchi, D.; Snyder, R.; Mauriac, L.; Tubiana-Hulin, M.; Chan, S.; Grimes, D.; Anton, A.; Lluch, A.; et al. Randomized phase II trial of the efficacy and safety of trastuzumab combined with docetaxel in patients with human epidermal growth factor receptor 2-positive metastatic breast cancer administered as first-line treatment: The M77001 study group. *J. Clin. Oncol.* **2005**, *23*, 4265–4274. [CrossRef]

21. Hassler, M.R.; Vedadinejad, M.; Flechl, B.; Haberler, C.; Preusser, M.; Hainfellner, J.A.; Wohrer, A.; Dieckmann, K.U.; Rossler, K.; Kast, R.; et al. Response to imatinib as a function of target kinase expression in recurrent glioblastoma. *SpringerPlus* **2014**, *3*, 111. [CrossRef] [PubMed]
22. Bender, R.; Lange, S. Adjusting for multiple testing–when and how? *J. Clin. Epidemiol.* **2001**, *54*, 343–349. [CrossRef]
23. Welch, D.R. Tumor Heterogeneity—A 'Contemporary Concept' Founded on Historical Insights and Predictions. *Cancer Res.* **2016**, *76*, 4–6. [CrossRef] [PubMed]
24. Meacham, C.E.; Morrison, S.J. Tumour heterogeneity and cancer cell plasticity. *Nature* **2013**, *501*, 328–337. [CrossRef] [PubMed]
25. Kim, S.T.; Lee, J.; Hong, M.; Park, K.; Park, J.O.; Ahn, T.; Park, S.H.; Park, Y.S.; Lim, H.Y.; Sun, J.M.; et al. The NEXT-1 (Next generation pErsonalized tX with mulTi-omics and preclinical model) trial: Prospective molecular screening trial of metastatic solid cancer patients, a feasibility analysis. *Oncotarget* **2015**, *6*, 33358–33368. [CrossRef]
26. Stockley, T.L.; Oza, A.M.; Berman, H.K.; Leighl, N.B.; Knox, J.J.; Shepherd, F.A.; Chen, E.X.; Krzyzanowska, M.K.; Dhani, N.; Joshua, A.M.; et al. Molecular profiling of advanced solid tumors and patient outcomes with genotype-matched clinical trials: The Princess Margaret IMPACT/COMPACT trial. *Genome Med.* **2016**, *8*, 109. [CrossRef]
27. Andre, F.; Bachelot, T.; Commo, F.; Campone, M.; Arnedos, M.; Dieras, V.; Lacroix-Triki, M.; Lacroix, L.; Cohen, P.; Gentien, D.; et al. Comparative genomic hybridisation array and DNA sequencing to direct treatment of metastatic breast cancer: A multicentre, prospective trial (SAFIR01/UNICANCER). *Lancet Oncol.* **2014**, *15*, 267–274. [CrossRef]
28. Le Tourneau, C.; Delord, J.P.; Goncalves, A.; Gavoille, C.; Dubot, C.; Isambert, N.; Campone, M.; Tredan, O.; Massiani, M.A.; Mauborgne, C.; et al. Molecularly targeted therapy based on tumour molecular profiling versus conventional therapy for advanced cancer (SHIVA): A multicentre, open-label, proof-of-concept, randomised, controlled phase 2 trial. *Lancet Oncol.* **2015**, *16*, 1324–1334. [CrossRef]
29. De Rubis, G.; Rajeev Krishnan, S.; Bebawy, M. Liquid Biopsies in Cancer Diagnosis, Monitoring, and Prognosis. *Trends Pharmacol. Sci.* **2019**, *40*, 172–186. [CrossRef]
30. Bartsch, R.; de Azambuja, E. I-SPY 2: Optimising cancer drug development in the 21st century. *ESMO Open* **2016**, *1*, e000113. [CrossRef]

Publisher's Note: MDPI stays neutral with regard to jurisdictional claims in published maps and institutional affiliations.

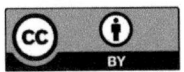

© 2020 by the authors. Licensee MDPI, Basel, Switzerland. This article is an open access article distributed under the terms and conditions of the Creative Commons Attribution (CC BY) license (http://creativecommons.org/licenses/by/4.0/).

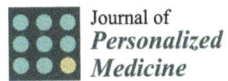

Review

Patient-Derived Tumor Xenograft Models: Toward the Establishment of Precision Cancer Medicine

Taichiro Goto

Lung Cancer and Respiratory Disease Center, Yamanashi Central Hospital, Kofu, Yamanashi 4008506, Japan; taichiro@1997.jukuin.keio.ac.jp; Tel.: +81-55-253-7111

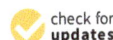

Received: 28 June 2020; Accepted: 17 July 2020; Published: 18 July 2020

Abstract: Patient-derived xenografts (PDXs) describe models involving the implantation of patient-derived tumor tissue into immunodeficient mice. Compared with conventional preclinical models involving the implantation of cancer cell lines into mice, PDXs can be characterized by the preservation of tumor heterogeneity, and the tumor microenvironment (including stroma/vasculature) more closely resembles that in patients. Consequently, the use of PDX models has improved the predictability of clinical therapeutic responses to 80% or greater, compared with approximately 5% for existing models. In the future, molecular biological analyses, omics analyses, and other experiments will be conducted using recently prepared PDX models under the strong expectation that the analysis of cancer pathophysiology, stem cells, and novel treatment targets and biomarkers will be improved, thereby promoting drug development. This review outlines the methods for preparing PDX models, advances in cancer research using PDX mice, and perspectives for the establishment of precision cancer medicine within the framework of personalized cancer medicine.

Keywords: patient-derived tumor xenograft (PDX); anti-cancer drug development; immunodeficient mice; precision medicine

1. Introduction

Tumor cells have high proliferative activity, and they actively undergo DNA synthesis. DNA damage is more likely to occur in tumor cells than in normal cells, and this damage can lead to the loss of cell viability [1]. By closely examining these features of tumor cells, compounds with the following mechanisms of action have been developed as anti-cancer drugs: (1) direct damage of DNA through adduct formation; (2) suppression of DNA synthesis through the inhibition of nucleic acid metabolism or DNA–protein complex formation; (3) suppression of cell division through the inhibition of the function of proteins involved in cell division (e.g., tubulin). Numerous standard methods of tumor treatment, each of which is designed to suppress tumor cell proliferation and induce the loss of tumor cell viability, have been established by combining two or more of these compounds [2–5]. These treatment methods are based on the concept "one size fits all," which aims to use the same treatment method for many patients [6]. Although these methods have displayed some level of therapeutic efficacy, their effects are sometimes insufficient because of adverse reactions or drug resistance. For this reason, treatment methods matching individual patients, i.e., "personalized treatment", have been explored [1,6].

Following advances in methods for studying molecular biology, thorough gene analysis of tumor cells has been conducted in recent years, leading to the detection of driver mutations involved in the acquisition of traits promoting tumor cell survival (e.g., enhanced cell proliferation, resistance to apoptosis) [7–9]. Furthermore, molecular targeted drugs, which aim to specifically eradicate tumor cells, have been newly developed by targeting these gene mutations [8–11]. These drugs are transforming cancer therapy, as observed for the HER2 inhibitor trastuzumab in breast cancer, c-Kit inhibitor imatinib in chronic myelogenous leukemia and gastrointestinal stromal tumor, and epidermal growth factor receptor inhibitor cetuximab in colorectal cancer [8,12]. Furthermore, "immune checkpoint blockade" therapy designed to eradicate tumor cells through the reactivation of tumor-suppressed immune function has proven effective in select patients. Drugs in this class, such as ipilimumab (anti-CTLA-4 antibody) and pembrolizumab (anti-PD-1 antibody), have already been introduced clinically [12–16].

Following such remarkable advances in the field of tumor treatment, active research has been conducted at a global scale to facilitate the development of additional molecular targeted drugs. However, in the research and development of molecular targeted drugs, the results of non-clinical studies rarely predict clinical efficacy. This paradox is largely attributable to the lack of appropriate non-clinical models reflecting the diversity and complexity of tumors [17,18]. In other words, the existing DNA-damaging anti-cancer drugs are based on a relatively common and simple mechanism, namely the high proliferative activity of tumor cells. These drugs have been analyzed using models involving the constant proliferation of tumor cells [14]. However, the development of molecular targeted drugs, which target specific molecules in diverse and complex tumors, requires a model that permits the appropriate expression and function of the target molecule in tumor cells [19,20]. In this context, the xenograft model, which involves the implantation of cultured tumor cell lines established from tumor tissue into immunodeficient mice, has been often used as an in vivo model for cancer research [19,20]. As is the case for in vitro models, constant tumor cell proliferation is maintained in xenograft models, and the validity of anti-cancer drugs based on the results of non-clinical studies has been assured to some extent [21]. Furthermore, the correlation of the outcomes of preclinical studies using xenograft models of cell lines possessing certain driver mutations with clinical efficacy is known [19,22]. However, because cultured cell lines consist only of specific tumor cells adapted to culture conditions that differ markedly from the in vivo environment, xenograft models of cultured cells are not considered, at present, to reflect the diversity and complexity of tumors [19,22]. One model type expected to resolve this open issue is the patient-derived xenograft (PDX) model, which involves the direct implantation of tumor tissue into immunodeficient mice without in vitro incubation (Figure 1) [18]. In the PDX model, the molecular, genetic, and histological characteristics of tumors are preserved, and it is also possible to compare PDX models among multiple cases [23–27]. Thus, this model is expected to be immediately applicable to research because it reflects the diversity and complexity of tumors [23,25,28]. Furthermore, it is possible to confirm the findings of PDX models using the patient tumor tissue from which the PDX model originated. This model type is thus expected to represent a tool used for translational research, serving as a bridge between non-clinical and clinical studies [18,28,29].

The development of novel anti-cancer drugs is an important task for prolonging the survival of patients with cancer and curing cancer itself. In recent years, active efforts have been made toward the development of new types of anti-cancer drugs (e.g., molecular targeted drugs, immune checkpoint inhibitors) in addition to the existing cytotoxic anti-cancer drugs. However, the probability that a novel anti-cancer drug will reach clinical use after the successful completion of clinical trials (Phases I through III) is as low as 5%. It is particularly common that the investigational new drugs cannot enter Phase III development after Phase II trials. This issue slows the pace of new drug development, thereby markedly increasing the expense of drug development [30]. In other words, many drugs that exhibit efficacy in preclinical studies fail to demonstrate sufficient efficacy in patients.

Compared with cell line-derived xenograft models, PDX models are expected to feature high predictability of therapeutic efficacy while preserving the inhomogeneity of the patient's tumor [31]. Large-scale PDX libraries are currently being established in Europe and the USA. In 2016, the US National Cancer Institute announced plans to switch its anti-cancer drug screening system from the "NCI-60 Human Tumor Cell Lines Screen" to PDX-based models [32]. The precise prediction of responses to treatment cannot be achieved by simply measuring the expression of proteins or mutation of genes. Furthermore, when treatment in individual patients is decided on the basis of genomic information, beneficial effects are achieved in only a limited number of patients. In addition, the identification of biomarkers based on information about the molecular background is time-consuming and insufficient for the speed of anti-cancer drug development. Under such circumstances, the PDX model is anticipated as a means for supplementing or replacing molecular biomarkers.

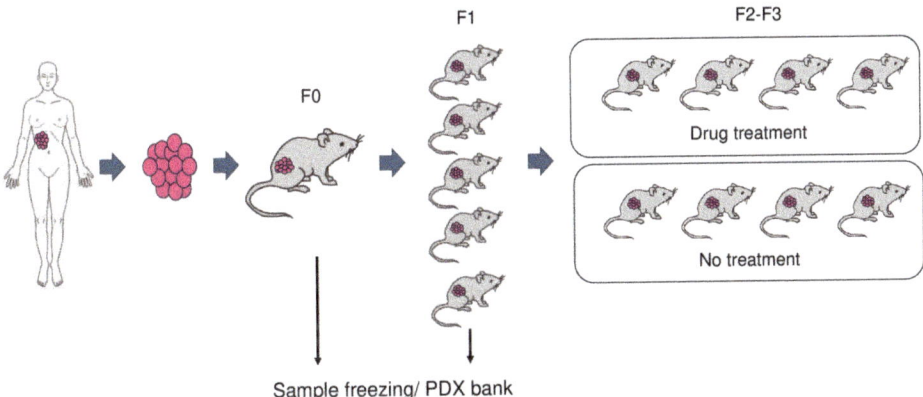

Figure 1. The grafting of patient-derived tumor cells into intensely immunodeficient mice leads to tumor growth in the mice within several months. The expanded tumor is excised. Part of the tumor is frozen, and the other part is grafted into intensely immunodeficient mice. These tumors are grafted again into intensely immunodeficient mice to conduct pathophysiological studies and evaluate drug efficacy. If the frozen patient-derived xenograft (PDX) tumor is registered with the PDX bank and a database of genetic analysis data and drug sensitivity data is created, it is expected to facilitate precision cancer medicine corresponding to the characteristics of the tumor in a given case.

2. Development and Modification of Immunodeficient Animal Models

To create a PDX model, immunodeficient mice are indispensable. Human tumors will initiate a graft versus host reaction, leading to rejection in immune-competent mice. In practice, the idea of the PDX model was triggered by the discovery of immunodeficient mice. The first generation of immunodeficient mice consisted of nude mice lacking T cells [33]. These mice were discovered early in the 1960s. Dr. Rygaard (Denmark) reported a nude mouse lacking the thymus and T lymphocytes, and it displayed a defect in T-cell-mediated immune responses and antibody formation that requires helper T cells [34]. The use of this mouse stimulated remarkable progress in basic research on immunity and cancer [35]. In addition, they remain an important resource for PDX establishment because nude mice have benefits including a relatively high engraftment ratios of gastrointestinal tumors, easy observation of subcutaneous tumors due to lack of hair, and relatively low price [31,36,37]. Later, a wide variety of immunodeficient mice were developed and modified [38]. Table 1 summarizes the lineage and characteristics of immunodeficient mice used specifically for PDX models.

Via repeated efforts to improve the efficacy of grafting, severe combined immune deficiency (SCID) mice lacking T and B cells were developed, making it possible for the first time to successfully graft human blood cells [39–41]. This was initially termed the "SCID-hu system". However, sufficient grafting required fetal tissue, and the manifestation of acquired immunity (leakiness) occurred over time in theoretically immunodeficient mice [42]. Thus, the graft survival rate was not sufficient in this model. In the 1990s, SCID mice were crossbred with non-obese diabetic (NOD) mice, yielding NOD/SCID mice with composite immunodeficiency (e.g., T/B cell defect + NK cell malfunction) [43–46]. NOD/SCID mice have a markedly improved human hematopoietic cell graft survival rate, and they remain in extensive use. However, NOD/SCID mice have several shortcomings, including the lack of T cell graft survival, the absence of long-term observation (because of the high incidence of thymoma and a short lifespan), and the lack of graft survival for stem cell systems other than the hematopoietic system.

Table 1. Development and characteristics of immunodeficient mice used in animal models.

Characteristic	Nude	SCID	NOD/SCID	NOG
Reporting year	1966	1983	1995	2002
Mutated gene	Foxn1	Prkdc	Prkdc	Prkdc, Il-2rg
T cell	×	×	×	×
B cell	○	×	×	×
NK cell	○	○	△	×
Engraftment of human cells				
Normal HSC	–	+	++	+++
Tumor cell	+	++	+++	++++
Success rate of PDX	Low	Low	Moderate	High

○: intact, △: deficit, ×: none. HSC: human hematopoietic cells. The Success rate of engraftment is represented by – (negative) or + (positive), with more + indicating higher possibility.

To further improve the graft survival rate, in the 2000s, a new trait (common gamma chain knockout) was introduced into NOD/SCID mice, yielding NOG mice [47,48]. NOG mice were created by crossbreeding NOD-scid (NOD/Shi-scid) mice with IL-2Rγc^{null} mice, and they exhibit composite immunodeficiency (T, B, and NK cell defects and dendrocyte/macrophage malfunction; Table 1) [38,49,50]. Because of these characteristics, NOG mice are considered the best immunodeficient animals for human tissue graft transplantation [18,50]. In essence, engraftment ratios are higher in more immunocompromised mice (Nude < SCID < NOD/ SCID < NOG) (Table 1) [36].

3. Creation of PDX Models

A PDX model is created by grafting a patient-derived tumor sample into immunodeficient mice (Figure 1) [37,51]. Usually, tumor growth begins within several months after grafting (F0). At that time, part of the graft is used for genetic analysis, such as whole-exome sequencing, RNA sequencing, and copy number alteration, to analyze the genetic characteristics of the tumor, and another part of the graft is stored in the PDX tissue bank. Part of the tissue is grafted into immunodeficient mice (F1), and the tumor after proliferation is frozen in a large quantity. If these tumor samples are grafted simultaneously into numerous mice and candidate drugs are administered to the mice, it is possible to screen and identify drugs that are effective against the patient's tumor. If the results of gene analysis are compared with the clinical data, it is possible to cultivate the path for personalized treatment. With the PDX model, tumor growth in vivo in mice accelerates as passaging is repeated. In the F3 generation, the patient-derived sample is approximately identical to the genetic expression profile. Thereafter, the genetic profile changes with further passaging [18]. For this reason, it has been recommended to use tumor of F3 or earlier generations in PDX model-based evaluation.

PDX tumors possess the genetic characteristics and tumor heterogeneity that are more similar to the patient's derived tumor than to the tumor cell line. These tumors contain patient-derived cells such as stromal cells/cancer-associated fibroblast and tumor-associated macrophages before they are gradually replaced by mouse cells as the passage increases. PDX models, especially in the early passages, are therefore expected to be applicable to clinical and pathophysiological analyses of tumor and anti-tumor drug development because the models most closely resemble the clinical environment. PDX models have already been created for many cancer types. Reports are available concerning their creation for solid cancers (e.g., breast cancer, lung cancer, pancreatic cancer, colorectal cancer, melanoma, head and neck cancer, prostate cancer, renal cell carcinoma, glioblastoma, ovarian cancer) and blood tumors (e.g., leukemia, lymphoma) [18].

Following the recent development of intensely immunodeficient mice presenting with various types of immunodeficiency, the grafting efficiency of PDX models has been remarkably improved (Table 1). However, the long-term rearing of intensely immunodeficient mice requires an SPF (specific pathogen free) setting, and the breeding of such mice is difficult. It is therefore desirable to use mouse strains that are suitable for the target type of tumor by precisely assessing the advantages and shortcomings of individual mice. It must be considered that 3–6 months are usually required to establish a PDX model.

The graft survival rate of PDX models varies depending on the type of tumor involved (Table 2). Colorectal and pancreatic cancers have high graft survival rates, and a favorable outcome to some extent may be expected even when nude mice are used. Conversely, ultra-intensely immunodeficient mice such as NOG, NSG (NOD/Scid/IL2Rγ-null), and NOJ (NOD/Scid/Jak3-null) mice are required to establish PDX models of hematopoietic tumors [52]. The grafting efficiency usually tends to be higher in mice with more intense immunodeficiency, but mice with intense immunodeficiency are more difficult to rear. Furthermore, the probability of the successful establishment of PDX lesions is higher for metastatic foci than for the primary lesion, and this tendency is more marked for tumors with greater malignant potential [53]. Regarding the shape of the tumor used for this model, a square tissue section of several millimeters in size, excised from the patient's tumor via biopsy or surgery, is usually used. In recent years, reports have described the creation of PDXs using circulating tumor cells or bodily fluids (e.g., cancerous hydrothorax, cancerous ascites) [54]. Regarding the recipient site, subcutaneous tissue is generally used because subcutaneous grafting is simpler and it permits the easy evaluation of tumor growth after grafting. However, the efficiency of subcutaneous grafting is low for breast and prostate cancers. For this reason, breast cancer is grafted into the mammary glands of female mice to enable the efficient creation of PDXs, and prostate cancer is grafted into the prostate glands of male mice (orthotopic implantation) [55]. It is also known that the grafting efficiency of hormone-dependent tumors (e.g., breast cancer, prostate cancer) increases if human hormones are replenished [18,53]. Thus, four essential elements for the establishment of PDX models are as follows: (1) properties of the tumor (primary lesion/metastatic foci or surgical specimen/biopsy specimen/humoral cells); (2) selection of recipient mice; (3) recipient site; (4) replenishment based on tumor characteristics (hormone treatment).

In practice, the graft survival rate varies greatly depending on the tumor type. High graft survival rates (80% or higher) have been reported for malignant melanoma and colorectal cancer, whereas the rate is as low as approximately 30% for breast cancer (the mean graft survival rate for 18 tumor types was approximately 50%; Table 2) [56,57]. Furthermore, in the case of triple-negative breast cancer, the graft survival rate following orthotopic implantation is 60–86% (more than twice the rate after subcutaneous implantation). This also suggests the importance of recipient site selection.

Table 2. Comparison of patient-derived xenograft graft survival rates based on the primary lesion site.

Tumor Type	Engraftment Rate
Melanoma	88% (n = 8)
Colorectal	85% (n = 112)
Head and neck	68% (n = 53)
Pancreatic	65% (n = 62)
Sarcoma	63% (n = 161)
Gastroesophageal	62% (n = 42)
Liver and biliary duct	54% (n = 35)
Lung	50% (n = 129)
Bladder	43% (n = 30)
Brain and neurological	40% (n = 15)
Ovarian	37% (n = 138)
Mesothelioma	36% (n = 11)
Breast	30% (n = 155)
Renal cell carcinoma	25% (n = 114)

Quoted from Ref Izumchenko et al. [57].

In recent years, active efforts have begun to be made toward the development of new methods of cancer treatment focusing on human immunity (e.g., immune checkpoint inhibitors). The PDX model uses immunodeficient mice, i.e., mice with markedly compromised immune function. Therefore, the balance of hematopoietic and immune cells remains different from that in humans and theoretically, the immune cell–tumor cell interaction may be totally missing in this model. If these drugs are administered to immunodeficient mice, then reactions of immunocompetent cells differing from those observed in humans are anticipated. These issues require attention for the development of a patient-similar immune response PDX model. For this reason, humanized mice (intensely immunodeficient mice implanted with human immunocompetent cells or umbilical cord-derived hematopoietic stem cells) are sometimes used to create PDX models. In some studies, humanized mice were created using immunocompetent cells derived from patients with cancer, and these mice were implanted with the patient's tumor to create PDXs and evaluate drug efficacy [58,59]. However, this approach is not yet extensively applicable because of problems as follows: (1) there is no model completely reflecting the human immune system; (2) intense host rejection occurs frequently, making long-term evaluation difficult; and (3) the costs are high [38].

4. Prediction of Cancer Response to Treatment Using the PDX Model

Large-scale PDX libraries are being established in Europe and the USA and utilized for drug development and biomarker screening. In 2013, "EurOPDX" was organized by 16 universities and public institutions in Europe. To date, more than 1500 PDX types, including rare cancers, have been established [56]. Furthermore, the Jackson Institute (USA) has begun to publicize the genetic and histopathological information of more than 450 types of PDXs established on its website. At the same time, the institute has initiated the industrial utilization of PDXs by commercializing various PDX mice.

The greatest advantage of PDX use is the high predictability of treatment response. When the efficacy of 129 drugs was evaluated using 92 PDX types, the response rate evaluated using PDX models had 87% agreement with the clinical response rate (112/129), and the variance depending on the site of the primary lesion was also small (81–100%) [57]. In another study designed to compare the efficacy of treatment using approximately 1000 types of PDXs with the clinical efficacy, the rate of agreement was as high as 66% [60]. This agreement rate was excellent compared with that of conventional tumor cell grafting models (approximately 5%). If drugs targeted for clinical development and the subjects anticipated to respond to them can be selected efficiently using PDX models in preclinical studies, the mental/physical stress on clinical trial participants and the cost of clinical development will be reduced. Furthermore, because PDX models enable tumor collection over time (e.g., before and after drug efficacy evaluation), PDXs may contribute to clarifying the pharmacokinetics, response, and resistance development mechanisms of tumors.

PDX models are also expected to play important roles in the development of treatments for rare cancers. As the definition suggests, the number of patients with rare cancers is extremely small. This feature is usually considered disadvantageous from the viewpoints of diagnosis and treatment. Furthermore, because the collection of clinical specimens and implementation of large-scale clinical trials are difficult for rare cancers, the development of treatments generally does not proceed smoothly. Therefore, the creation of PDX models using specimens from patients with rare cancers may permit the collection of samples needed for drug efficacy evaluation and pathophysiological analysis. In addition, this strategy will enable the confirmation of proof of concept during preclinical or early clinical studies, thus promoting remarkable advances in the development of treatments and clarification of the mechanisms of carcinogenesis (e.g., genetic factors).

5. Cancer Stem Cells and PDXs

Previously, cancer was considered to be a group of single cells that deviated from the normal mechanism for preserving the living body, resulting in permanent proliferation. However, it has been increasingly recognized that a group containing a small number of cells called "cancer stem cells" is present in both blood tumors and solid cancers [61]. According to this cancer stem cell hypothesis, stem cells similar to normal tissue are also present in tumor tissue, and they have the potential for self-renewal, accompanied by the ability to form a tumor similar to the original tumor tissue despite being small in number [62]. Cancer stem cells are considered to maintain stemness for a long period, similarly to tissue stem cells. They divide more slowly than daughter cells, and thus, they are resistant to conventional anti-cancer drugs or radiotherapy (Figure 2) [63]. Furthermore, it has been suggested that these cells exhibit relatively strong resistance to molecular targeted drugs [64]. Therefore, the risk for recurrence or metastasis is considered high if cancer stem cells are not eradicated, even in cases in which the tumor is not clinically detectable after treatment. Furthermore, recurrent or metastatic cancer usually has high resistance to drugs, and therefore, it has been highlighted as a major factor for poor prognosis. Under such circumstances, treatment methods targeting cancer stem cells are anticipated as a promising therapeutic strategy.

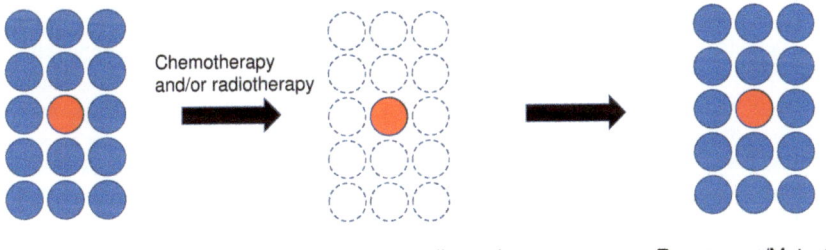

Figure 2. Schematic diagram of cancer stem cells responsible for recurrence/metastasis. Cancer stem cells are likely to remain after treatment because they are resistant to anti-cancer drugs or radiotherapy. They are considered to serve as a cause for recurrence/metastasis.

It has been reported that a specific subpopulation within a tumor is more likely to form a tumor than the other subpopulations when grafted into mice [61]. Following this finding, the concept of cancer stem cells became widely accepted. To reveal that specific cells have the nature of stem cells in a study of cancer stem cells, it is necessary to demonstrate in vivo that a tumor composed of heterogeneous cell groups can be formed. When such an analysis is conducted, PDX are more informative than cell lines, which have been maintained for a long periods in two dimensions, on a non-natural surface, which may have led to genetic drift and selection [31]. Because cancer stem cells are present in tumors in extremely small quantities, there may be cases in which the tumor is too small to secure the quantity of stem cells needed for analysis via flow cytometric sorting. In such cases, new PDXs having undergone a few rounds of passaging are sometimes used [65]. If the nature of cancer stem cells is further clarified using PDX models, then the development of effective treatments, either selectively targeting cancer stem cells or simultaneously targeting both cancer stem cells and other cancer cells, will be facilitated.

6. Open Issues Related to PDX Models

PDX models are considered promising tools for tumor research, but several open issues have been identified. PDX models cannot be established from all patient-derived tumors. It has been stated that the models are difficult to establish from some tumor tissues [18,20]. Furthermore, substantial resources (e.g., money, time, labor) are needed to create PDX models [18,20]. To extensively use PDX models in tumor research, it is indispensable to improve the efficiency of model creation by using greater amounts of tumor tissue [18–20].

If genetic analysis and drug sensitivity testing are conducted and the tumor characteristics and clinical information are analyzed simultaneously, established PDX models, as well as the databases constructed from the collected data and information, are expected to be useful in the personalization of treatment corresponding to the characteristics of tumors in individual patients. The EurOPDX and Jackson Institute databases contain large numbers of samples, and they have started to make samples publicly available [52,56]. Some pharmaceutical companies are also creating their own PDX libraries. Novartis reported the results of drug screening using more than 1000 PDX types [60]. The tumor characteristics differ by ethnicity and region. For this reason, it is desirable that such large-scale libraries are established globally.

As mentioned previously, a considerably large number of PDXs have already been established and utilized in various studies (e.g., drug efficacy evaluation) and the promotion of personalized treatment. However, the methods and evaluation of PDX creation and studies using PDX have not yet been sufficiently standardized. For example, the appropriate frequency of PDX passaging differs among investigators. "EurOPDX" recommends the use of PDXs after five or fewer passages for studies such as drug efficacy evaluation because the tumor stroma derived from the patient is increasingly replaced with mouse stroma with increasing passaging, possibly causing discrepancy of the clinical interactions between tumor cells and the stroma [56]. A study by the Broad Institute demonstrated that genomic mutations present in patients' tumors are lost with increasing passaging, resulting in the loss of the genetic characteristics of the tumor [66]. Furthermore, it is plausible that dynamic changes of genes occur during the course of growth and infiltration of patients' tumors, occasionally leading to the appearance of mutations not present in PDXs. For this reason, it is difficult to set certain conditions for each PDX unilaterally. It appears essential to store patients' specimens and the tissue/specimens obtained during passaging in close linkage with data including treatment history, genomic information, and other data collected from various studies (e.g., omics analysis). In addition, it is critical to use the PDX for each study after sufficient assessment concerning whether the model satisfies the requirements for a given setting of use.

The maintenance of PDX libraries results in the accumulation of large amounts of data from clinical practice and studies, and these data should be maintained with high levels of privacy. According to the current main practice in Europe and the USA, the collected data are made public on websites and other media, after anonymization, to permit the free use by researchers and clinicians. However, the control and disposal of such data requires significant labor and financial expenditure. It is therefore difficult for an individual or single institution to establish and maintain a PDX library. It is desirable to form a consortium of multiple institutions, clearly defining to whom the PDX, as well as the patent and financial rights related to its research, should belong at the stage of planning.

Furthermore, crossreactivity between human and mouse proteins (e.g., humoral factors) can occur in PDX models. Regarding the genetic homology between frequently used experimental animals and humans, the homology between mice and humans has been reported at approximately 92% (versus 99.9% between humans). Thus, even proteins with the same function can differ slightly in terms of amino acid structure between humans and mice, leading to the lack of binding between a ligand and its receptor and the absence of signal transduction [67]. To resolve this problem, attempts have been made to achieve a more faithful reproduction of diseases by introducing human cytokine and HLA genes into various immunodeficient mice and creating next-generation immunodeficient mice capable of producing human proteins (e.g., cytokines) [68–70].

7. Application to Personalized Treatment

In the case of cancer, heterogeneous cell groups are present within a single tumor, and furthermore, tumors located at the same site exhibit many differences between patients [71,72]. For this reason, the need for personalized treatment is being emphasized. Identification of the gene mutation serving as a driver via target or exome sequencing provides a useful tool for predicting an effective treatment method in silico, and this strategy is expected to be adopted actively in the age of personalized treatment [73–75]. If the prediction of treatment methods using bioinformatics is combined with the evaluation of responses to drugs in vivo using PDX models, integrated personalized treatment will be enabled. The PDX model created using tumor tissue derived from individual patients can supply information regarding the response of tumors to various drugs, thus enabling evaluation of the efficacy of treatments prior to clinical use (Figure 3). Thus, PDXs are expected to contribute to advancing the personalization of treatment.

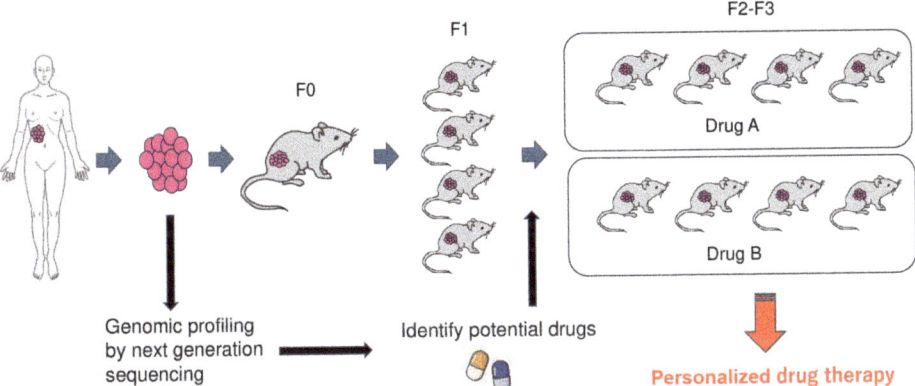

Figure 3. Grafting of patient-derived tumor cells into intensely immunodeficient mice leads to tumor growth within several months. The expanded tumor is excised. Part of the tumor is frozen, and the other part is again grafted into intensely immunodeficient mice. Multiple candidate drugs are selected corresponding to the genetic profile of a given tumor, and each drug is administered to the PDX mice to evaluate its efficacy. If drug sensitivity data collected using these are utilized for patients, then precision cancer medicine may become possible.

Meanwhile, PDX models can also take significant time to create, which may pose a challenge to patients with advanced stages of cancer. For example, growth rates of prostate cancer PDX are slow, needing many months to generate models [76]. The time to initial growth is reported to be from four up to over 12 months, and time from implantation to initial growth of secondary passage ranges from 6 to 36 weeks, partly due to the differences in androgen levels between human and mouse [26,77]. This time-consuming process is clearly beyond the period that would be useful to define the best treatment modality. If problems such as the low graft survival rate and the time required for tumor formation can be resolved, PDX models will be extremely helpful in tailoring treatment to individual patients.

8. Conclusions

Following the recent development of intensely immunodeficient mice that permit the grafting, proliferation, and differentiation of human cells, it is currently possible to create PDXs of various tumors. PDX models faithfully reproduce human tumors. If drug screening is extensively conducted, then the number of new drug candidates that fail to proceed beyond phase II development may be reduced, thereby improving the efficiency of anti-cancer drug development. This will undoubtedly serve as an extremely valuable tool for translational research. In the near future, further modification of intensely immunodeficient mice and the enrichment of PDX libraries are expected to stimulate further advances in the application of PDX models to precision cancer medicine.

Funding: This research received no external funding.

Acknowledgments: We greatly appreciate the contributions of Yosuke Hirotsu, Yoshihiro Miyashita and Kenji Amemiya in helpful scientific discussions.

Conflicts of Interest: The author declares no conflict of interest.

References

1. Cheung-Ong, K.; Giaever, G.; Nislow, C. DNA-damaging agents in cancer chemotherapy: Serendipity and chemical biology. *Chem. Biol.* **2013**, *20*, 648–659. [CrossRef] [PubMed]
2. Chabner, B.A.; Roberts, T.G., Jr. Timeline: Chemotherapy and the war on cancer. *Nat. Rev. Cancer* **2005**, *5*, 65–72. [CrossRef] [PubMed]

3. Dasari, S.; Tchounwou, P.B. Cisplatin in cancer therapy: Molecular mechanisms of action. *Eur. J. Pharm.* **2014**, *740*, 364–378. [CrossRef] [PubMed]
4. Minotti, G.; Menna, P.; Salvatorelli, E.; Cairo, G.; Gianni, L. Anthracyclines: Molecular advances and pharmacologic developments in antitumor activity and cardiotoxicity. *Pharm. Rev.* **2004**, *56*, 185–229. [CrossRef]
5. Wilson, P.M.; Danenberg, P.V.; Johnston, P.G.; Lenz, H.J.; Ladner, R.D. Standing the test of time: Targeting thymidylate biosynthesis in cancer therapy. *Nat. Rev. Clin. Oncol.* **2014**, *11*, 282–298. [CrossRef]
6. Kalia, M. Personalized oncology: Recent advances and future challenges. *Metabolism* **2013**, *62* (Suppl. 1), S11–S14. [CrossRef]
7. Goto, T.; Hirotsu, Y.; Amemiya, K.; Mochizuki, H.; Omata, M. Understanding intratumor heterogeneity and evolution in NSCLC and potential new therapeutic approach. *Cancers* **2018**, *10*, 212. [CrossRef]
8. Martini, M.; Vecchione, L.; Siena, S.; Tejpar, S.; Bardelli, A. Targeted therapies: How personal should we go? *Nat. Rev. Clin. Oncol.* **2011**, *9*, 87–97. [CrossRef]
9. Torkamani, A.; Verkhivker, G.; Schork, N.J. Cancer driver mutations in protein kinase genes. *Cancer Lett.* **2009**, *281*, 117–127. [CrossRef]
10. Higuchi, R.; Nakagomi, T.; Goto, T.; Hirotsu, Y.; Shikata, D.; Yokoyama, Y.; Otake, S.; Amemiya, K.; Oyama, T.; Mochizuki, H.; et al. Identification of clonality through genomic profile analysis in multiple lung cancers. *J. Clin. Med.* **2020**, *9*, 573. [CrossRef]
11. Nakagomi, T.; Goto, T.; Hirotsu, Y.; Shikata, D.; Amemiya, K.; Oyama, T.; Mochizuki, H.; Omata, M. Elucidation of radiation-resistant clones by a serial study of intratumor heterogeneity before and after stereotactic radiotherapy in lung cancer. *J. Thorac. Dis.* **2017**, *9*, E598–E604. [CrossRef] [PubMed]
12. Arnedos, M.; Soria, J.C.; Andre, F.; Tursz, T. Personalized treatments of cancer patients: A reality in daily practice, a costly dream or a shared vision of the future from the oncology community? *Cancer Treat Rev.* **2014**, *40*, 1192–1198. [CrossRef] [PubMed]
13. Kunimasa, K.; Goto, T. Immunosurveillance and immunoediting of lung cancer: Current perspectives and challenges. *Int. J. Mol. Sci.* **2020**, *21*, 597. [CrossRef] [PubMed]
14. Moffat, J.G.; Rudolph, J.; Bailey, D. Phenotypic screening in cancer drug discovery—Past, present and future. *Nat. Rev. Drug Discov.* **2014**, *13*, 588–602. [CrossRef] [PubMed]
15. Postow, M.A.; Callahan, M.K.; Wolchok, J.D. Immune checkpoint blockade in cancer therapy. *J. Clin. Oncol.* **2015**, *33*, 1974–1982. [CrossRef]
16. Goto, T. Radiation as an In Situ Auto-Vaccination: Current perspectives and challenges. *Vaccines* **2019**, *7*, 100. [CrossRef]
17. Stock, J.K.; Jones, N.P.; Hammonds, T.; Roffey, J.; Dillon, C. Addressing the right targets in oncology: Challenges and alternative approaches. *J. Biomol. Screen* **2015**, *20*, 305–317. [CrossRef]
18. Tentler, J.J.; Tan, A.C.; Weekes, C.D.; Jimeno, A.; Leong, S.; Pitts, T.M.; Arcaroli, J.J.; Messersmith, W.A.; Eckhardt, S.G. Patient-derived tumour xenografts as models for oncology drug development. *Nat. Rev. Clin. Oncol.* **2012**, *9*, 338–350. [CrossRef]
19. Ruggeri, B.A.; Camp, F.; Miknyoczki, S. Animal models of disease: Pre-clinical animal models of cancer and their applications and utility in drug discovery. *Biochem. Pharm.* **2014**, *87*, 150–161. [CrossRef]
20. Williams, S.A.; Anderson, W.C.; Santaguida, M.T.; Dylla, S.J. Patient-derived xenografts, the cancer stem cell paradigm, and cancer pathobiology in the 21st century. *Lab. Investig.* **2013**, *93*, 970–982. [CrossRef]
21. Kerbel, R.S. Human tumor xenografts as predictive preclinical models for anticancer drug activity in humans: Better than commonly perceived-but they can be improved. *Cancer Biol.* **2003**, *2*, S134–S139. [CrossRef]
22. Wilding, J.L.; Bodmer, W.F. Cancer cell lines for drug discovery and development. *Cancer Res.* **2014**, *74*, 2377–2384. [CrossRef] [PubMed]
23. Burgenske, D.M.; Monsma, D.J.; Dylewski, D.; Scott, S.B.; Sayfie, A.D.; Kim, D.G.; Luchtefeld, M.; Martin, K.R.; Stephenson, P.; Hostetter, G.; et al. Establishment of genetically diverse patient-derived xenografts of colorectal cancer. *Am. J. Cancer Res.* **2014**, *4*, 824–837. [PubMed]
24. DeRose, Y.S.; Wang, G.; Lin, Y.C.; Bernard, P.S.; Buys, S.S.; Ebbert, M.T.; Factor, R.; Matsen, C.; Milash, B.A.; Nelson, E.; et al. Tumor grafts derived from women with breast cancer authentically reflect tumor pathology, growth, metastasis and disease outcomes. *Nat. Med.* **2011**, *17*, 1514–1520. [CrossRef] [PubMed]

25. Dong, X.; Guan, J.; English, J.C.; Flint, J.; Yee, J.; Evans, K.; Murray, N.; Macaulay, C.; Ng, R.T.; Gout, P.W.; et al. Patient-derived first generation xenografts of non-small cell lung cancers: Promising tools for predicting drug responses for personalized chemotherapy. *Clin. Cancer Res.* **2010**, *16*, 1442–1451. [CrossRef] [PubMed]
26. Lin, D.; Wyatt, A.W.; Xue, H.; Wang, Y.; Dong, X.; Haegert, A.; Wu, R.; Brahmbhatt, S.; Mo, F.; Jong, L.; et al. High fidelity patient-derived xenografts for accelerating prostate cancer discovery and drug development. *Cancer Res.* **2014**, *74*, 1272–1283. [CrossRef]
27. Monsma, D.J.; Monks, N.R.; Cherba, D.M.; Dylewski, D.; Eugster, E.; Jahn, H.; Srikanth, S.; Scott, S.B.; Richardson, P.J.; Everts, R.E.; et al. Genomic characterization of explant tumorgraft models derived from fresh patient tumor tissue. *J. Transl. Med.* **2012**, *10*, 125. [CrossRef]
28. Malaney, P.; Nicosia, S.V.; Dave, V. One mouse, one patient paradigm: New avatars of personalized cancer therapy. *Cancer Lett.* **2014**, *344*, 1–12. [CrossRef]
29. Doroshow, J.H.; Kummar, S. Translational research in oncology—10 years of progress and future prospects. *Nat. Rev. Clin. Oncol.* **2014**, *11*, 649–662. [CrossRef]
30. DiMasi, J.A.; Reichert, J.M.; Feldman, L.; Malins, A. Clinical approval success rates for investigational cancer drugs. *Clin. Pharm.* **2013**, *94*, 329–335. [CrossRef]
31. Xu, C.; Li, X.; Liu, P.; Li, M.; Luo, F. Patient-derived xenograft mouse models: A high fidelity tool for individualized medicine. *Oncol. Lett.* **2019**, *17*, 3–10. [CrossRef] [PubMed]
32. Ledford, H. US cancer institute to overhaul tumour cell lines. *Nature* **2016**, *530*, 391. [CrossRef] [PubMed]
33. Flanagan, S.P. 'Nude', a new hairless gene with pleiotropic effects in the mouse. *Genet. Res.* **1966**, *8*, 295–309. [CrossRef]
34. Rygaard, J. Immunobiology of the mouse mutant "Nude". Preliminary investigations. *Acta Pathol. Microbiol. Scand.* **1969**, *77*, 761–762. [CrossRef] [PubMed]
35. Rygaard, J.; Povlsen, C.O. Heterotransplantation of a human malignant tumour to "Nude" mice. *Acta Pathol. Microbiol. Scand.* **1969**, *77*, 758–760. [CrossRef]
36. Collins, A.T.; Lang, S.H. A systematic review of the validity of patient derived xenograft (PDX) models: The implications for translational research and personalised medicine. *PeerJ* **2018**, *6*, e5981. [CrossRef]
37. Okada, S.; Vaeteewoottacharn, K.; Kariya, R. Establishment of a patient-derived tumor xenograft model and application for precision cancer medicine. *Chem. Pharm. Bull.* **2018**, *66*, 225–230. [CrossRef]
38. Shultz, L.D.; Ishikawa, F.; Greiner, D.L. Humanized mice in translational biomedical research. *Nat. Rev. Immunol.* **2007**, *7*, 118–130. [CrossRef]
39. McCune, J.M.; Namikawa, R.; Kaneshima, H.; Shultz, L.D.; Lieberman, M.; Weissman, I.L. The SCID-hu mouse: Murine model for the analysis of human hematolymphoid differentiation and function. *Science* **1988**, *241*, 1632–1639. [CrossRef]
40. Mosier, D.E.; Gulizia, R.J.; Baird, S.M.; Wilson, D.B. Transfer of a functional human immune system to mice with severe combined immunodeficiency. *Nature* **1988**, *335*, 256–259. [CrossRef]
41. Bosma, G.C.; Custer, R.P.; Bosma, M.J. A severe combined immunodeficiency mutation in the mouse. *Nature* **1983**, *301*, 527–530. [CrossRef] [PubMed]
42. Bosma, G.C.; Fried, M.; Custer, R.P.; Carroll, A.; Gibson, D.M.; Bosma, M.J. Evidence of functional lymphocytes in some (leaky) scid mice. *J. Exp. Med.* **1988**, *167*, 1016–1033. [CrossRef] [PubMed]
43. Koyanagi, Y.; Tanaka, Y.; Kira, J.; Ito, M.; Hioki, K.; Misawa, N.; Kawano, Y.; Yamasaki, K.; Tanaka, R.; Suzuki, Y.; et al. Primary human immunodeficiency virus type 1 viremia and central nervous system invasion in a novel hu-PBL-immunodeficient mouse strain. *J. Virol.* **1997**, *71*, 2417–2424. [CrossRef] [PubMed]
44. Lowry, P.A.; Shultz, L.D.; Greiner, D.L.; Hesselton, R.M.; Kittler, E.L.; Tiarks, C.Y.; Rao, S.S.; Reilly, J.; Leif, J.H.; Ramshaw, H.; et al. Improved engraftment of human cord blood stem cells in NOD/LtSz-scid/scid mice after irradiation or multiple-day injections into unirradiated recipients. *Biol. Blood Marrow Transpl..* **1996**, *2*, 15–23.
45. Pflumio, F.; Izac, B.; Katz, A.; Shultz, L.D.; Vainchenker, W.; Coulombel, L. Phenotype and function of human hematopoietic cells engrafting immune-deficient CB17-severe combined immunodeficiency mice and nonobese diabetic-severe combined immunodeficiency mice after transplantation of human cord blood mononuclear cells. *Blood* **1996**, *88*, 3731–3740. [CrossRef]
46. Ueda, T.; Yoshino, H.; Kobayashi, K.; Kawahata, M.; Ebihara, Y.; Ito, M.; Asano, S.; Nakahata, T.; Tsuji, K. Hematopoietic repopulating ability of cord blood CD34(+) cells in NOD/Shi-scid mice. *Stem Cells* **2000**, *18*, 204–213. [CrossRef]

47. Ito, M.; Hiramatsu, H.; Kobayashi, K.; Suzue, K.; Kawahata, M.; Hioki, K.; Ueyama, Y.; Koyanagi, Y.; Sugamura, K.; Tsuji, K.; et al. NOD/SCID/gamma(c)(null) mouse: An excellent recipient mouse model for engraftment of human cells. *Blood* **2002**, *100*, 3175–3182. [CrossRef]
48. Ito, M.; Kobayashi, K.; Nakahata, T. NOD/Shi-scid IL2rgamma(null) (NOG) mice more appropriate for humanized mouse models. *Curr. Top Microbiol. Immunol.* **2008**, *324*, 53–76. [CrossRef]
49. Hiramatsu, H.; Nishikomori, R.; Heike, T.; Ito, M.; Kobayashi, K.; Katamura, K.; Nakahata, T. Complete reconstitution of human lymphocytes from cord blood CD34+ cells using the NOD/SCID/gammacnull mice model. *Blood* **2003**, *102*, 873–880. [CrossRef]
50. Zhou, Q.; Facciponte, J.; Jin, M.; Shen, Q.; Lin, Q. Humanized NOD-SCID IL2rg-/-mice as a preclinical model for cancer research and its potential use for individualized cancer therapies. *Cancer Lett.* **2014**, *344*, 13–19. [CrossRef]
51. Morton, C.L.; Houghton, P.J. Establishment of human tumor xenografts in immunodeficient mice. *Nat. Protoc.* **2007**, *2*, 247–250. [CrossRef] [PubMed]
52. Shultz, L.D.; Goodwin, N.; Ishikawa, F.; Hosur, V.; Lyons, B.L.; Greiner, D.L. Human cancer growth and therapy in immunodeficient mouse models. *Cold Spring Harb. Protoc.* **2014**, *2014*, 694–708. [CrossRef] [PubMed]
53. Cho, S.Y.; Kang, W.; Han, J.Y.; Min, S.; Kang, J.; Lee, A.; Kwon, J.Y.; Lee, C.; Park, H. An integrative approach to precision cancer medicine using patient-derived xenografts. *Mol. Cells* **2016**, *39*, 77–86. [CrossRef]
54. Lallo, A.; Schenk, M.W.; Frese, K.K.; Blackhall, F.; Dive, C. Circulating tumor cells and CDX models as a tool for preclinical drug development. *Transl. Lung Cancer Res* **2017**, *6*, 397–408. [CrossRef] [PubMed]
55. Sia, D.; Moeini, A.; Labgaa, I.; Villanueva, A. The future of patient-derived tumor xenografts in cancer treatment. *Pharmacogenomics* **2015**, *16*, 1671–1683. [CrossRef] [PubMed]
56. Byrne, A.T.; Alferez, D.G.; Amant, F.; Annibali, D.; Arribas, J.; Biankin, A.V.; Bruna, A.; Budinska, E.; Caldas, C.; Chang, D.K.; et al. Interrogating open issues in cancer precision medicine with patient-derived xenografts. *Nat. Rev. Cancer* **2017**, *17*, 254–268. [CrossRef] [PubMed]
57. Izumchenko, E.; Paz, K.; Ciznadija, D.; Sloma, I.; Katz, A.; Vasquez-Dunddel, D.; Ben-Zvi, I.; Stebbing, J.; McGuire, W.; Harris, W.; et al. Patient-derived xenografts effectively capture responses to oncology therapy in a heterogeneous cohort of patients with solid tumors. *Ann. Oncol.* **2017**, *28*, 2595–2605. [CrossRef]
58. Holzapfel, B.M.; Wagner, F.; Thibaudeau, L.; Levesque, J.P.; Hutmacher, D.W. Concise review: Humanized models of tumor immunology in the 21st century: Convergence of cancer research and tissue engineering. *Stem Cells* **2015**, *33*, 1696–1704. [CrossRef]
59. Morton, J.J.; Bird, G.; Refaeli, Y.; Jimeno, A. Humanized mouse xenograft models: Narrowing the tumor-microenvironment gap. *Cancer Res.* **2016**, *76*, 6153–6158. [CrossRef]
60. Gao, H.; Korn, J.M.; Ferretti, S.; Monahan, J.E.; Wang, Y.; Singh, M.; Zhang, C.; Schnell, C.; Yang, G.; Zhang, Y.; et al. High-throughput screening using patient-derived tumor xenografts to predict clinical trial drug response. *Nat. Med.* **2015**, *21*, 1318–1325. [CrossRef]
61. Liu, Q.; Luo, Q.; Ju, Y.; Song, G. Role of the mechanical microenvironment in cancer development and progression. *Cancer Biol. Med.* **2020**, *17*, 282–292. [CrossRef] [PubMed]
62. Ayob, A.Z.; Ramasamy, T.S. Cancer stem cells as key drivers of tumour progression. *J. Biomed. Sci.* **2018**, *25*, 20. [CrossRef] [PubMed]
63. Marin, J.J.G.; Macias, R.I.R.; Monte, M.J.; Romero, M.R.; Asensio, M.; Sanchez-Martin, A.; Cives-Losada, C.; Temprano, A.G.; Espinosa-Escudero, R.; Reviejo, M.; et al. Molecular bases of drug resistance in hepatocellular carcinoma. *Cancers* **2020**, *12*, 1663. [CrossRef] [PubMed]
64. Rahman, M.A.; Saha, S.K.; Rahman, M.S.; Uddin, M.J.; Uddin, M.S.; Pang, M.G.; Rhim, H.; Cho, S.G. Molecular insights into therapeutic potential of autophagy modulation by natural products for cancer stem cells. *Front. Cell Dev. Biol.* **2020**, *8*, 283. [CrossRef]
65. Lai, Y.; Wei, X.; Lin, S.; Qin, L.; Cheng, L.; Li, P. Current status and perspectives of patient-derived xenograft models in cancer research. *J. Hematol. Oncol.* **2017**, *10*, 106. [CrossRef]
66. Ben-David, U.; Ha, G.; Tseng, Y.Y.; Greenwald, N.F.; Oh, C.; Shih, J.; McFarland, J.M.; Wong, B.; Boehm, J.S.; Beroukhim, R.; et al. Patient-derived xenografts undergo mouse-specific tumor evolution. *Nat. Genet.* **2017**, *49*, 1567–1575. [CrossRef]

67. Katano, I.; Takahashi, T.; Ito, R.; Kamisako, T.; Mizusawa, T.; Ka, Y.; Ogura, T.; Suemizu, H.; Kawakami, Y.; Ito, M. Predominant development of mature and functional human NK cells in a novel human IL-2-producing transgenic NOG mouse. *J. Immunol.* **2015**, *194*, 3513–3525. [CrossRef]
68. Ashizawa, T.; Iizuka, A.; Nonomura, C.; Kondou, R.; Maeda, C.; Miyata, H.; Sugino, T.; Mitsuya, K.; Hayashi, N.; Nakasu, Y.; et al. Antitumor effect of Programmed Death-1 (PD-1) blockade in humanized the NOG-MHC double knockout mouse. *Clin. Cancer Res.* **2017**, *23*, 149–158. [CrossRef]
69. Hanazawa, A.; Ito, R.; Katano, I.; Kawai, K.; Goto, M.; Suemizu, H.; Kawakami, Y.; Ito, M.; Takahashi, T. Generation of human immunosuppressive myeloid cell populations in human interleukin-6 transgenic NOG mice. *Front. Immunol.* **2018**, *9*, 152. [CrossRef]
70. Yoshimi, A.; Balasis, M.E.; Vedder, A.; Feldman, K.; Ma, Y.; Zhang, H.; Lee, S.C.; Letson, C.; Niyongere, S.; Lu, S.X.; et al. Robust patient-derived xenografts of MDS/MPN overlap syndromes capture the unique characteristics of CMML and JMML. *Blood* **2017**, *130*, 397–407. [CrossRef]
71. Goto, T.; Hirotsu, Y.; Mochizuki, H.; Nakagomi, T.; Oyama, T.; Amemiya, K.; Omata, M. Stepwise addition of genetic changes correlated with histological change from "well-differentiated" to "sarcomatoid" phenotypes: A case report. *BMC Cancer* **2017**, *17*, 65. [CrossRef]
72. Higuchi, R.; Goto, T.; Hirotsu, Y.; Nakagomi, T.; Yokoyama, Y.; Otake, S.; Amemiya, K.; Oyama, T.; Omata, M. PD-L1 expression and tumor-infiltrating lymphocytes in thymic epithelial neoplasms. *J. Clin. Med.* **2019**, *8*, 1833. [CrossRef]
73. Nakagomi, T.; Goto, T.; Hirotsu, Y.; Shikata, D.; Yokoyama, Y.; Higuchi, R.; Amemiya, K.; Okimoto, K.; Oyama, T.; Mochizuki, H.; et al. New therapeutic targets for pulmonary sarcomatoid carcinomas based on their genomic and phylogenetic profiles. *Oncotarget* **2018**, *9*, 10635–10649. [CrossRef] [PubMed]
74. Goto, T.; Hirotsu, Y.; Mochizuki, H.; Nakagomi, T.; Shikata, D.; Yokoyama, Y.; Oyama, T.; Amemiya, K.; Okimoto, K.; Omata, M. Mutational analysis of multiple lung cancers: Discrimination between primary and metastatic lung cancers by genomic profile. *Oncotarget* **2017**, *8*, 31133–31143. [CrossRef] [PubMed]
75. Dancey, J.E.; Bedard, P.L.; Onetto, N.; Hudson, T.J. The genetic basis for cancer treatment decisions. *Cell* **2012**, *148*, 409–420. [CrossRef] [PubMed]
76. Shi, C.; Chen, X.; Tan, D. Development of patient-derived xenograft models of prostate cancer for maintaining tumor heterogeneity. *Transl. Urol.* **2019**, *8*, 519–528. [CrossRef] [PubMed]
77. Nguyen, H.M.; Vessella, R.L.; Morrissey, C.; Brown, L.G.; Coleman, I.M.; Higano, C.S.; Mostaghel, E.A.; Zhang, X.; True, L.D.; Lam, H.M.; et al. LuCaP prostate cancer patient-derived xenografts reflect the molecular heterogeneity of advanced disease an–d serve as models for evaluating cancer therapeutics. *Prostate* **2017**, *77*, 654–671. [CrossRef]

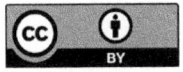

© 2020 by the author. Licensee MDPI, Basel, Switzerland. This article is an open access article distributed under the terms and conditions of the Creative Commons Attribution (CC BY) license (http://creativecommons.org/licenses/by/4.0/).

MDPI
St. Alban-Anlage 66
4052 Basel
Switzerland
Tel. +41 61 683 77 34
Fax +41 61 302 89 18
www.mdpi.com

Journal of Personalized Medicine Editorial Office
E-mail: jpm@mdpi.com
www.mdpi.com/journal/jpm

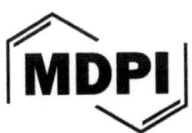

www.ingramcontent.com/pod-product-compliance
Lightning Source LLC
LaVergne TN
LVHW070708100526
838202LV00013B/1052